BODY FAILURE

Medical Views of Women, 1900–1950

In this energetic new study, Wendy Mitchinson examines medicine's perceptions and treatment of women in Canada in the first half of the twentieth century. It is based on in-depth research in a variety of archival sources, including Canadian medical journals, textbooks used in many of Canada's medical faculties, popular health literature, patient records, and hospital annual reports, as well as interviews with some of the patients themselves.

Each chapter covers aspects of a woman's life cycle: puberty, menstruation, sexuality, marriage, and motherhood – and the health problems connected to them: infertility, birth control and abortion, gynaecology, cancer, nervous disorders, and menopause. Mitchinson provides a sensitive understanding of the physician/patient relationship, the unease of many male doctors with the bodies of their female patients, and overriding concerns about the relationship between female and male bodies. Throughout the book, Mitchinson takes care to examine the roles and agency of both patients and practitioners as diverse individuals.

WENDY MITCHINSON is Canada Research Chair in Gender and Medical History and a professor in the Department of History at the University of Waterloo.

Body Failure

Medical Views of Women, 1900–1950

WENDY MITCHINSON

UNIVERSITY OF TORONTO PRESS
Toronto Buffalo London

© University of Toronto Press 2013
Toronto Buffalo London
www.utppublishing.com
Printed in Canada

ISBN 978-1-4426-4626-1 (cloth)
ISBN 978-1-4426-1431-4 (paper)

Printed on acid-free, 100% post-consumer recycled paper with vegetable-based inks

---

Library and Archives Canada Cataloguing-in-Publication

Mitchinson, Wendy, author
Body failure : medical views of women, 1900–1950 / Wendy Mitchinson.

Includes bibliographical references and index.
ISBN 978-1-4426-4626-1 (bound). – ISBN 978-1-4426-1431-4 (pbk.)

1. Women patients – Canada – History – 20th century. 2. Women – Health and hygiene – Canada – History – 20th century. 3. Physician and patient – Canada – History – 20th century. 4. Medicine – Canada – History – 20th century. I. Title.

RA564.85.M58 2013   613′.04244097109041   C2013-904523-6

University of Toronto Press acknowledges the financial assistance to its publishing program of the Canada Council for the Arts and the Ontario Arts Council.

University of Toronto Press acknowledges the financial support of the Government of Canada through the Canada Book Fund for its publishing activities.

Canada Council   Conseil des Arts
for the Arts   du Canada

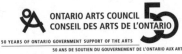

ONTARIO ARTS COUNCIL
CONSEIL DES ARTS DE L'ONTARIO
50 YEARS OF ONTARIO GOVERNMENT SUPPORT OF THE ARTS
50 ANS DE SOUTIEN DU GOUVERNEMENT DE L'ONTARIO AUX ARTS

This book has been published with the help of a grant from the Canadian Federation for the Humanities and Social Sciences, through the Awards to Scholarly Publications Program, using funds provided by the Social Sciences and Humanities Research Council of Canada.

In Memory of Daphne Lingwood

Contents

Abbreviations

AMB	Alberta Medical Bulletin
AMJ	Alberta Medical Journal
BAM	Bulletin of the Academy of Medicine Toronto
BOHI	Bulletin of the Ontario Hospitals for the Insane
CC	Canadian Child
CD	Canadian Doctor
CFW	Child and Family Welfare
CH	Canadian Health
CJMH	Canadian Journal of Mental Hygiene
CJMS	Canadian Journal of Medicine and Surgery
CJP	Canadian Journal of Psychology
CJPH	Canadian Journal of Public Health
CL	The Canada Lancet
CLNH	The Canada Lancet and National Hygiene
CLP	The Canada Lancet and Practitioner
CMAJ	Canadian Medical Association Journal
CMR	The Canada Medical Record
CN	The Canadian Nurse
CPHJ	Canadian Public Health Journal
CPMR	Canadian Practitioner and Medical Review
CW	Canadian Welfare
DMJ	Dalhousie Medical Journal
DMM	Dominion Medical Monthly and Ontario Medical Journal
HW	The Hospital World
JPMS	The Journal of Preventive Medicine and Sociology
ManMR	Manitoba Medical Review
McMJ	McGill Medical Journal

MHR   Montreal Homeopathic Record
MMAR   Manitoba Medical Association Review
MMB   Manitoba Medical Bulletin
MMC   Modern Medicine of Canada
MMJ   Montreal Medical Journal
MMN   Maritime Medical News
MMR   Montreal Medical Record
MS   Medical Sentinel
NHPW   National Hygiene and Public Welfare
NSMB   The Nova Scotia Medical Bulletin
OJNP   Ontario Journal of Neuro-Psychiatry
PHJ   The Public Health Journal
QMQ   Queen's Medical Quarterly (New Series)
SMJ   Saskatchewan Medical Journal
UTMJ   University of Toronto Medical Journal
UWOMJ   University of Western Ontario Medical Journal
WCMJ   The Western Canadian Medical Journal

Acknowledgments

Much of the primary research for this book was done at the same time as that for *Giving Birth in Canada, 1900–1950* so separating the list of people and institutions who supported me for both projects is impossible. Early parts of the manuscript appeared in various venues and I acknowledge this and thank the various editors and readers for their input and the publishers for giving me the opportunity to work out some my ideas in a public forum.[1] The manuscript that follows, however, has been rewritten significantly. One of the most rewarding aspects of writing a book is seeing how chapters feed into one another and how themes that seemed minor in an article become more significant when all the research is put together.

Funding allows historians to research. Despite the increasing number of sources available online, most historians still need to go to archives and libraries to access the wealth of material that is connected to their projects. I have been incredibly fortunate in the financial support received from the Social Sciences and Humanities Research Council (SSHRC), the Hannah Institute for the History of Medicine through Associated Medical Services, the Thérèse Casgrain Fellowship, the University of Waterloo, and most recently the Canada Research Chair program. In addition, two residencies have provided wonderful environments and collegial support over the years: the Rockefeller Study Center, Bellagio, Italy, and the Fundación Valparaiso, Almeria, Spain.

Archivists and librarians have always been willing to help in finding material for me and easing my access to it. Dr Badley, Victoria General Hospital, Halifax, gave me permission to look at patient records and Lynn Molloy helped in accessing and explaining the records themselves. The McGill University Archives, the Public Archives of Nova

xii   Acknowledgments

Scotia, the BC Archives, Queen's University Archives, Women's College Hospital, Toronto, and the Kitchener-Waterloo Hospital were generous in allowing me access to their collections. Susan Mavor of the Doris Lewis Rare Book Room, Dana Porter Library, University of Waterloo, was always helpful. Jane Forgay of the Dana Porter Library would track down articles and patiently explain how to wend my way through the ever-changing "upgrades" of the library's ordering system.

Over the years I have benefitted from the work of wonderful research assistants, many of whom have gone on to their own successful careers: Linda Ambrose, Megan Davies, Marlene Epp, Mona Gleason, Barbara Holzmark, Susan Johnston, Mary MacDonald, Julia Roberts, and Danielle Terbenche. Many of the interviews were done by Helen Harrison. Working collaboratively with the following scholars has also had an impact on my perspective: Françoise Baylis, Marilynne Bell, Maria DeKonick, Jocelyn Downie, Abby Lippman, Margaret Lock, Kathryn Morgan, Janet Mosher, Barbara Parish, Susan Sherwin, Peggy Spencer, and Ariella Pahlke, all part of a SSHRC Strategic Research Network Grant entitled the Feminist Health Care Ethics Research Network. And then there are my co-authors of the second edition of *Canadian Women: A History*: Alison Prentice, Naomi Black, Paula Bourne, and Gail Cuthbert Brandt. Last but certainly not least is my co-editor for *On the Case*, Franca Iacovetta.

Other scholars have also been willing to share their work with me: David Gagan, Dr Charles Hayter, Janet McNaughton, Dr Stuart Houston, Dr Robert Macbeth, Laura Shanner, Dan Bender, Cheryl Krasnick Warsh, and Jane Rothstein. Dr Murray Enkin and Dr Kate Bailey read the whole manuscript and it is a better one for their reading. Both gave up significant time from their own busy lives to do this and I am very grateful. The late Dr Charles Roland always was a supporter of those of us who worked in the field of medical history. I benefitted both from that support and his friendship. I miss him. I also owe thanks to Camilla Blakely for acting as a structural editor on a manuscript that was more than twice the length it should have been and advising where the cuts could be made so it became a length that a publisher would consider. As I became involved in the publishing process I enjoyed comparing the experience with Susan Armstrong Reid.

Colleagues may not realize how important they are in creating an environment that enriches the often lonely process of doing research. I have been fortunate in that the Department of History, University of Waterloo, is a collegial one inhabited by scholars constantly working on a wide variety of projects. The department also had incredible support staff for the period I was working on this book: Irene Majer, Nancy Birss, and Donna Lang. Not surprising given my university's orientation towards computer science, the support system for those of us in the arts faculty is excellent. Vic Neglia and Keith McGowan coped with my basic questions and were patient when I would get frazzled by something my computer did that I didn't understand. My usual comment was, "But I didn't touch anything!" – not a particularly helpful explanation of what might have caused a specific problem.

The process of getting work into print can sometimes be long and stressful. I thank Len Husband, editor for Canadian history at the University of Toronto Press for his calming emails to me and for his encouragement. The anonymous readers' comments were both helpful and challenging. And despite a delay due to an incorrect email address, the actual copyediting process was straight forward and I thank Frances Mundy of the University of Toronto Press, David Zielonka, account manager of APEX for UTP, and the anonymous copy editor whose sharp eyes caught inconsistencies in the manuscript.

Experiences with the medical system impinged on my life throughout 2009 and 2010. I saw many aspects of our health care system, both negative and positive, as my husband's health problems remained undiagnosed for a year. Diagnosis, however, was followed by immediate treatment. During that time friends and relatives were my support. They are too many to list but I need to thank my ongoing daily drivers to the various hospitals in London, Ontario: Patrick Harrigan, Tracy Penny Light, Carol Cole, and Mary Wybrow. Jean and Ray Rivers would care for our dogs at a moment's notice. Janice Dickin flew in from Calgary to be with me. A special debt is owed to Ross Baker who interceded with the medical system when necessary. And my brother Michael and my sister-in-law Donna were always there for me. As for the person at the centre of this coming together, for the vast majority of my life Rex has given me his time, support, and love. I can only feel deep gratitude that he is still with me.

BODY FAILURE

Medical Views of Women, 1900–1950

Introduction

Body Failure: Medicine's View of Women, 1900–1950 is in many respects a sequel to *The Nature of Their Bodies: Women and Their Doctors in Victorian Canada.* As with the earlier book, it focuses predominantly on English Canada and examines the life cycle of women and some of the perceived health problems connected with it. In this study, however, I do not address childbirth per se, having done so in a previous study.[1] What I do examine is the medical ideal of motherhood and how it was visited on women according to the most up-to-date medical information on breast feeding. While the structure of the two books is similar, both the changing lives of women and the practices of medicine in a later period introduced new medical concerns and altered the perception of some old ones.

Unlike many studies that focus on the "firsts" of medicine as temporal divides, I have chosen a more traditional chronological division within chapter themes: from 1900 to and including World War I (WWI) and from after the war to mid century, or depending on the topic, using the interwar years and WWII and afterwards as separate divisions. The years before the war were very much influenced by Victorian perceptions of women, albeit with recognition that significant changes in many women's lives had taken place. But WWI changed the world Canadians had known. Loss of life was significant – almost 60,000 dead – and if the influenza epidemic that followed is taken into account the number almost doubles. Those losses had long-lasting repercussions for individual families and for the nation as a whole. The society that emerged from war appeared modern and even its music, dances, and clothing signalled shifting values. Women, excepting those in marginalized groups such as the Japanese, Chinese, Aboriginals, and Indo-Canadians, had gained the right to vote. More than had been the case in prior years, women extended their educational experience, entered the work force, and saw their roles within the family change. For doctors, too, the war and its end seemed to coincide with significant changes in the practice of medicine. The standards for medical education rose and the commitment to scientific medicine gained ascendancy and confirmation with Frederick Banting and Charles Best's discovery of insulin. Medicine became increasingly specialized and extended its sway over the lives of Canadians (especially women). Medical advances in the understanding of the female cycle occurred with the isolation of the hormone estrogen in the late 1920s and its synthetic production in 1938. Such changes gave the medical profession in Canada more confidence, as reflected in the engagement of many practitioners with the medical literature of the time. Combine the changing context of general society – two world wars, a depression, and the reality of and concern about modernity – with the changes in women's lives and in medical practice, and the first half century provides a fascinating period in which to examine medicine's perceptions and treatment of women.

Historiography

One of the strengths of the discipline of history is its eclectic nature. There is no one way to answer the questions historians raise. Using primary sources from the past but writing in the present, historians are constantly applying and testing analytic frameworks or theories originating in other disciplines to illuminate our understanding of the past. While they cannot be overlaid on the past, they often provide both different ways of looking at our sources and questions to ask of them. The theoretical and analytical influences in researching and writing this book are multitudinous, adopted and adapted over several decades. When I first began to study history as an undergraduate student in the late 1960s, the concept of finding "the" truth about the past was no longer fashionable. The sureness of our predecessors had disappeared with increasing numbers of historians acknowledging that there was no ultimate history; each generation wrote its own past.[2] The decentring of history had begun and it only intensified. The New Left and feminist movements of the 1960s and 1970s brought with them an awareness of the need for what became known as the new social history, a history that many historians believed could be written from a qualitative or quantitative perspective from the bottom up, to incorporate not only Canadians whose lives had been ignored, but also seeing in those Canadians a form of identity politics through class, sex, and race.[3] To that trinity were added others – among them religion, place, age, and eventually gender. It was an exciting time of new subjects and approaches introduced.

Part of the excitement, and at times the frustration, were on-going theoretical challenges. The linguistic turn as represented in structuralism and poststructuralism raised questions about how to read a text and the underlying meaning of words, exhibited in binaries such as man/woman.[4] Their influences are evident in approaches to the meanings of medical terms throughout *Body Failure*; for example, the rather wide variability in definition of words such as infertility and menopause. Compared to structuralism, the mutability of poststructural perspectives reflected the broader attraction of postmodernism[5] to a society in which many of its verities were under attack. Critics noted that binaries were hierarchal in nature – man/woman, white/black, West/East – and value ladened with the unexpressed favouring of one aspect of the binary compared to the silencing of the other. Canada in the years 1900 to 1950 was filled with binaries, reflecting how society was thought to be and thus should be. The medical system was predicated on women's bodies being seen as significantly different from men's, the other to men's norm. The challenges to the way in which historians thought about their sources, how to read these sources, how to figure out meaning(s), came at a furious rate. The new social history was no longer new. The emergence of gender history, for some, disputed the underlying premises of women's history.[6]

In writing a book on medicine and women as patients, both sex and gender become defining variables. Feminist scholars introduced the concept of gender to lessen the emphasis on what they saw as a biological determinist view of women. But as with any dichotomy, the more it is used, the less clear the line of division becomes.[7] Physicians did not have to worry about such a dichotomy. For them sex was paramount; indeed, for them gender, as we consider it, was collapsed into sex, itself a gendered way of thinking. But that conflation allowed some practitioners to see the lives of women as limited, not because of their bodies, but because of the ways the wider society and the medical profession collectively perceived those bodies. Underlying the meaning of gender was the concept of social/cultural construction. But social construction has limits when applied to the body. As Susan Bordo has cogently argued, "commitment to cultural constructionism has gone far beyond notions that the biological body ... is always historically and politically *inscribed* and shaped ... to the much more radical position that the very notion of the biological body is itself a fiction."[8] Our understanding of bodies may be constructed, but the pain and distress bodies can cause and experience are real. The material body is more than gender.

Challenging women's history as well was a critique from third wave feminists who complained that too often the category of women overlooked the differences among them based on class, race, and ability. Others went further and stressed the ambiguity of what the concept of "woman" meant.[9] Out of the decentring and destabilizing challenges of various theories came a willingness to accept and even expect instability. Identities were multiple, not a new idea but one emphasized by postcolonial scholarship. As applied to Canada, the usefulness of this approach has been vis-à-vis marginalized "racial" and "ethnic" groups, especially salient with respect to First Nations peoples. Underlying it, as with so many of the postmodern critiques, is the concept of power – who has it and who does not – and the rejection of essentialism, the generalization of those without the power. But as some critics of postcolonial theory have argued, the same rejection of generalization needs to be applied to those in power as well.[10]

What all the theoretical, conceptual, and analytic upheaval of the past half century has emphasized is the problematic nature of generalizing the past, especially when that past views its own society in terms of binaries that by their nature are generalizations. Part of the challenge for historians is not only to make some sense for the reader out of the past but also to note the silences of the past. Those silences often reveal deep-seated beliefs on race, class, and gender, each of which has its own hierarchy. Seldom do practitioners address their own whiteness or that of most of their patients, but it is integral to their concept of the ideal body.[11] Nevertheless, underneath the silence on race are signs that concerns about it existed. Various racial references weave their way throughout concerns about modernity and fear for the future of the "human race," or the "race." Race was very much a contingent term. In "racial suicide" it could mean a threat from a class, a nondesignated group based on a perceived specific behavioural trait, or more often based on a nonwhite, non-Anglo, non-middle-class "other." As the reader will see, the racialized idea of the primitive or uncivilized in the guise of women of ethnicity or "colour" emerges in discussions about breast feeding and pelvic shape. In the chapter on puberty, I point out the cultural and racialized specificity of Western medicine to remind readers of other ways of looking at bodies and their experiences. Those scholars using a postcolonial approach to the health of minority women have focused largely on puberty customs, the changing nature of childbirth, the devastation of infectious diseases, and the delivery of hygiene. But few have addressed the medical topics covered in *Body Failure* except in a generic way, stressing the ways in which various groups of women kept to their own traditions.[12] The reasons for this are numerous, but essentially the contact zone, if you will, was very limited between the vast majority of Canadian practitioners and women who were deemed "racialized." Yet there was no denying that medicine was "a cultural system itself, and an appendage of the colonial state structure."[13] As for the "racialized" women themselves, silence on certain aspects of their bodily experience is strong. For the women of the First Nations, the menopausal experience as a physiological change did not loom large in their lives; as a marker of a power shift, however, it did.[14]

Class is less silent than race in the medical discourse – being acknowledged in patients and to a lesser extent in the physicians themselves. Practitioners' own interest in being part of a respectable profession was class based. Status came from where they had trained – Canada or in one of the major schools/hospitals in the United States, Britain, or Europe. Physicians were divided as well depending on the nature of their practices (general or specialties) and where they were based (urban/rural, small towns/isolated areas). As for patients, while they self-selected whether they would seek help from a physician, increasing numbers did so over the period 1900–1950. The poor were often carried as charity cases both in private practices and in hospitals. Patient records reflect a wide variety of patients treated. Where the middle-class woman dominates is in the textbooks, when physician authors discuss the normative way for a body to work and recommend standard treatment modalities. Physicians' views of class as they pertained to their women patients were filled with tension. They were concerned about the plight of working-class women in the domestic sphere but particularly in the conditions of their paid employment and how it undermined their health. They recognized that standard treatment modalities were not always practical for women who had to work to survive. At the same time, they could be quite judgmental about the behaviour and morals of working-class women and antagonistic about the challenge their employment represented to physicians' view of the proper place and role of women in society. As for middle-class women, they often saw in them the negativity of modernity – a frivolousness in behaviour and thought – that belittled care of family and threatened traditional mores. It was those mores that practitioners associated with their idealized view of a middle-class woman and the normative view of what a woman was and should be.

The silence of gender revolves around the gender of the male practitioners themselves. Their masculinity is tied up with their expertise, their professionalism, their ability to diagnose and treat. But that masculinity is tinged with affective traits – caring for patients, their own fear of failure, and their hesitancy about the ability of science to deliver certainty in their professional lives. Scholars of the affective turn have considered it as part of the decentring of specific disciplines, a recognition of emotion, feelings, and what appears to be nonrational or intuitive thinking. Historians have long addressed many of these aspects in the past, but without using the specific terminology of affectiveness.[15]

The historiography on medicine has mirrored many of the conceptual shifts in the discipline of history and elsewhere. Social historians of medicine in the latter decades of the twentieth century studied medicine with a critical eye and challenged the triumphal view of its progress. They did so in ways similar to the broader field of social history, using numerous interpretative perspectives, among them Marxist, gender, and postmodernist. Such approaches altered significantly how scholars saw the medical past.[16] Poststructuralism especially had a powerful impact on historians of medicine, largely through the work of Michel Foucault.[17] Foucault put forth the notion of a disciplinary society in which specific technologies had decentred the state as a seat of power through the control and use of knowledge. Medicine was one of those technologies. And feminists quickly adapted Foucault's ideas of power and knowledge to examinations of women's bodies.[18]

As will be obvious in this study, I see medicine as a bedrock of societal norms, sometimes in their creation and more often in their maintenance. While many historians of medicine took up the notion of social control (Americans more than Canadians), it was a rather blunt interpretation that recognized neither the complexity of doctor/patient relationships nor the agency of the patient and the insecurity of the physician. While the power of the medical profession outweighs that of the patient, I argue in this book, as I have elsewhere, that the individual practitioner was not always able to feel that control vis-à-vis his patients as he faced insecurities about the efficacy of his own role and expectations of it. And I use the term 'he' deliberately as men dominated the profession.

No matter what the interpretive perspective taken, the common theme of medicalization has come to dominate the historiography of medicine. Medicalization refers to the way in which physicians comment on actions of the body or the behaviour of an individual and link them to potentially harmful physical and/or mental repercussions.[19] Historians have argued that doctors medicalized issues not traditionally considered medical and co-opted them in a way that extended the medical area of expertise. In doing so they have taken the social and cultural and reduced them to the biological, thus enabling them to ignore the original broader context. This tendency has brought medicine under attack for it reduces the patient to body parts divorced from the person the patient is and from her/his environment. Yet a closer historical study of medicine reveals that in some respects, physicians have long been aware of the cultural influences on the body.

For feminists, medicalization of women's bodies refers to the ways in which physicians have made the female body problematic. Out of a vast literature, both historical and current, a general consensus has emerged about the reasons. First, doctors who, until recently, were predominantly male, have tended to view the male body as the norm and the female body as other than the norm.[20] The male body was the body physicians knew. Deviations from that body – menstruation, childbirth, menopause – appeared suspect and prone to weakness. In addition, few physicians or even nurses were from nonwhite, non-European groups, so that women from those groups were even more at a disadvantage.[21] Second, women's disadvantage in society was reflected in medicine. When a woman patient faced a male physician who saw her body as "other," she was in a less powerful position than a male patient would have been; the societal context, in which both the physician and the female patient lived, invested status to men over women. Third, the tendency of physicians has been to generalize the problems of sick women to healthy women.[22]

Recent literature on the history of the body has critiqued the emphasis scholars have given to the body as a singular whole. In doing so we have created an "opaque" understanding of how it works and how it was seen in the past. Needed as well are examinations of body parts and their specific histories.[23] *Body Failure* focuses largely on the various parts of the reproductive system and in doing so illuminates its centrality for physicians in their dealings with women patients and how the parts and the whole were in a dynamic relationship.

All of the above and other influences appear in *Body Failure*. Historians try to make sense of the past, which means we will use concepts to make the complex understandable, while not necessarily adopting a complete theory, approach, or even methodology out of which a concept or interpretation emerges. Questions come from varying perspectives, analytical methods, and theories. In the words of Anne McClintock, adherence to one perspective "begs the question of rethinking the global situation as a *multiplicity* of powers and histories, which cannot be marshalled obediently under the flag of a single theoretical term."[24]

Body Failure is about the medical profession in Canada, seen from a national perspective, and its perception and treatment of women in the first half of the twentieth century. In these years the profession was expanding its power and increasingly Canadians were using their services – in private practice; in hospitals as paying, subsidized, or charity patients; through public health provisions; through private companies in the workplace; through the responsibility of the federal government in providing health care to specific groups such as the First Nations peoples; and through welfare programs at the provincial or local level. The vast majority of practitioners, however, were involved in the first two and it is those on which I focus. As Foucault argued, medicine had the disciplinary power of scientific/medical knowledge. In the years under study, regular medicine dominated in terms of prestige within the health pyramid. It does not mean Canadians did not look elsewhere for health support, but that the meaning of "medicine" for most meant what licensed medical doctors did. As a profession it had its accepted standards, which, it could be argued, were generally accepted within the broader geographical boundaries of the West. Believing that place matters, however, I am looking at the profession in Canada. This does not mean there were not regional differences as well, but they would largely be consequences of wealth, rural/urban splits, patient/doctor ratios, and culture.[25] The beliefs underlying most treatment would be within a fairly small range.

The book is an overview. As with *The Nature of Their Bodies* I see each chapter as potentially a topic for a book, a spark to encourage further research on subjects that time and space have prevented me from pursuing and debate on the generalities I make as a result.[26] After one of her lectures on contemporary literature, Gertrude Stein was asked, "What about the woman's question?" Her reply was one with which I sympathize writing amidst the turmoil of theories and multiplicity of identities – "Not everything can be about everything."[27] Medicine has been my research conduit to the past. The interest in practitioners' treatment of women highlights attitudes about sex, gender, age, sometimes class, and to a lesser extent race. It reflects normative and sometimes not so normative beliefs of an increasingly powerful profession about the most personal aspect of women's lives – their bodies.

Themes

Several themes underlie the following chapters. One is the power of medicine. Medicine can define a social problem and how it should be discussed; that is, it can create the limits of discussion or the basis of discussion and by doing so determine its outcome. It prevents the possibility of a wider view and keeps the discourse within the realm that doctors control through their specialized language and their description of normality. Heightening medicine's power is that our engagement with it most often occurs when we are at our most vulnerable. Strengthening it as well is our belief that, as a science, medicine can give us a sense of the health risks we face and how to judge them. In recent years, however, activists and scholars have challenged such views, emphasizing instead the cultural relativity of certain medical practices and providing a litany of areas in which medicine has supported various practices and technologies long after information was available about their danger or lack of efficacy.[28]

Central to any study of medicine is the relationship between patients and physicians. Modern critics of medicine have expressed concerns about the kind of surveillance that patients undergo from their physicians, the fear being that the monitoring of the body can result in losing sight of the patient.[29] In modern language, doctors read the text (body) and lose sight of the context (person). Physicians tell us how to behave, what to do, and what not to do in order to maintain health. Our physicians at times know more about us than we do ourselves. They see parts of our bodies that we do not see. What is it that they see? What does it mean? Does it give away secrets of our lives to those doctors?

Throughout the years 1900 to 1950, the influence of the medical profession in Canadian women's lives increased significantly. Doctors, in their own medical journals and in the popular literature women were reading, proffered women advice on issues seemingly not medical: education, clothing, cosmetics, and marriage. But they gave women more than advice; they also intervened in some of the central experiences of women's lives from puberty to menopause. Underlying much of the medical advice was the suspicion that women could not achieve the same standard of health as men. What health they did have could be maintained only if they remained within clearly defined social roles; if women went outside those roles they would endanger their health, a variant of the "biology is destiny" argument.

Given the above, it is not surprising that modern feminist literature on medicine has made autonomy, choice, and agency watchwords, but they are difficult concepts with which to deal. The difference between them is often unclear and certainly they may not mean the same thing in the past as they do today. Historians of women, racial minorities, and workers have emphasized the issue of agency to take away the image of passiveness that being a "victim" portrays. But only recently have scholars started to look seriously at the issue of agency (and/or autonomy) to see the problems that it presents.[30] Agency is limited, confined, influenced, and shaped by so many different factors that it is impossible for any person to have total agency. Within medicine the limits on the patient with respect to agency are twofold. One stems from medicine and its practitioners. Within conventional medicine (the focus of this study) the difference in power between a patient and physician compromises the agency of the patient. The patient comes to the physician for advice and in doing so expresses her/his belief in the medical system. The patient also pays for the advice and it goes against rational commercial standards to reject it. The image of medicine as a rescuer also means that to refuse to be rescued or to debate the nature of the rescue attempt seems irresponsible, especially when your life might be at risk. Patients have refused and do refuse to be rescued, but in the medical literature, until very recently, physicians have viewed this as aberrant behaviour, especially when the patient was a woman with little social capital compared to a man. And remember, physicians were not just any kind of man; most were white, middle-class, and largely Anglo in heritage.[31]

The limits on patient agency also stem from the patient. We are all bounded by limits, so choice is never open. How we see ourselves and how others see us will partially determine what options we are willing to consider for ourselves. We do not live in isolation but are enmeshed in relationships that define our identity. We are constrained by our social place. With choice comes responsibility and patients are not always able to accept that responsibility. They need to share it with their medical advisers, friends, and family. Nevertheless, patient case records remind us that women patients did exert agency even if they did not have much autonomy.[32] Their refusal to see a physician until absolutely necessary, their rejection of suggested treatment, their refusal to stay in hospital as long as advised, and their willingness to seek medical advice from alternative caregivers were acts of noncompliance that suggest the need and determination to be other than a patient. Neither were women necessarily overwhelmed by the prestige of medicine. Many women saw the medical profession not only as a source of help but also a source of injury.

Less discussed in the critical literature on medicine are the constraints members of the medical profession experience. The law, the norms of their profession, and the medical institutions in which they work all place limitations on physicians' actions. Like their patients, they, too, are limited by their own personal morality, by the mood they are in at the time of the patient encounter. Medicine and its practice can be capricious masters for the individual practitioner. In his study of causality, Stephen Kern argues that a major shift took place from the "positivism, reductionism, determinism, and materialism" of the nineteenth century to an "increasing specificity, multiplicity, complexity, probability, and uncertainty of causal understanding" of the twentieth century.[33] People don't like living with uncertainty, however, and so they turned to science and technology for answers to some of modernity's problems and challenges. Science provided the explanation and technology provided the means; together they made life easier, more comfortable, and, at times, safer. While physicians basked in and shared those beliefs, they were also unsure of their individual ability to live up to the expectations of their patients, their profession, and its science. Some physicians found themselves torn between what they saw as the scientific advantages that came with modernity and what they saw as worrisome social changes that also accompanied it. The tension between the two could be significant and in medicine was reflected between an older more person-oriented practice of medicine and a newer one that was increasingly laboratory based. In addition, the profession was not always able to speak with one voice. As Paul Komesaroff has concluded, "There is not one 'medical gaze,' but many."[34]

Many practitioners were uneasy about living in what they and many other Canadians believed was a modern world that was changing too quickly and challenging the received wisdom (or what was thought to be the received wisdom).[35] To that source of uncertainty add professional concerns of status. They worried about what they considered their lack of training and what the increasing power of hospital care meant for individual practitioners. Medical competitors still existed – alternative caregivers, healers, abortionists, home and proprietary remedies – all of which had an allure not provided by practitioners and reminders that not all Canadians had embraced belief in mainstream medicine. Although members of a profession, physicians were spread across a huge land mass, caring for a relatively small population, both of which led to a sense of isolation on the part of those outside the major urban centres. Often physicians were not paid enough for the work they did. As well, a diversity among physicians kept them from being able to speak with one unified voice divided as they were by where one was trained; where one practiced; and whether a physician was a specialist and, if so, what kind of specialist. Bolstered by the prestige of science, the profession was secure; the individual practitioner did not always share that sense of security.[36]

Physicians work in an arena of uncertainty much of the time. Medication may work but the reasons for it are unclear. What should work may not. It is difficult for any person to deal with uncertainty, especially when people's lives may be at stake. As a way of dealing with responsibilities that are overwhelming, physicians try to turn uncertainty into certainty. They gloss over what is unknown for what they think is known, what is accepted as fact by the profession as a whole. They accept the wisdom of medical expertise. They tend to deal with absolutes and not process and to work for answers in a world that constantly changes. To survive the uncertainty they have to convince themselves that they are choosing between good and bad, treatment and suffering, even when they may be choosing between levels of harm. Uncertainty is integral to medicine simply because the body is so complex.

Woman's body has been considered especially so. The medical literature of the first half century, both in Canada and elsewhere in Western society, exposed a fairly mechanistic image of how the body worked. The body as machine was how physicians wanted the body to be, which is understandable for it would make their work much easier. What frustrated physicians about a woman's body was its unpredictability. It was the lived body of women that many physicians had difficulty seeing as normal, healthy, and acceptably different from a man's body. What physicians saw in a woman patient was a body that was not regular, a body with which they could not identify. In addition, for male practitioners that body was surrounded by cultural taboos. By 1900 most medical texts insisted on the need to view and examine the female body in the interests of providing better medical care. When this occurred, it signalled a perceived separation for doctors between their professional being and their sex; that is, in their professional guise they were physicians, not men. The Victorian reticence about men viewing the female body, however, never totally disappeared, and sometimes resulted in uneasiness on the part of physicians when treating female patients.

Social Context and Doctors' Response

The medicalization of women's bodies in the first half of the twentieth century was a reflection of the value system of the time and the reality of woman's place in that system. Canadians and physicians alike perceived men as the superior sex. Such a view was part of the ideology of separate spheres, which although never a reflection of reality, had enough connection to it to bolster its continuation on an ideological level. For Canadians of the first half century, differences between the sexes mattered. Nonetheless, Canadians were well aware that the world women inhabited had changed. In the 1900s and 1910s the evidence was there for all to see. Women were employed in doing work they had never done before and doing traditional work in increasing numbers. But not all Canadians were accepting of the changes. In a 1903 article on women in business life, Annie Merrill detailed how such a life altered woman. It made her "cynical," lessened "her sweet faith," and "clouded" her "sunny disposition."[37] Merrill wrote as if an endangered species had lost its battle for survival. Canadians believed the roles of woman as wife and mother were natural, but society had changed over time and so while the original "instincts" could direct women to those roles, they could not assist in how to engage with them in a modern society.

Physicians, too, were aware of the influence of society. Dr Jennie Drennan of St Thomas, Ontario, looked to a past when mating with the primitive woman followed nature's design – at sexual maturity she married and "entered on the generative cycle of a mammal," feeding her young for two years and then starting the cycle over again. In the present, however, Drennan saw woman's body as somehow estranged from what nature had meant it to be. Ovulation had become more frequent and "a pernicious environment" was the culprit.[38] In changing biology, Drennan recognized how incredibly powerful environment was. Physicians were well aware that bodies were not stable. After all, much of the physician's job was responding to a biology (body) that was not functioning well. Since nature's or God's design could not fail, it must be human society that had damaged what had been designed. That in itself was worrisome since it challenged the fixedness of nature and opened it up to change. How serious the challenge was unclear. For some, it confirmed the threat of modernity. For others, it became integrated into a belief in first principles of creation, whether through God or some more distant process. In either case, it appears that culture could change "basic nature"; whether it could change the "essence" of what had been designed was less certain.

The irony of woman's role being seen as preordained by her body was that anthropologists were becoming aware of different ways of seeing body and societal place. Franz Boas was publishing in the early twentieth century about the "Eskimo" of Baffin Island and Hudson Bay. According to him, those near Cumberland Sound believed in a mythological woman, Sedna. Here was a society, then, with a female deity. Also different among some groups was the lack of "fixedness" of body. Many Inuit believed that the body could change its sex during the birth process, depending on how difficult the labour was. Some First Nations peoples were accepting of a third gender in their belief in the bedarche, when a person born one sex could take on the roles of another. Thus body had a permeability that was missing in the belief structure of Euro-Canadians. Nonetheless there were strong similarities between cultures. Most cultures saw women as closer to nature than men and the general roles of each sex were differentiated.[39]

The years following WWI only deepened the changes in society and in women's lives. Fear was that women were becoming more like men and if that happened, the underlying basis of society was in jeopardy. Byrne Hope Sanders wrote about the difficulty of judging what to do: "We have trained ourselves to think that it is a far, far better thing for a daughter to sit in a crowded office all day and pound a typewriter, than live at home and help her mother with the cares of the house and the younger children. In the past years we thought she was 'expressing' herself; living her own life."[40] But expressing yourself was more than some could accept. Doing so suggested putting yourself first, being selfish, and, for some, endangering the well-being of the race. While the changes that were occurring and revolving around women were not the only ones in society, Canadians often viewed them as the most significant. Taken together they represented the loss of what some saw as the "politeness and decencies of life."[41] With respect to married women, as late as 1950, a Catholic marriage course made clear that a wife and mother's place was in the home, not in "an endless round of women's clubs and teas."[42] The modern world too often was an enticement that many feared middle-class women in particular could not resist. Much of the medical literature also engaged in complaints about the modern woman. Dr Woods Hutchinson from New York, who often wrote for *Maclean's*, was clear that woman had changed physically and that her emotional and psychological attributes had shifted for the worse. Underlying his diatribe was a vision of what he thought woman should be: healthy, so she could perform her household tasks; unselfish, so she would put the needs of others before her own and enjoy doing so; instinctual in her mothering, so that the children raised would be of credit not only to her and the family but also to the race. Dr Albini Paquette warned that women could not have it all. If they shared in the rights of men then they would lose their God-given place in the home.[43] Unlike Paquette, H.B. Atlee reveled in the changes in women and their lives: "The flapper ... has broken down the petty, irritating, rasping claims that bound women to the wheel of an oft time unfair convention for many years. With a jaunty bravado ... she displays breezily her maiden charms in public."[44] Atlee believed such changes were for the better and made such women appealing. Of course, the woman he described was the young, unmarried woman. The changes for most commentators, however, were disturbing because they directed women to a different place, a different goal than what had existed in the past. Change acknowledged the so-called inherent or natural instincts of woman's make-up were not so inherent after all, at least if inherent meant immutable. With World War II more willingness to accept behaviour that traditionally had not been acceptable was evident. Dr J.J. Heagerty, the head of the division of industrial welfare, commented on the adjustments needed to ensure the health of women in war production factories and recommended that "the girls should be allowed to relax in whatever manner they see fit – including smoking."[45] Mores were changing and in the case of smoking would eventually affect health and life expectancy.

Change called into question long-held ideas about women and, while most Canadians were not troubled enough to face the implications of change, many railed against it, almost as an instinctive response. Some also recognized how the changing context and changing experience of women's lives altered what they had seen as woman's "nature" and the healthy functioning of her body. Throughout the following chapters, we will see physicians grappling with both in an attempt to prevent ill health and to understand its origins. Underlying those attempts remained a vision of woman's place as the leitmotif of women's lives.

1 Woman's Place

"Woman ... is not man at all." She differs from man "structurally [and] functionally ... In physical origin she is an animal and human as man is but in ... variational tendency so differs from man as to be unique in kind."[1] With those words, J.D. Logan in the January 1913 issue of *Canadian Magazine* encapsulated the thinking of many Canadians, both lay and medical, on women. They compared woman to man and by seeing woman as *not* man, emphasized the differences between them. Biology was *the* determinant of those differences and, consequently, of women's and men's social destinies.

Thomas Laqueur has suggested that the perceived physical differences between the two sexes became accentuated by the end of the eighteenth century. Until then, Western commentators had perceived woman's body as a similar but lesser version of man's. Subsequently, the differences became ones of kind, contributing to the creation of what has become known as the ideology of separate spheres, the belief that woman's domain was the private and man's, the public.[2] Not that the separation of spheres was only a Western phenomenon. Most cultures separate activities into those men do and those women do; for some, it may not be an ideology per se, but rather a practical way of surviving.[3]

What follows is an examination of how medical practitioners viewed women. The chapter begins by examining the perceived physical and nonphysical differences between women and men. From such listings the centrality of viewing the sexes as destined for particular social roles and the priority that physicians gave to the body in determining those roles becomes clear. With respect to women, the potential for motherhood dominated. Yet the stability of sexual differences seemed in peril, increasingly acknowledged in the fear that many experienced about modernity and the changes that accompanied it. What seemed stable – the body – was not, a destabilizing thought in itself. Beliefs about body and the fear of instability had consequences for women's lives in physicians' advice on topics that at first glance don't appear medical: exercise, food consumption, fashion, and paid employment.

Physical Differences

In the early years of the twentieth century, lay Canadians had a very strong sense of what the physical differences between the sexes were. As Logan's quote suggests, they existed at every level and the most obvious were the external. Physicians were not restricted in such a discussion. Through their specialized writings, they communicated with one another about the details of women's bodies, both external and internal. While Laqueur has argued that the vision of woman as a lesser version of man had its heyday by the end of the eighteenth century, it did not disappear. In his 1908 *The Principles and Practice of Gynecology for Students and Practitioners*, E.C. Dudley pointed out, "The development of the external genitalia follows the same lines in both sexes, except the development in the male is more extensive than in the female, being arrested in the female with the formation of the clitoris, nymphae, and labia majora, but going on in the male to the development of the penis and scrotum." Female development was on the same curve as the male, but stopped sooner, with the conclusion, not having to be said, that the large penis was more significant than the smaller clitoris. Size mattered. Woman's body was the one that differed from the norm, differed from man's. Dudley examined the different phases of a man's life and concluded the transitions between them were "gradual and even processes, relatively free from special outlay of energy, unmarked by specially critical periods." Women's phases – puberty, childbearing, menopause – were "critical turning-points" demanding "greater expenditure of energy"[4] Fortunately, nature had made accommodations for the needs of women as girls, wives, and mothers. But ignoring those "provisions" could only undermine women's health.[5] Medical books were written on the "diseases peculiar to women,"[6] a phrase used frequently in the medical literature and which suggested more than anything else that women's bodies deviated from men's and in ways that suggested they were not well designed.

The intrinsic nature of sexual differences was reinforced by the awareness in the 1910s of substances from the ovaries of women and the testes of men, which scientists labelled as female and male sex hormones. For many, they were what made women female and men male. Nelly Oudshoorn has argued that by naming the female hormones "estrogens," a term which refers to "the cyclic changes in the vagina characteristic of estrus," endocrinologists defined femaleness by reproduction and cyclicity.[7] Body and the language describing that body, then, in the first decades of the century determined differences between the sexes. Physicians noted the differences and as a result the differences became significant.

While physicians viewed the reproductive differences between the two sexes as primary, they didn't overlook the significance of secondary sexual attributes. These, too, favoured men: greater muscular strength and a voice that commanded attention.[8] More significant, man's brain was larger than woman's. While relative to body size the female brain was not smaller than that of man's, it was absolute size that mattered. Physicians seldom discussed the implications of the difference in brain size, but they didn't have to – they were obvious. What could be measured – brain size – was important.[9] The consequences of brain size went beyond intelligence. The belief was that a larger brain size resulted in larger head size for male babies. The trauma of such babies being born could affect both them and their mothers. Fortunately, medical assistance (largely male) could help.[10] If females had an easier time surviving birth because of their smaller brain size, it must have been the last time that it was considered an advantage.

Women did have some secondary advantages. Women were "naturally quick of eye and deft of wrist." Unlike men, they did not go bald. In his 1913 textbook, Woods Hutchinson gave a fascinating explanation for the latter. Men went bald because it didn't matter if they were bald; certainly it didn't prevent them from attracting a spouse. For women, the situation was different. If a woman became bald she would have difficulty attracting a mate and keeping him.[11] Thus it was nature's way (or the Darwinian interpretation of it) of ensuring that women who were bald would not reproduce their own kind. The combination of a societal bias (about which women could attract a mate) and the application of some version of selection of the fittest was telling about how hazy the understanding of heredity and scientific theories of it were at the time.

For many practitioners, the science of hormones remained key to understanding the differences between the sexes throughout the 1920s, '30s, and '40s. But understanding the relationship between the two became more complicated. By the end of the 1930s, studies revealed that each sex had within them both "male" and "female" hormones.[12] That awareness, however, did not lessen perceived differences between the sexes. Practitioners were aware that the biological edge females had in utero and as infants. And it continued past infancy. The president of Dalhousie University reported to the readers of *Canadian Medical Association Journal* that women students were healthier by far than men students. And mortality statistics revealed that women's life expectancy was greater than men's.[13] Nevertheless, physicians were convinced that women's biological edge was offset by a physiological disadvantage. Men still had more muscle strength than women. Women were "enslaved and tortured" by menstruation and menopause and were prone to health problems.[14] H.B. Atlee argued that women's bodies wore them down and were simply not as strong as men's given the "outrageous physiology" that was woman's. Medical science could help women, but Atlee made clear that medical science was "male directed."[15] Tensions between body strength and fragility were not unique to Western society or medicine. As Mary-Ellen Kelm has argued, the First Nations' perspective after contact had similar tensions between belief in their bodily power and the risk posed to them by infectious diseases. The difference was that in the latter the strain came from an outside threat whereas in the former they were deemed sexed in nature.[16]

Several themes emerge from the perception and discussion of bodily differences in the first half of the twentieth century. First was the belief that differences between men and women were significant to list, even if the implications of those differences were not always apparent. By listing them, physicians made them important. Second, while most of the differences seemed to favour men, not all of them did and recognition was given to areas of superiority in women. Third, the interwar period and beyond came to recognize the biological advantage of females in conceptual and survival rates of embryos and newborns as well as in life expectancy. Still, the underlying fragility of women because of their reproductive destiny was not something doctors were willing to rethink; physicians looked to the reproductive system of women to bolster the age-old view of women being less strong physiologically than men.

Nonphysical Differences

The physical aspects of sex differences dominated the lay and medical view of woman. They reinforced biological determinism, the belief that the differences were formed in nature. But while the physical differences between the two sexes were primary, the nonphysical that often sprang from them were also a significant focus. For Canadians, the society around them and their own experiences convinced them of the truth of female and male personality/social characteristics. Even medical writers detailed the nonphysical differences, at times linking them to the physical, at others simply pontificating about woman's nature in a way that brooked no opposition. Opposition to such views would have been limited in any event, since physicians' views were more often than not the conventional wisdom of the day.

While medical expectations of behaviour applied to both sexes, the specific expectations of women were more fundamental than the social expectations placed on men, linked as they were to woman's "instinctual life."[17] As most Canadians, medical practitioners saw women as caregivers; it was something on which all could agree. It was the expected role and, thus, the natural one for them. Dr James S. Sprague could easily publish an article entitled "Woman" in a medical journal and explain to his medical readers that "a woman's crown of glory should be her family, her throne – home; and her sceptre – affection" and not feel that he was going outside the expertise of medicine. Because physicians had the influence to label women who did not conform as physically or mentally ill, such descriptions went beyond prescription. A.T.B. Hobbs, surgeon at the asylum for the insane, London, Ontario, in an article entitled "The Relation of Ovarian Disease to Insanity and Its Treatment" argued that the mental life of woman corresponded to her physical so that as a young girl she could be "romping and hoidenish"; after puberty and throughout her menstrual life, however, she should exhibit "all the instincts of vigorous motherhood"; and at the end of her life display "placid contentment and sedateness."[18] Hobbs was describing what he saw as normative behaviour. In fact it was an idealized version of what the norm should be, very much attuned to the social expectations of the time. It went without saying that individual women outside the normative description could find themselves at risk.

The interwar period did not lessen medicine's focus on what doctors deemed natural for a woman and man to do and be. As with physical characteristics, physicians in the interwar years were trying to understand the origins of different attributes. In 1927 A.B. Chandler explained women using an analogy between plant and animal life. The former conserved energy, the latter consumed it. As Chandler explained, biologists had concluded "that woman comes nearer to the metabolism of the plant than does man." Thus analogies with the natural world explained differences between the sexes. But with women being analogous to plants and men to animals, they were being aligned to different species. Of the two, the belief was that animals were more fully evolved. For his part, Melville C. Watson of Toronto told readers of the 1936 *Canadian Medical Association Journal* that the hormone estrogen created the "feminine demeanour"[19] and thus gendered differences all came down to chemistry.

But the urge to understand was not always present. "A Medical Man" writing in *Canadian Magazine* in 1927 stated that it was "natural" for women to want to pursue a mate. Thus specific actions were simply sexed. In the *Manitoba Medical Bulletin*, C.C. Ferguson, the General Manager of the Great West Life Assurance Company, Winnipeg, told his medical readers something he assumed they agreed with, that "women are more emotional and hysterical than men." Placing this next to his main point that women outlived men, he concluded that "Pope's dictum 'woman's at best a contradiction still'" remained true.[20] Thus a specific difference in psychology seen as a weakness and a specific difference in biology seen as a strength came down to the contradictory nature of women. And in case any particular attribute challenged gendered roles, there was always an explanation that circumvented any necessity to confront it. While apparently men had a superior sense of taste and smell, such a perception did not lead to the conclusion that they should be the general cooks in society, but rather the ones who could best appreciate good cooking. The sense of smell and taste, however, did make men "more fastidious and discriminating critics of the 'bouquet' of wines than are women."[21] Why any of this mattered in the medical sense is unclear. Nevertheless, differences, or the interpretation of them, did matter in a social sense. The point of looking at the medical literature is to suggest the willingness or perhaps even the reasonableness of practitioners taking up the social perceptions of women as significant to mention in medical textbooks and journals. In doing so, they linked those social perceptions with body and with scientific understanding.

Differences wouldn't matter so much if the perception of them was neutral. What is clear from the above is that they were not; they had consequences. Perceived differences in male and female bodies led to the assumption of differences in attributes, which, in turn, led to assumptions about roles to be played by each sex. Underlying both the biological and the nonbiological differences was the sense of naturalness, which had no fixed meaning. The biological differences were more fixed whereas the nonbiological tied to them were more adapt-able, even if the preference was that they shouldn't be. What emerged in discussions of both kinds of difference was the sense that they existed for a reason and that the culture/society must adapt to allow for those differences.

Motherhood

The reason for women's differences was belief in motherhood as woman's central role, her raison d'être. Her body dictated that destiny and as experts on the body physicians' views of woman shored up those beliefs. The discussion of woman's place and women's bodies reflected the unwavering belief, at least in the early years of the century, that women were meant to be mothers.[22] It wasn't just that their bodies had the potential for childbearing; those bodies *needed* to bear children. Women who did not have children were pitied, those who limited the number of children were criticized. Motherhood was woman's destiny.

Montreal physician A. Lapthorn Smith *knew* that woman's destiny was to marry and have children:

> We need hardly spend any time in arguing that the cheerful and happy performance of these duties is the manifest destiny of woman, and that any general disinclination to undertake them, or any attempt to shirk them when undertaken, will inevitably throw the whole world's machinery out of gear, and bring disaster upon her and upon the race. Nature indeed has a summary way of punishing either men or women, who from motives of selfishness, or from physical inability, to not marry and raise a family; she simply extinguishes that breed and replaces it on the earth by a race of people less highly educated, but which knows enough to propagate itself.[23]

Smith's quote is rich in beliefs, prejudices, and fears. Nature, in his view, was a conscious entity; it had a goal in mind and for women their "manifest destiny" was to be wife and mother. Accepting one's destiny would assure happiness; if too many rejected it, the repercussions went beyond the individual (in the assumption of unhappiness) and had an impact on and for the broader society. One "breed" declined to be replaced by an inferior "race," which, at least, understood its bio-logical reproductive destiny. Lapthorn Smith was not concerned with the survival of the species, but rather a particular race or class within the human species. He used "breed" and "race" as interchangeable and with the former referred to an animal analogy that all would under-stand. His worry was clear – if the "better class" of women denied their destiny, then the society of Canada as he knew and wanted it to be would decline. His attitudes were more blatant than those of many physicians but based on the racialized science that was predominant at the time.[24]

The medical literature continually reflected belief about the normality of women wanting children and a home. In 1923 Eugene St Jacques, professor of clinical surgery, University of Montreal, reminded his colleagues of women's destiny and wrote that "the heart and soul of a woman lie in her pelvis."[25] In 1949 D.E. Cannell exclaimed, "Childbirth is the summation or climax of achievement in any woman's life."[26] Being able to conceive and bear a child provided woman with a specific prestige that no man could rival and was present in many cultures.[27] With respect to many physicians, however, it also limited the ability to see women in any other role than an instinctual one, which any healthy woman could perform.

For proof of woman's role, physicians looked to science, nature, and God. All three came together and reinforced notions of women as other, similar to the way in which Europeans saw the "exotics" of other lands. As some postcolonial theorists have suggested, the discourse of colonialism made the colonizers feel significant.[28] In a similar way, looking at women through the lens of medicine and body did the same for physicians. The rhetoric of scientific/medical/ technical language and its apparent precision created a sense of knowledge, understanding, and sureness for practitioners. As we have seen in his description of the "development of the external genitalia" in both sexes, E.C. Dudley was careful to refer to the various parts that emphasized the differences between males and females.[29] His detailed description provided exactness and, thus, credibility and weight to the differences, offsetting any sameness. Science, or its interpretation, gave practitioners the explanation to confirm their societal beliefs. In turn, preconceived notions could influence science as in the referencing of hormones as male or female.

Physicians and others also looked to nature to determine the essence of sexual differences. Of course, science, in some respects, was the study of nature so the two were closely bound. In the early years of the century, animal analogies were popular. Dr Jennie Drennan of St Thomas, Ontario, depended on animal analogies to establish what should be.

Arguing that because in nature mammals did not menstruate, it was not natural for women to do so, she worried that woman was becoming further separated from how nature wanted her to function. But nature still held some influence. Ovulation occurred in animals at only certain times of the year and, although women ovulated every month, "the fact that even in civilization more births occur in the spring and autumn, indicates an adherence to natural law." And if nature or science wasn't enough to convince people how things should be, physicians were quite willing to bring in God. Explaining why health was so important for women, Lapthorn Smith noted, "in God's providence she has to furnish all the material for the growth of the child before birth and for a year after."[30] For those who believed, nature was simply a reflection of God's design. Science, in turn, was an attempt at understanding God's creation.

The appeal to science was even stronger after WWI and in some respects subsumed nature and its creator. By the end of the nineteenth century there was the belief on the part of some biologists that at the level of the cell two different processes were at work: "upbuilding, constructive, synthetic processes" and "disruptive, descending series of chemical changes."[31] We have seen this above in regard to mammals and plants, with the former being seen as analogous to the male and the latter the female. A.B. Chandler was using this same kind of analogy in the late 1920s to both explain and emphasize sexual differences. Others chose to appeal to the "sex glands" with their "sex specific action." In 1936 Melville C. Watson of Toronto saw in the hormone estrogen an explanation of both the body and nature of women. While he understood that estrogen was also found in the urine of male animals and had recently been found in the tissue of stallions' testicles, it was its female nature that was significant.[32] Hormones were part of woman's nature and her body. Nature determined what the body was and needed and medical science's role was to confirm how nature worked. Rejecting a natural role, physicians believed, could cause ill health either physically or emotionally. Medicine's responsibility was to cure and to cure was to make normal. For one young woman psychotherapy brought a cure, but her subsequent marriage was its confirmation.[33] Indeed, the psychological inclination of the period from the 1920s to mid century saw the denying of motherhood both as a source and evidence of psychological problems.[34]

Being a mother, however, was not enough. Women had to be good mothers. Yet as many scholars have argued, the meaning of motherhood is a contested concept. In the contact between Aboriginal and newcomer women, for example, the latter undertook the role of mother vis-à-vis the former, seeing their understanding of motherhood as the universal template of good motherhood for First Nations women to emulate.[35] A good mother put the responsibilities of mothering before her own needs and in doing so set an example for her daughters. Good motherhood was the solution for life's ills. In the 1908 *Queen's Medical Quarterly*, J.E. Hanna argued the need for women to concentrate on their maternal duties. If they did "there will be less drinking, and fewer men's clubs, and more happiness, and less disease and sorrow, and less cause for anxiety and worry." It was mother who gave birth to the child, who suckled the child, and who was physically present more often than the father as the child grew older. No wonder at the opening of the Women's College Hospital and Dispensary in 1915, one speaker repeated what for her was a truism: "When we are sick, we want mother, not father, tho' we love him; but he is not 'mother,' and in this hospital will be found the mother element."[36] Physicians contrasted a good mother with one who was bad. A bad mother limited the number of children she had, leaving Canada's future to those born of a "weaker" and "corrupt" heritage. The fashionable woman, who thought more of her image than her responsibility to have children, was condemned as setting a poor example. A bad mother was one who did not prepare her daughters to be future wives and mothers.[37] Bad mothers challenged belief in the "naturalness" of motherhood.

The interwar and postwar years continued to contrast the good mother with the bad. But the definition of a good mother didn't remain static. While the preferred mother should be married, there were hints of change. An article in the 1946 *Canadian Medical Association Journal* was sympathetic to the unwed mother and the role the physician could play to help her make an informed decision about whether to keep her child or not. Such a view is a far cry from the earlier dismissal of such women as morally corrupt or mentally deficient. It also presents the role of the physician as protector and guide. We should not exaggerate, however, the sympathy towards unmarried women. While some practitioners were willing to think about the situation of such women, society as a whole did not shift in its condemnation.[38]

What did becoming a mother mean? In the early years of the century most women who became pregnant and gave birth experienced considerable wear and tear on their bodies. The patient records of hospitals detail many women who in their reproductive lives had gone through tremendous stress, pain, and hardship and did so many times. Not all of these women, however, were able to bear a live child. Many miscarried or lost a full-term baby. Given the emotional trauma the death of a child caused, the statement by some physicians that maternal ignorance was a significant cause of the high rates of infant deaths was uncaring to say the least. The high maternal mortality rates also testify that the life of the child was not the only one at risk.[39] If the birth went well and both mother and child survived, women in all cultures faced the physically demanding work of motherhood. Once the child had arrived, few women received physical relief; in working-class homes many mothers limited their food intake in order to ensure that their husbands and children were adequately fed, and they and other women often delayed medical care for themselves because they were needed at home and unwilling to leave.[40]

The hardship of pregnancy, childbirth, and mothering did change over time. Infant mortality declined. The birth rate also declined and with it the wear and tear on many women's bodies. Nonetheless, some women still found their experiences of becoming a mother stressful. Dorothy Atkinson gave birth to her first child at age nineteen, breast fed for nine months, had one period, and then became pregnant again. She breast fed that child for nine months and a year later was pregnant for the third time and breast fed that child for five months. She remembers, "I just felt that my body had been assaulted, I wanted it back again."[41] Women still faced death, although better maternal care, new drugs, and improved medical practices had resulted in significant decline in maternal mortality by the end of the 1930s. But being a mother still meant sacrifice. As Dr Janet K. Lang exclaimed, "The mother of the family is the constant companion of her children and the central figure in every family group. She bears the greatest strain and runs the greatest risk to life and health in bringing children into the world. She cares for her infant and growing children, her husband and their household."[42] Some physicians even recognized that maternity made it difficult for women to function as individuals in society and to pursue their own goals and aspirations. E.C. Menzies, from Verdun, Quebec, queried what happened to these women when they reached their fifties and sixties and their children had left home and had lives of their own.[43]

Several themes emerge from the medical perception of motherhood. First, by seeing the desire to be a mother as instinctual, it aligned motherhood with the biological and thus removed it from women's agency.

The instinctual view of motherhood also ignored social, political, and cultural influences that were part of the construction of motherhood. In motherhood, women became grouped and generalized. Second was the problematic nature of becoming and being a mother. Physicians more than other Canadians understood the significant dangers and hardships that childbirth posed in high maternal mortality and morbidity rates and in the high infant mortality rates. For something that was "natural," becoming a mother was problematic. Third was the total aspect of motherhood itself. It was hard work and had (or should have) priority over other needs and interests of women. If not, the repercussions for the well-being of the family and the state could be dire.

Advice to Women

Physicians considered themselves as the guardians of the body and, as a result, were obliged as part of preventive medicine to let healthy women know what was best for them in order to maintain their health. They told women what physical activity was safe, how they should eat or diet, and what kinds of clothing to avoid, and advised on the dangers of paid employment. In doing so they extended medicine's influence. Underlying their advice were concerns about gendered differences and the social role of women in society. Some physicians were somewhat understanding and supportive of women stepping outside traditional activities, but whether supportive or not, they tended to see certain activities of women as barometers of the wider society and its values and felt, as citizens, the need to speak out and, as physicians, to warn about the possible physiological repercussions.

Exercise

Historians of physical education have tended to be very critical of physicians and their attitudes towards women's involvement in sport.[44] While physicians believed limits on women's sporting activities should exist, by the turn of the twentieth century, physicians had embraced exercise for women, seeing it as necessary for health and arguing that too much study or too many indoor activities were not conducive to general well-being.[45] Support of physical activity was, in many respects, a recognition of reality as Canadian women in the early years of the century increasingly involved themselves in sports of a varied and sometimes surprising nature: hockey, swimming, golf, bicycling, riding, and baseball, to name only a few. Physicians, however, differentiated between sporting activities. Dr David Tod Gilliam took a rather modern view and argued that solitary diversions such as walking were "too funereal." John Joseph Cassidy, editor of the *Canadian Journal of Medicine and Surgery*, debated the pros and cons of the side-saddle versus the astride position in horseback riding and concluded that there was no objection to women riding astride. Of special concern were the physical activities open to pregnant women, with one 1915 editorial in the *Canadian Journal of Medicine and Surgery* extolling the virtues of golf.[46] Exercise and sporting activities did more than build up the strength of women; they eased some of the physical consequences of being female. Practitioners recommended exercise as a way of offsetting the gynaecological disorders they believed women often experienced. D. Gilbert Gordon, associate professor of clinical surgery at the University of Toronto, told readers of the *Canada Lancet* that the use of the bicycle was therapeutic for neuralgic dysmenorrhoea and indeed for most women's diseases. Using hyperbole to make his point he exclaimed, "I think the bicycle has done more to lessen the amount of fees paid to gynaecologists than all drugs on the market put together." His was a far cry from the ambivalence about cycling expressed by some physicians of an earlier generation.[47]

Modern activities challenged the opinion of physicians. Motoring had joined golf and cycling as a favourite activity. But was it healthy? The author of a *Public Health Journal* editorial expressed concern that it could result in nervous disorders in women largely due to "speeding and to the fear of accidents." If women had to drive, they would be better off doing so in less crowded areas since they were "more excitable and of less steady judgment than men." Also the strength needed for "cranking" up the car and for putting in a clutch was beyond most women. The author didn't provide any specific medical proof to back up his concerns, but instead appealed to the conventional image of women as being more nervous and emotional and less rational than men. True, their muscle physical strength was less than men's, but even this author admitted that with modern changes in car design, such as the self-starter, the strength issue would disappear.[48] As for organized sport, the central issue was how women played it. The medical literature agreed that amateur and noncompetitive activities were best for women.[49] Amateurism was the respectable norm of sport of the time; competitiveness was perceived as a male attribute.

If gender differences were to be taken into account, class distinctions were not. Seldom did the medical literature acknowledge that certain sports were only accessible to certain classes. There was only one exception to this and it occurred early in the century and revolved around the lack of access of working-class housewives to any form of leisurely exercise. The solution for some was not to advocate more strongly for the need for exercise but to see housework as a form of exercise. It was not the specific nature of the activity that was key to making it exercise but the "pleasurable zest" with which it was engaged and that could occur, it was rather optimistically believed, while doing housework.[50] All women could participate. Noteworthy is that unlike some "sports" there was little discussion of the dangers of doing too much housework. Neither did the linkage between housework and exercise survive the second decade of the century. It was as if in the first two decades of the century the meaning of exercise was not clear and any physical movement could come under its rubric. Since women already did exercise in the form of housework, for those women who were younger, unmarried, etc., exercise could be seen as a preparation for their future role and thus legitimized.

The postwar period saw a greater expansion of women's athletic prowess. Stressed in the medical literature, more than it had been, was the pleasure of exercising and being active. Physicians accepted that sports had become "the modern enthusiasm,"[51] and enjoined on their readers that women who were physically active when they were young were building a good foundation for health in their later years when they would face the stresses of pregnancy and childbirth. Exercise and sport, then, would help the young woman fulfill her biological destiny in a way that would ease its physical demands. Among the benefits of riding, walking, swimming, motoring, and rowing were that they kept women outdoors and were especially beneficial for young women trying to overcome menstrual difficulties. Physical health was primary, but a healthy and fit woman was also a more attractive woman. Exercise that involved voluntary contractions of the abdomen, for example, could help eliminate its "prominence."[52]

Competitive sport remained an issue. In an anonymous commentary in the 1936 *Canadian Medical Association Journal*, the author quoted one expert as saying that the excessiveness of some activities posed more of a danger for women than men. While admitting that exercise did not appear to hurt child-bearing abilities, "violent exercise" might harm uterine development and "subsequent fertility." For one 1940 text it was the "sudden force being applied to the abdomen" that was the problem in certain activities such as "riding, cycling, tennis, diving and surf bathing." The irony was that the reproductive organs of women were

more protected than those of men and yet the same concern with protecting male reproductive organs from injury was seldom expressed.[53]

Physicians were sensitive to the changing society around them and
changes in women's lives. They would have had to be blind not to be
aware of the increasing involvement of women in leisure activities and
sport. That such activities involved the body meant physicians could
interpret them as deserving of medical evaluation. Their comments
on exercise and sport reflected social concerns described in a medical
rhetoric. They saw exercise and sport as potentially healthy for women
in that they could overcome some of the liabilities of their sex and gain
a greater sense of well-being. Physicians didn't always agree with one
another on what specific sports or activities were best for women, but
they certainly believed in their right to express their opinion based on
their medical expertise. That their expertise was based, in part, on their
own perceived notions of woman's place in society is not surprising,
nor was their willingness to use those perceptions as part of their medical argument about health.

Eating Habits

What women ate also became a concern. The early years of the century
saw critical comments on what some women consumed, mostly off-
the-cuff remarks about women who ate and drank to excess. J. Clifton
Edgar in his 1907 text, was more specific, noting that "soda-water, ice-
cream, and candy are most harmful if taken to excess, as they very often
are," and concluded that "indigestible and non-nutritious foods" could
produce anaemia and general ill health.[54] Linked to concern about what
women were eating was the perception that women were dieting to
excess. Of special note were the use of patent medicines and folk remedies with one author regaling medical readers with the exploits of factory girls eating six lemons a day in order to appear "emaciated" and
to lose weight. Physicians' worries about dieting were understandable.
Even if it wasn't as common as it later became, anorexia nervosa was
a disease with which some were familiar.[55] They also were well aware
of the danger of malnutrition that could occur with dieting. Less mentioned was the malnutrition of many Canadians, both men and women,
caused by poverty.

While there was some concern about eating habits in the early years,
it was the interwar years and beyond that brought it to the fore. The

emergence of food science gave physicians something concrete as a measure of health. Nutrition was no longer to offset hunger but became a complex balance between nutrients and between carbohydrates, protein, and fat. The new concern over nutrition led to the recognition that many women were undernourished. In the 1920s, a Toronto study revealed that whereas men received 77.5 percent of the dietary standard deemed healthy for them, women received only 70 percent. Similar studies in Quebec City and Halifax concluded the same – within families, mothers and wives received the least nourishment.[56] Survival of the family demanded that the main wage earner remain healthy and for children who were growing to have adequate food. The result was that women paid the price of their place within the family structure.

Of special concern was women's desire to appear thin and what doctors viewed as the unhealthy lengths to which some would resort in order to accomplish it. The fashions of the 1920s were designed for the slender, boyish, and youthful figure, which was often difficult for mature women to achieve without some serious dieting and exercising. While some historians have suggested that the 1930s and '40s emphasized "the look of maturity," the discussion of and concern about dieting to control body image remained strong.[57] Pundits blamed the search for the slender figure by women for the declining birth rate and the difficulty many women had in giving birth. One practitioner accused women of being "suckers" for being taken in by the advertisements for dieting aids; all that could be said for the best of the nostrums advertised was that they were ineffective and harmless.[58] If women needed to diet, medical practitioners believed they had the expertise through food science to advise women to do so safely. But even eating well and properly could be dangerous as one public health article pointed out, reminding readers that fruit was often sprayed with insecticides.[59]

While some physicians worried about the health of women who took dieting too far and criticized them for being taken in by extravagant ads, some sympathized with their desire to control their weight and indeed helped them do so. In 1933, J.H. Duncan, a physician from Sault Ste Marie, Ontario, described to his colleagues a case of a woman who had had an ovarian fibroma. She was 35 years old and rather stout. In describing the surgery Duncan noted, "In making the skin incision consideration was given to the desire of the patient to reduce and so a transverse ellipse of skin and fatty tissue, weighing about two pounds, was removed, and then the peritoneum was incised."[60]

Fashion

Linked to the desire to control body image through dieting were women's fashion trends. The disquiet about the kind of clothing women wore and its connection to health in the pre–WWI years was a continuation of what had gone on in the nineteenth century – the focus being on tight-lacing and the wearing of corsets. The danger of wearing corsets was obvious to practitioners. William Benham Snow saw tight-lacing as contributing to a vast array of "derangements" including "nervous exhaustion, ... insomnia, ... perversions innumerable," as well as indulgence in luxuries. Tight-lacing was not simply a misguided fashion, but a part of a social life found wanting. It was the perceived downside of modernity among the social set. Others were not as vehement as Snow; nevertheless, they pointed to pelvic disorders, uterine displacement, circulation difficulties, pelvic weakness in young women, weakening of the abdominal wall, bulging of the vulva, headaches, and obstetrical problems.[61] Physicians advised women, or at least one another, that more sensible dress was required. Women had to wear fewer garments around the waist and had to ensure that those garments worn should hang from the shoulders rather than pressure the abdominal area.[62] At the same time that critics were lamenting the wearing of corsets, an editorial in a 1910 edition of *Public Health Journal* argued "a properly constructed corset gives the woman wearing it the most artistic figure possible."[63] Perhaps the editor's concession to the critics was to suggest that women consult their physicians on what corset was best to wear. Clearly the only women who could do so and have "the most artistic figure" were those with enough money to seek out advice on what most women would see as a nonmedical subject.

The discussion of tight-lacing, at times, became part of a broader discussion. L.W. Jones in the *Queen's Medical Quarterly* of 1905 in an article entitled "Ojibiway Obstetrics" discussed the issue within an evolutionary context. He queried, "Why, then, do our Caucasion women suffer the agonies incidental to motherhood?" and noted that various obstetric textbooks suggested that, in part, "the wearing of corsets and tight-lacing deforms the figure, malplaces the abdominal viscera, and weakens the strength of the wearer," that is, modernity in fashion was the cause. In contrast, the textbooks depict First Nations "squaws" as suffering very little. But contrary to what the common wisdom of most texts was, the author refuted such a racial separation. Describing being called to attend two Ojibway women in labour, he was adamant that they experienced pain as much as "the ordinary robust white woman."

He was impressed by the various aspects in birthing techniques among the Ojibway, but was clear that not wearing a corset did not lessen birth pains.[64]

Other aspects of clothing fashion also came under scrutiny. Clothing was not evenly layered over the body so that some parts of the body were covered well and some not at all. Tight collars constricted blood supply to the brain. Wearing high heels was problematic[65] with some physicians managing to make wearing such shoes the breaking of a woman's health. J. Clifton Edgar warned of foot distortion, neuralgic leg pains, alteration in the shape of the pelvis, and curvature of the spine. He associated wearing fashionable shoes with other aspects of girls' and women's lives that he found problematic such as "social pleasures entailing later hours."[66] Altogether it was part of a vision of a woman who was not a domestic animal, but, rather, a social one, a vision many found disturbing. Women were to wear clothing that kept them graceful and when they did not, some physicians felt they had to speak out. One anonymously written article in the 1914 *Canadian Practitioner and Medical Review* bemoaned the new fashions of the tight skirt, which made it difficult for women to climb onto street cars, forcing them "to march along the street in a very crippled manner very much after the style of a lame Jap."[67] The racial slur was one that the author knew most readers would understand and take to heart.

The years after the First World War saw significant change in clothing. There was less of it and it was lighter. The change in fashions removed the corset from medical purview except with regard to pregnant women.[68] Nevertheless, M.A.R. Young, a Lamont, Alberta, physician, compared modern Canadian women's dress with that of Ukrainian-Canadian women whom Young saw as wearing loose clothing and using little "breast support," and whose activities consisted largely of "out-door work in the garden, fields and farmyard." He considered such women healthier than most Canadian women.[69] Young compared the "modern" woman with her sense of fashion to women he saw as suggestive of an earlier era. His was a yearning for a past that for most women no longer existed, assuming it ever had. What bothered others was women blindly following the dictates of fashion whether it be in the shoes they wore; their fascination with beauty contests, which attacked the moral and spiritual underpinnings of young women and put the physical well-being of the contestants at risk; or their increasing use of make-up and other complexion aids that were physically harmful because of the chemicals in them.[70] Physicians didn't reject women's search for beauty – they admired beautiful women – but they did worry about how beauty was achieved. Physicians' interest in and willingness to comment on the various aspects of women's attempts to improve their appearance were only a sidelight, however, to an even larger concern about women's health.

Employment

Paid employment raised the contradiction of women remaining healthy while doing heavy physical labour or work that placed stress on their bodies. It went against what physicians believed and had learned about women's bodies. This, despite the visible hard and difficult work that women did successfully on farms, in factories, and in the home. Medical views did not vary significantly from the views of other Canadians about their concerns with women entering the paid labour force,[71] except physicians appealed to what they considered was their expertise concerning the physical and mental strength (or lack thereof) of women. Underlying their discussions of women's employment in the pre–WWI period was their belief that women were different from men, physically weaker and emotionally more sensitive. Each by itself or in combination, they argued, made women's health vulnerable. As the author of one 1914 hygiene text put it, women were "less resistant to weakening influences" and "more delicately organized."[72] Young, single women could work outside the home, but in different jobs than men. Married women were not to take paid employment outside the home. The class dimension of such beliefs were obvious.

Many practitioners advised that menstruating women needed to be given extra consideration even to the point of taking time off from work during their menstrual cycle.[73] Bodies had finite energy and energy expended as a result of menstruation necessitated the conservation of energy expended elsewhere. Of course, if women had followed such dictates, they would have had difficulty being employed at all (most likely the point). Central to the concern about the health of working women was the worry that any breakdown in health would lead to their inability to give birth or to give birth to healthy babies.[74] Overlooked was that childbirth itself was hard work and that the conditions of that work were often not very good. Given worry about the health of future generations, the prospect of married women working was particularly upsetting for many medical commentators. Of particular concern were those women who continued to work up to and even after the birth of their children and in doing so caused medical commentators to blame them for high infant mortality rates.[75] Such a stance, of course, relieved physicians from looking at their own childbirth practices as a contributing factor in those rates.

A few physicians went beyond the generalities of women working and focused on specific conditions of work. Especially problematic were the inadequate "hygienic and sanitary conveniences."[76] The poor washroom facilities of many industrial and clerical environments in particular were worrisome. If the facilities were uncomfortable or unsuitable, women would simply try to delay voiding their body wastes, potentially leading to dyspepsia, anaemia, neuralgia, cystitis, and uterine displacement.[77] Working-class women faced even worse problems Some work places exposed them to the dangers of lead poisoning, which could result in miscarriage for those who were pregnant. Close confinement in factory or office also meant that women did not get the fresh air deemed necessary for health. Audrey Goudre, 24 and single, entered the Royal Victoria Hospital, Montreal, on 3 February 1905 suffering from menorrhagia (excessive bleeding when menstruating), leucorrhea (discharge from the vagina or uterine cavity), and pain in her back. Her medical file noted that "about eight mos ago began stenography this led to close confinement to house with very little outdoor exercise."[78] Physicians, like most Canadians, considered work gendered and by participating in what men had traditionally done, women were transgressing their natural sphere and their bodies paid the price. Occasionally some physicians recognized that the traditional work that women did also posed health problems.[79] But in the concerns expressed about farm work and housework there was a sense of women not really suffering physically from their jobs, at least nowhere comparable to the physical breakdown that conditions of paid employment were believed to cause.

Linked to physical health was mental health. The pressure of working resulted in many women's nerves being frayed. The 1907 Bell Telephone Strike in Toronto brought such concerns to the fore. An editorial in *Canadian Journal of Medicine and Surgery* pointed out that being a telephone operator was nerve wracking. Not everyone could do the job without risk and so those who applied to do so needed to undergo a medical examination with subsequent biannual check-ups. Many of the physicians called on to give testimony at the Royal Commission into the 1907 strike were experts in nervous and mental disorders who believed that women were particularly prone to such problems because of their sensitive "nature." Such women workers needed to be protected, if necessary, by the state.[80] In the investigation of the strike, medical testimony made clear that the conditions of work for these telephone operators was poor and that the health of many of the workers had been broken. Indeed, what was interesting about the investigation is that whereas 21 women were asked to give testimony (including strikers, former workers, supervisors, and strikebreakers), 33 physicians were invited. Even before the medical testimony, then, there already was a general preconception that such work was harmful for young women and that officials were seeking the opinions of physicians to confirm it.

While physicians sympathized with conditions working women, and especially working-class women, faced, sympathy did not support labour action. The business manager of *Canadian Journal of Medicine and Surgery*, W.A. Young, responding to the "plight" of telephone operators, argued that going on strike was more stressful for the nerves of women than the actual job they did. He belittled women's concerns about their health by sarcastically pointing out, "'Tis marvellous how health often improves when wages go up." Worker response would have been clear – yes, of course it did.[81] For Young, however, there was little sympathy for such a view. A living wage for a woman was an individual wage whereas for a man it was a family wage (whether married or not), the assumption being women workers did not have families to support and would not remain in the work force for long.

Practitioners were reacting to changes they saw in society when they addressed the paid employment of women. Change is often uncomfortable to deal with and in delineating the problems posed by working women, Canadian physicians were acknowledging their unease with change and concerns about what it meant. The future was at stake in the possible repercussions of paid employment on women's reproductive health. But at times physicians were clear that more than health was at risk – traditional gender identity and separation was as well. As an article in a 1910 *Public Health Journal* feared, the desire of business girls for financial comfort could lead them to "falling victims to the violent temptations of business life" and eschewing marriage.[82]

World War I presented practitioners with an even greater challenge to their opposition to paid employment for women. The war was a national crisis and, consequently, Canadians had to accept that the normal gender division hoped for was not possible. The physical strength of women, or rather its lack, reared its head. Ignoring the influence of social custom in determining worth, Liverpool physician W. Blair Bell explained that differences in body strength led to the different jobs that men and women held (or should hold) and thus the differences in wages. Society did not discriminate against women, their own bodies did. Even when women themselves testified to their stamina, both mental and physical, during menstruation, Bell was unwilling to take their word at face value.[83]

Some of the negativity about women and paid employment continued. This was particularly evident in the 1920s. C.K. Clarke of the Psychiatric Clinic of the Toronto General Hospital could have been W. Blair Bell when he reported on several hundreds of women who had come to the clinic and were factory operatives. He raised the issue of the low wages they received as a potential reason for their mental health problems, but concluded that the wages reflected their "simple" work. Neither did low wages lead to immorality as some had suggested; rather, in his opinion, the immorality was a result of the low mental capacity of many of the workers. As a result of this situation, he argued that the immorality of the factory setting was "rife" and it was clear to him, that such women should "be under rigid and careful supervision, and that social service should recognize that here prevention has a true place."[84] Clarke's view was one of the most antagonistic against working-class women and did not bode well for them being treated well or with sympathy.

J.S. Fairbairn reported a survey of British women in industry that provided a raft of statistics proving that menstruation was a liability for women. Yet when the figures are examined carefully they suggest that most women were not bothered by their menstrual cycle and even more were not affected in a way that interfered with their employment. But by raising the issue, the report lent credence to seeing menstruation as a problem. Fairbairn certainly drew his own conclusions in that he turned the argument around and appealed to the *possibility* of employment causing menstrual problems. He ignored whether similar work conditions could cause harm in women workers after menopause or in male workers. Neither group was of interest to him. His focus was the menstruating woman who, he believed "had" to be at a disadvantage in the work world. For Fairbairn, the psychological stress of work, the fatigue caused by employment, and the sedentary occupations and resultant lack of exercise, were all unhealthy and conducive to neurasthenia and depression. What is more, women had the pressure of being responsible for domestic chores in addition to paid work, a recognition of the way gendered divisions of societal roles discriminated against women.[85] Other practitioners worried about women working with lead and other poisons in industry because of their harm to reproductive capacities.[86] Compared to the earlier part of the century, however, the stridency of criticism of women in paid labour had decreased. The reality of women's involvement in the labour force was a trend in the modern world and as long as those workers remained predominantly unmarried the trend was easier to accept.

Traditional gender roles meant that married women and especially those with children should not be in the paid labour force. In the province of Ontario and elsewhere, studies in the 1920s reported that employed women experienced more stillbirths than their unemployed counterparts and that the infant mortality rate was higher for their children.[87] Despite his concern about the problems menstruation posed to working women, Fairbairn provided a more nuanced look at the topic of married women working. He reported that women doing manual labour tended to have easier births than those in sedentary work. He argued that fatigue as a result of "continued brain work" resulted in "weak uterine action" and women doing such work should be relieved of it. Thus, acceptance of married women in the work force depended on what kind of work they did. Fairbairn, however, did not approve of working women returning to work after childbirth if it interfered with nursing their children.[88]

Intriguing is that during the Depression, when many in society were concerned about women working and taking jobs from men, there was little discussion of women's paid employment in the medical literature. The arguments had been put forward about the problems and there was little to add that was new. Some supportive voices were even heard. H.B. Atlee understood young women's yearning for happiness, but feared that chasing after employment in a man's world was not going to give it to them. At the same time, Atlee expressed his sympathy for the plight of married women with children and how they were encouraged to remove themselves from the waged world. He advocated day care centres and good domestic help as a way around the problem of childcare. Of course in doing so, it was clear that he had middle-class career women in mind rather than the vast majority of women who worked at "jobs." While not willing to engage in the kind of support for working mothers that Atlee was, Grant Fleming, a Montreal physician in the 1930s, was also unwilling to dismiss them out of hand as earlier generations had. His concern, as that of many others, was the high maternal mortality rate, which he felt was the result of many factors of which working was only one and not even the central one.[89] Looking beyond the biological, Fleming argued that poverty was a significant factor in forcing married women to continue working.

The solution did not seem to be within the grasp of women or society. The result was an uneasy maintenance of the status quo that had consequences for those in most need. In 1938, the Province of Quebec ensured that women who had young children and were the heads of their families were removed from the relief rolls; such women were considered unemployable because of their maternal responsibilities.[90]

World War II raised the issue of working women to the fore again, but little discussion of their ability or inability to work occurred. Women's health was not as central an issue as their productivity. The perception of gender differences had not disappeared, only the need to respond to them as simply another aspect of doing business. And if smoking, which had been anathema in earlier years, helped working women relax, then so be it. If people were worried about the morality of women working at night, some industries made adjustments to ensure that most night workers would be men.[91] As for the common belief in women's menstrual disadvantage in the workforce, it could be overlooked when women as workers were needed to win a war. An advertisement in *Canadian Hospital* focused on the menstrual problems that women faced, but in this case, women and their physicians were not to worry: "'Riona' Capsules can improve the efficiency of female workers by combatting the physiologic 'slow-down' periodically experienced by most normal women between the ages of fourteen and forty-five."[92] Even though the "normal" woman experienced a lessening of energy during menstruation, relief was at hand. Some worried about pregnant women continuing to work or women with specific gynaecological conditions, but generally the concerns were fairly pragmatic.[93] At the end of the war the societal and government push to get women back in the home and to open up jobs for returning veterans meant that the attention paid to women in paid labour had lessened even more in the medical literature. But its lack also signalled a shift in attitudes that had occurred in the previous decades. Women were in the labour force and any debate about it was not over whether they could work but what kind of work they should do and when.

While a shift in attitudes among medical practitioners about women in the work force took place in the first half century, certain concerns remained. Unmarried working women were not an issue except in the early years of the century and largely with respect to the effect of work on their childbearing capabilities. Such concern was focused more on working-class women because of the conditions faced in their work environments. Married women were another issue. They were not to be in the work force. WWI and WWII, however, were crisis periods when the normative hostility towards married women working gave way to the needs of a nation at war. The decline in the economy in the Depression has focused historians' attention on the efforts to get married women out of the work force in order to privilege male employment. Practitioners were not involved much in such arguments. Their area of expertise was the health of the body and the Depression did not lend itself to arguments about married women working and health. Indeed, the contrary was probably true. Employment would guarantee enough food for a family, which led to good health. The postwar period was the time when attitudes might have changed but the short period between the end of WWII and 1950 was not long enough to note much except an apparent willingness not to reject married women working out of hand.

Conclusion

That some practitioners went to the trouble of making their beliefs known on what we might see as nonmedical issues – exercise, dieting, fashion, and employment – reflects the expansion of the medical gaze. Such expansion is not surprising. Other professions experienced the same broadening, but physicians, because their mandate was to care for the body, were able to forge a wider swathe through societal issues than most. Much medical advice could easily be categorized as preventive medicine, trying to offset physiological harm before it began. And some practitioners' concerns were pragmatic. Excessive exercise does change physiology, excessive dieting can result in harm, and some employment practices were harmful. The truth of some of their concerns were underlined by the strong beliefs of the society of which they were a part – of women's special needs – and their own medical understanding of women's bodies. The two tended to go hand in hand and mutually reinforced one another. But as is evident, change was possible. The situation of women by mid century was quite different from what it had been at the beginning. And the medical discourse adjusted to those changes in making arguments more nuanced and narrowing its focus. But no matter what the changes, physicians saw limitations to women's bodies and those limitations were based on how women's bodies differed from men's.

2 Growing Up and Facing Puberty

Contemplating the birth of her first child in 1912, Lucy Maud Montgomery wrote of her secret desire, "And will it be a little son or a daughter? Of course I want a boy first."[1] But how did she envision a boy or girl – physically or psychologically? What were the differences that made her prefer a boy for her first child? At what age did the differences between the sexes become significant or were they so from birth? For medical practitioners looking at such questions, the dividing line was puberty. They recognized differences at birth and throughout childhood, but compared to what occurred at puberty, they saw the physical differences of childhood as minor, although endowed with future significance. The psychological differences presented a more complex and less united understanding. From them, some commentators suggested a "natural" predisposition whereas others introduced the idea that socialization had to be taken into account. Reflecting the changing mores of the time was the willingness of practitioners from the 1920s to mid century to discuss more than they had the sexual aspects of infants and children.

Compared to childhood, puberty was a transformative experience.[2] Despite individual physicians defining it in a way that used the preciseness of scientific language, no consensus emerged. Practitioners often disagreed with one another about what terms should be used to describe or denote puberty and/or the meaning of these terms. Most agreed, however, that because menstruation in girls provided a clear marker of puberty's onset, female puberty posed singular challenges. Practitioners were intrigued by the age at which menstruation began and the influences that determined that age. Some influences were fixed, such as climate and race; others were more social, such as class or sexual experience. Whatever they were, physicians endowed them, and thus the age of puberty, with moral overtones. But age of puberty was in some respects a curiosity for physicians. What really fascinated them were the physical and psychological changes that accompanied it. Their discussions of those changes exposed how imbued most physicians were by belief in the natural determination of both the physical transformations that occurred and the psychological attributes they saw accompanying them. Both determined what made a girl a woman and a boy a man, and what separated the two. Of most interest to practitioners were the differences in sexual urges between the two sexes; of most concern was the perceived need to contain those urges.

Childhood

Physicians in the early years of the century did not address childhood to any significant extent except in trying to offset infant mortality. The situation changed significantly after WWI and in a way that emphasized nurture over nature. In these years, Canadian child psychologists and physicians such as Samuel Laycock, William Blatz, Alan Brown, and Alton Goldbloom, and the American Benjamin Spock, became household names, in part because many of them proselytized their ideas through the popular press and through their students. Historians have traced the increased focus on children and the advice that bombarded women on how to raise them. Not many, however, have examined how physicians talked to one another about what they saw as the biological given of infants and children.[3]

Much of the medical literature of the first half century generalized child development in a way that remained relatively consistent. Experts on children and childhood believed a child went through stages of development in order to achieve mature adulthood. One popular view was the recapitulation theory introduced by psychologist G. Stanley Hall in the late nineteenth century, which suggested that just as "mankind" had progressed from the primitive to the civilized over millennia, children replicated that development in their own lives. In the 1930s and 1940s, physicians were still using various stages of life as a way to understand child maturation. J.C. Connell in his 1935 text, for example, referred to the third stage of life, beginning at age 6 and ending at age 10, as "the time of sex awakening in children."[4] No matter when physicians believed various stages occurred, the belief in them suggests the desire to generalize all children and their development, at times glossing over gender differences in the interests of creating a comprehensive and understandable schema of childhood growth. When the schema is examined more closely, however, the details of it, more often than not, suggest gender separation.

The most obvious differences between boys and girls were physical. In 1913 Joseph B. DeLee, a prominent American obstetrician, acknowledged that at birth the two sexes were very much alike and then listed in detail how they differed:

> A close study will show small differences; the boy weighs, on the average, one-fourth of a pound more, the head is a little harder and larger, absolutely and also relatively to the body; a difference in the pelvis is also discernible: the female pelvis is larger and shallower than the male, and this is also true of the lower animals. More boys are born than girls – 105 to 100, a proportion that prevails the world over, and for all the years, but since more boys die during labor – 1 in 16 – and during the first years of life, this proportion is reversed, so that later the females preponderate.
>
> During the first years the characteristics of the sexes gradually become more marked, and as soon as the child walks the differentiation becomes apparent. The girl develops mentally and physically earlier than the boy, and one can sooner discover in her those traits of the female that distinguish it in later life.[5]

Underlying the text is a tone that insists the differences between the sexes must be there for some reason; that is, they are functional in nature. It also reveals the firm belief in biology as destiny, that social roles are a given, determined by whether a body is female or male. Even as a child, a girl has characteristics that will separate her as a woman from man. By listing the differences, even in infants, the author endows them with significance, although he leaves it to the reader to draw conclusions about what that significance is.

Noting differences continued in the postwar period and beyond. As DeLee had, Thomas Watts Eden and Cuthbert Lockyer, authors of a major 1928 gynaecology text, stressed the pelvic differences between female and male infants and in doing so called attention to that part of the body. The text pointed out that there were differences in the weight of the "long bones" and speculated on the existence of endocrine distinctions, a reference to the newly "discovered" hormones that to physicians were clarifying the fundamental differences between the sexes. Differences noted could lead to divergent skills that became part of gender identity. The 1943 *Encyclopedia of Child Guidance* explained that girls had superior "motor coordination and 'especially a more flexible rotation at the wrist.'" As a result, girls had better "dressing habits" even by the age of two or three.[6] While differences were possible to see, we shouldn't exaggerate them. Most medical commentators believed that childhood differences, compared to pubescent ones, were negligible. Nevertheless, they did see in the differences the path the child would (or should) take.

Physical differences were matched by psychological or mental differentiation, which evidenced at such an early age seemed predetermined. We have already seen that DeLee acknowledged that mentally girls developed sooner than boys. But physicians in the international literature of the early years of the century went beyond seeing intellectual differences as sexed. They recognized they were gendered, although they didn't use this term. One of the most interesting aspects of discussion in the textbook literature was sex assignment at the birth of an hermaphrodite. One 1907 text made clear that "in the absence of positive proof it is better to regard the subject as a male, both for the moral effect and because anomalies of this kind are more frequent among males than females." As the author of a 1912 text added, because it was assumed that an hermaphrodite would/should not marry, being gendered male would provide him more freedom and "larger opportunities" for employment thus limiting the need to "enter upon the marriage relation."[7]

Emphasis on the psychological differences in children was more evident in the interwar years and beyond. W.H.B. Stoddart in his 1919 text on mental disorders suggested how close to the surface primitive "man" was when he argued that "destructiveness is an instinct which appears in the fifth year."[8] In doing so, he was aligning himself with the recapitulation theory, but in using the word "man" he meant it literally: the five-year-olds he had in mind were boys. In putting the two together – recapitulation theory and a specific attribute of boys – Stoddart made the attribute a natural developmental stage. Not all postwar commentators, however, focused on natural differences. Some recognized that socialization played a major role in the development of personality. One gynaecology text pointed out that the apparent variability of girls in their affections compared to boys was not inherent, but a result of restrictions on girls' activities. Marion Hilliard linked her own interest in obstetrics to her experience at the age of five when her mother in a private moment showed Hilliard baby clothes for the child she was expecting. In effect, Hilliard was suggesting there was a learned element to what she became.[9]

A major area of medical interest in childhood was sexuality. By the early years of the century, Freudian theories of infant and child sexuality had emerged in the international medical literature. Stressed was sexual motivation in children, not sexual innocence. Seldom did Canadian physicians adopt a strict Freudian view, even in the decades leading up to mid century. But Freud's theories were not needed for physicians in the years following the turn of the century to recognize the existence of sexuality in young girls as exhibited in self-pleasure. Others discussed it in terms of determining whether a young girl had been raped or not.[10] But much of the medical literature gave more emphasis to the sexual feelings in boys, arguing that young boys were more disturbed by their sexual feelings and at a younger age than girls and exhibited them in the form of masturbation.[11]

The years following World War I saw an increased recognition of sexuality in infants and young children. Stoddart's text noted, "Pleasure obtained by rubbing the thighs together is frequently observed in quite young infants, especially in girls." As well, the author acknowledged that other erogenous zones existed – the mouth, the anus, the neck of the bladder, and the breasts. In 1937, G.K. Wharton from the Department of Medicine, University of Western Ontario, agreed that masturbation seemed to occur "during a certain stage of development" in almost all boys and most girls. According to Blatz, parents needed to treat children who showed an interest in sex with respect and answer their questions. If not, the child's sex life could be "warp[ed]." Therefore the way in which parents socialized their children was crucial for the development of an instinct that evidenced itself somewhat differently in boys than in girls. Noted by some were the "crushes" that girls often had on one another or on older women. Appealing to socialization to explain the crushes, Howard A. Kelly pointed to the lack of contact with boys that girls had traditionally had, the assumption being that as gender barriers broke down, the two sexes would have more to do with one another and as a result such crushes would not be as prevalent.[12] All such discussions were a far cry from the relative silence in the early years of the century.

While extreme negative reactions to infant/child sexuality were rare, they did exist. Betsy Mackenzie recalled that in 1926 at the age of 10 she underwent an operation for masturbation. She wasn't clear what it involved (it was not a clitoridectomy), but she was sure that Dr Alan Brown, Hospital for Sick Children, Toronto, was the physician who either saw her and advised it or who performed it. Whatever the procedure, it was done without anaesthesia. And if designed to stop her masturbating, she admitted that it failed. Mentioned as well was tying younger children's hands, although not with unanimous medical approval. Preferred was for parents to encourage their children to focus on other interests.[13]

Care must be taken that in acknowledging medical awareness of sexuality in the young, we don't exaggerate it. Most references to it were in passing and seldom the focus of much attention. Similarly, what is intriguing about the medical view of infancy and childhood is how little discussion on these topics occurred in most general texts and in the journal literature. The early years of development simply did not engage physicians' interest except as a prelude to what was to come – puberty with its physical, psychological, and sexual changes.

Understanding Puberty

The language physicians used to describe puberty and all the changes associated with it denoted a major turning point. The adjective most favoured in the early years of the century was "critical." Although practitioners did not use the word as much in the post – World War I period, most agreed that puberty signified a major shift in the lives of both sexes.[14] Compared to boys, pubescent changes in girls were more complex and numerous and central to puberty for girls was menstruation. At the same time, physicians considered puberty as a process of change rather than any discrete act; it was a multifaceted experience that could include the onset of menstruation, but was not limited by it. In addition, the words used to denote the phenomenon varied as did the meanings of the terms.

Two years into the new century, Dr J.A. MacKenzie, assistant medical superintendent of the Nova Scotia Hospital (a hospital for the insane), Halifax, distinguished between puberty and adolescence. For him, puberty included the years from 12 to 16 and centred on the "functional development of the reproductive organs," whereas adolescence came afterwards when the individual gradually reached maturity. For MacKenzie, puberty's definition was a limited physical one, although it extended over time; the meaning of adolescence was much broader. Four years later, J. Bland-Sutton and Arthur E. Giles in their popular textbook *The Diseases of Women: A Handbook for Students and Practitioners* stressed the physical meaning of puberty, which they labelled as "reproductive maturity." But they pointed out that the timing of "reproductive maturity" was not always clear, arguing that conception could occur before maturity had started and that the uterus continued to grow until about age 20, at which point a girl had reached sexual maturity. Thus they took puberty well beyond MacKenzie's limits. They did not equate sexual maturity with the ability to conceive but rather with the ability to do so at the best time, that is, when a girl's body had fully developed. Ability to conceive did not necessarily signify the readiness to conceive. Less oriented towards the physical, but very much focused on the process involved, was the definition of puberty as "the critical transition-period in which the child becomes the woman" used by E.C. Dudley in his 1908 gynaecology text.[15] By defining puberty in terms of process, it potentially encompassed all manner of changes – both physical and psychological. Puberty then included discrete physical changes that both sexes underwent during their sexual maturing. In girls, menstruation was central, in boys wet dreams were key,[16] although not holding the significance of menstruation for girls. Puberty was also a process of physical development and it was not always evident how long it lasted.

The meaning of puberty and its parameters remained unclear. Luigi Luciani, the author of the 1921 text *Human Physiology*, saw puberty as a "line of demarcation between ... *infancy, childhood,* and *adolescence* from *youth* and *virility* or *maturity.*" Milton J. Rosenau, in his text *Preventative Medicine and Hygiene,* conflated the meanings of adolescence and puberty. Others separated them. Referring to girls, one 1940 obstetric and gynaecology text deemed puberty or "menarche" as the "epochal transition from childhood to womanhood" and adolescence as "the transition heralded by the onset of menses." The American *Encyclopedia of Child Guidance* reversed that understanding for it saw adolescence as a stage that encompassed puberty.[17] Despite the lack of clarity or even agreement on the meaning of puberty, each medical authority spoke with a certainty that suggested agreement on the meaning of terms existed. In doing so, they manufactured an aura of general consensus – if not a specific one. Within the many physical changes associated with puberty in girls, menstruation held pride of place, and as perceived in the early years of the century did not have a male equivalent except for wet dreams.[18]

Age and Influences on Age of Puberty

Because they saw menstruation as the central marker of puberty in girls, physicians spent a great deal of energy discussing it. The age at which menstruation began intrigued them, as it had their nineteenth-century predecessors.[19] Given that physicians often viewed menstruation as a process of development, the determination of age was not straightforward – certainly they were not always clear about whether they were referring to the beginnings of menstruation or its establishment on a regular basis. Nonetheless, what emerges from the medical discussion of age was physician interest in establishing a physiological norm so that they could make an assessment when medical care was indicated; for physicians, menstruation too early or too late was problematic.

The different ways practitioners expressed estimates of age of menarche is striking. Textbooks tended to give three different types of ages: the average age, the average range of age, and the extreme range in age beyond which abnormality would exist. All three were used over the period 1900 to 1950. In his 1907 obstetrics text, J. Clifton Edgar estimated the average age for menstruation at 15, but the extreme range between 10 and 20. In 1902, J.A. MacKenzie provided an *average* range between 12 and 16. In the 1935 *Gynecology and Obstetrics* edited by Carl Henry Davis, estimates of average age based on a variety of gynaecological textbooks ranged from 12 to 14. The extreme range still remained between 10 and 20 and the average was between 10 and 16. One of the few Canadian estimates was age 13 as an average provided in a 1946 text.[20]

Several conclusions emerge from the discussion of age of menarche. First is the decline in average age of menstruation over time. Second, the difference between the extreme range and the average range was linked more to locale than anything else. In the textbooks used in Canadian medical schools, average ranges usually referred to those experienced by young women in North America or western Europe. The extreme range encompassed the world – not that this was always made explicit. Third, the age ranges and averages were significant in creating a standard. J.S. Fairbairn, author of the 1924 *Gynaecology with Obstetrics – A Text-Book for Students and Practitioners*, believed that "menstruation beyond the age of seventeen must be regarded as pathological." One 1935 text lowered the age limit of the pathological to 15 or 16. A 1946 text written by Canadian authors agreed, noting that menarche could be delayed, but warned it should not go beyond 15.[21] Seeing late menstruation as "pathological" meant physicians would need to examine, determine causation, and perhaps treat the young women who came to their attention. What is intriguing about the notion of the average age of menstruation is its arbitrary nature. Average simply meant a numerical calculation. Physicians gave it meaning by linking average with normality.

Although age of menstruation was significant and seemingly provided physicians with some "hard" data on which to focus, even if the data varied somewhat, what really fascinated them were the reasons for the variation in the age of menstruation between groups of girls. It was unclear what physicians thought they would do with the information, even assuming they agreed on the factors. If physicians hoped to use the information for diagnostic purposes they were to be disappointed. The perceived factors leading to early (or late) menstruation were so various and the relationship between them so vague that determining them became more of an exercise in data gathering than in illuminating the functioning of menstruation. In addition, seldom was there any attempt to prioritize or discuss which factors would be more influential than others in bringing about early (or late) menstruation, and under what conditions.

Two fixed factors dominated the discussion: climate and race. Both had been of interest to nineteenth-century physicians as well. A consensus existed that young women living in warm climates matured at an earlier age than those living in colder climates. The extremes fascinated, so often physicians compared women in the tropics to women in the Arctic regions. Edgar in his obstetrical text thought the influence of climate had "been exaggerated," although he admitted that girls did menstruate "somewhat earlier" in tropical compared to Arctic regions. "Somewhat earlier" could be significant. Dudley saw a difference of 5 to 6 years between the tropics and the Arctic (age 10 or 11 compared to age 16). DeLee saw the two extremes ranging between the ages of 12 and 23.[22] What is striking about the discussions of climate was the lack of attention paid to why there was a connection between a warm climate and early menstruation or what that connection meant.

Interest in the influence of climate continued, although to a lesser extent. By the 1930s and 1940s, physicians increasingly denied its importance or at the very least downplayed it in comparison to other factors such as race.[23] Some authors of textbooks simply repeated previous generations of textbooks. Each author (no matter what the argument) presented his position on climate with a degree of certainty that gave his comments the aura of conventional wisdom not requiring debate. There was little dialogue, however, between those whose stance on climate differed.

Race was also a factor in many of the discussions of age of menstruation. In the early years of the century, the medical literature often noted that Jewish women menstruated early, as did "Hindoo" women and Oriental women. Among the groups who menstruated later were Aryans, Slavs, and, of course, women of the extreme north.[24] The way in which physicians conflated race and religion revealed the central focus on the exotic rather than any clear understanding of racial groupings. They also spent more attention on groups who menstruated early as if it were more problematic. Physicians had long believed that mental development slowed down or ceased at puberty; in the words of one turn of the century text, "where men and women are so soon ripe ... so soon rotten."[25] Such a belief suggested a mental hierarchy with women menstruating earlier (and usually from a warmer climate) being perceived as more mentally deficient compared to other women. An intriguing aspect of the concentration on racial distinctions, however, was that physicians seldom saw them as a reflection of climate differences. As with climate, subsequent generations of physicians repeated what their predecessors had found with respect to race – "Jewesses" experienced early menstruation, Slavs late.[26] Some physicians were adamant that race was a stronger variable than climate, while others suggested that climate trumped race.[27] But, as in the earlier years, there was no dialogue between the proponents of the conflicting views.

Race and climate were not neutral variables in accounting for early or late menstruation, but other factors revealed even more value-laden judgments. Physicians linked their concern about early menstruation to young women living in cities, an environment often seen as overly stimulating. They also suggested that aspects of life associated with wealth, such as sedentary habits or too much social life and luxury, contributed to an early menarche, as did early mental and sexual stimulation.[28] In his 1912 text, Barton Cooke Hirst was one of the few practitioners who tried to explain the latter connection, although not in a way flattering to women. He believed that menstruation coming earlier in women who had been sexually stimulated was analogous to a phenomenon he saw in the animal world: "If a bull is admitted to the pasture of a herd of heifers, heat appears earlier in the latter than it would if they were segregated."[29] In conflating menstruation in women and estrus (time of fertility and sexual arousal) in animals, Hirst was seeing girls at puberty as sexual beings. Yet by making the link with estrus in animals, he kept sexual desire tied to procreation. In the early years of the century, physicians did not understand that menstruation was not equivalent to the estrus and was not a fertile period in a woman's cycle.

Factors delaying the onset of menstruation were the opposite of the ones that stimulated it. If city living stimulated early menstruation, country living delayed it. Working-class girls could not lead the lives that wealthy girls did with their intensity of social life and luxury and, thus, practitioners assumed they menstruated at a later age. At one level that could be seen as positive. At times, however, the class dimension was trumped by sexual experience. For example, Edgar reported one study that noted sexual excitement among "hard-working factory girls ... where, in the nature of the work, there is a promiscuous mixing of sexes," leading to early menstruation. Thus social biases about the morals of working-class girls and belief in the influence of a bad environment came together to offset any perceived advantage of working-class girls over those with more wealth. Country living and being a working-class girl were not the only factors delaying menstruation. Ill health or extreme exercise could as well.[30] But no matter what the factor, physicians presented each in a way that made them fixed, even those linked to lifestyle that might otherwise suggest belief in environmental causation. As such, these factors provided a predictability to the mystery of age of menstruation, albeit more wishful than anything else.

In the postwar period and into the early 1940s, the fascination with correlation factors other than climate and race continued. Emphasis on city and country life leading to early and later menstruation respectively continued, if not intensified. Physicians still saw class, mental and sexual stimulation, and ill health as influences on the timing of menstruation in the same way as they had done for decades.[31] For example, concern about working-class girls coming to menstruation later remained a concern.[32] Nevertheless, in the post – WWI years they clearly associated early menstruation with morally problematic causes and late menstruation with more morally neutral factors. As in the prewar years, when you look at the factors leading to early menstruation, the image they depict is of a wealthy girl, living in the city, tempted and stimulated by its excitement, and being able to afford to take advantage of that excitement. Her opposite is either the good clean country girl or the overworked working-class girl who is unable to get enough food. With the possible exception of health, physicians seldom explained the reasons for the correlations they made between specific factors and age of menstrual onset. Underlying the listing of factors, however, was a tone of a proper and healthy age of puberty and a fear about the development of an early (precocious) one.

What are we to make of these kinds of distinctions? Whether or not physicians used the factors contributing to early or late menstruation, such as climate and race, to assess the health of young women, they drew lines between groups of girls based on how their bodies worked. They were fascinated by the extremes of early and late menstruation, which pushed the boundaries of normality. The cultural mores of the time clearly influenced physicians. Not coincidental is that it was best not to be on the extreme end of menstrual age but somewhere in the middle where most middle-class, Anglo-Celtic girls were. Age of menstruation became one more feature that separated "racial" groups into a hierarchy of worth. The stress on climate privileged an environmental explanation and perhaps was not as judgmental as a racial explanation. The emphasis on race over climate gave precedence to nature through a deep-seated belief in the influence of heredity. Other factors such as class, sexual experience, health, etc., were more socially determined, but how they and factors such as race and climate worked together and which ones were more significant was unclear.[33]

Pubescent Changes and Restrictions

While menstruation was the most significant physical change for girls at puberty, it was not the only physical development. In his 1912 text, David Berry Hart was typical of the way physicians described the changes – a girl "becomes plumper and more rounded, the mammae develop, hair appears in the armpits and over the pubes and external genitals." Such descriptions were straightforward. They varied in their specificity and detail over time, but the sense of objective observation was present in all of them. At other times, however, physicians endowed such changes with cultural meaning. According to David Tod Gilliam in his 1904 text, puberty was the point at which the girl "takes on the lines and curves that distinguish the mature female from the male. The increased development of bust and hips and general fullness of contour add greatly to her attractiveness, and proclaim her readiness for motherhood."[34] Several themes emerge from Gilliam's quote. The first is the use of the male as the basis for comparison, the norm; puberty is when the female is distinguished from the male not when the male is distinguished from the female. Second, Gilliam linked the physical changes to attractiveness. They were no longer neutral changes. Third, the changes announce a woman's social role and her "readiness" for it. In this respect, the image raised is of a female animal in heat, attracting the male so that she can become pregnant. And fourth, the changes ushered in a new state of being for the young woman. But they also brought with them potential dangers to young women's health because the changes came more quickly than those in boys and were, consequently, more difficult to absorb. Among the problems of the pubescent crisis facing girls were the lessening of energy and circulation disorders. Even worse, the consequences of a bad puberty were future problems – the inability to lay the groundwork for a healthy adult stage that would permit a woman to bear healthy children.[35]

The internal physical changes young women's bodies underwent remained the medical focus in the interwar years. These were the ones hidden from sight, "known" only to physicians. Most Canadians, however, were more aware of and interested in the external changes and perhaps that is why Percy Ryberg in his best-selling *Health, Sex and Birth Control* emphasized them, stressing "a new femininity" that emerged. Similarly others referred to the "graceful contour" given to woman during puberty.[36] The tone of approval was evident. Indeed, physicians were very positive about the physical changes in pubescent girls, finding in them the basis for their own attraction to women. Nevertheless, concern about physical problems continued. One 1935 text referred to the "physiological disharmonies" that were "not uncommon,"[37] but compared to the earlier years, the negativity was not as pervasive. Alton Goldbloom, Canada's expert on teenagers, cautioned his colleagues not to be too quick to "embark" on what he characterized as a "fog-bound and poorly charted sea" of understanding. He insisted many of the problems that girls had would sort themselves out with no intervention. He also insisted that girls should not view menstruation as an illness.[38] Nonetheless, others stressed the emotionality that puberty caused in girls.[39] The young women readers of the 1946 *Gynaecology for Nurses* would certainly have taken away a mixed message about puberty. The authors were very clear that menstruation was normal. But at the same time they warned mothers and educators that "while apparently overlooking the event, consideration must be given to the girl's irritability which must never be actually blamed on the menstrual period." Thus the girl was not made to feel that menstruation was a problem, but the people around her were being warned that it was. The authors seemed to compare menstruating girls to some "ideal" that apparently was a nonmenstruating girl. In this way, physicians placed menstruating girls outside the normative model of girlhood even though they viewed menstruation as its central event.[40] Yet if emotionality and even irritability were experienced by most young women during this time, as some believed, then emotionality and irritability should have been seen as "normal." But they were not. Physicians and others viewed these attributes in a negative way and so they turned those attributes into something about which to be concerned.

Boys during puberty had their own changes to contend with – the growth in body size, the deep voice, hairs on the face and in the pubic area, and the angularity of the limbs. A boy's muscles developed and his hips narrowed.[41] And, as in girls, social expectations came with the physical changes. In *Sexual Knowledge*, his 1913 medically informed advice manual for young men, Winfield Scott Hall made clear what changes at puberty demanded of young men: "The spermin is carried to his central nerve system to his spinal cord, his medulla oblongata, and his brain, and hammered into these by his strong young heart; ... he is a man, every inch of him a man." But manhood meant virile manhood. Just as girls' bodies were preparing them for motherhood, boys' bodies were preparing them to become reproductive men. William Graves in his 1935 textbook was equally blunt about the sexual changes, "the appearance of the libido, powerful attraction toward the opposite sex, and a more or less periodic discharge of sexual products [semen]." The changes were ones leading to manliness.[42]

If the descriptions of physical changes at puberty at times incorporated social expectations and cultural meanings for both sexes, psychological changes attributed to puberty did so even more. Psychological changes, however, were less visible and hence more open to interpretation. Early in the century, physicians were interested in what they believed to be the creation of the normative woman – mentally and morally. At puberty the beginning of womanhood occurred with its purity, altruism, and modesty.[43] By believing that the physical changes brought about psychological changes in girls, physicians, and those who based their arguments on medical knowledge, saw such attributes as normal and necessary for adulthood, and the lack of them pathological. As with physical changes, some of the psychological shifts were problematic. In the early years of the century some physicians argued, for example, that because of the stresses placed on the body during puberty that young people, if hindered by a "hereditary predisposition," might succumb to mental instability;[44] this was especially true in the case of young women.[45]

While the specific psychological changes mentioned could vary somewhat from physician to physician, what remained common throughout the postwar decades was the link between puberty and the social and psychological separation of the two sexes, a separation based in nature. H.B. Atlee described what was happening best:

> At puberty a girl enters a troubled halfworld where, part child part woman, she has little more than the wits of the one to meet the problems of the other. While her brother faces a similar situation, he does not have to adjust to those cataclysmic changes that beset her ... every month. True, he will have the burden of the daily shave and the poser of the erect penis, but he does not have to contend with the loppy agitation of breasts that require a special harness, or the bewildering ebb and flow of monthly emotional tides produced by the endocrine glands.[46]

Puberty was a crisis for girls because of body. For most physicians who were male, the idea of the "loppy agitation of breasts" seemed more problematic than "the poser of the erect penis."

Not all cultures were as pessimistic about the problems puberty presented. An examination of the puberty rights of many Aboriginal peoples suggests a much more positive view for both sexes. Most seemed to have viewed it as a critical time, but not necessarily in a negative way. The puberty rites for women among the southern Kwakiutl, as with many indigenous peoples, included separating the menstruating girl from the rest of the tribe, a ritual that acknowledged the power of fertile women. Over time, however, some of the traditional customs weakened. Whereas once the Haida had publicly celebrated puberty, they did so less than they had, in part because of exposure to European society and the pressures of the missionaries.[47] Certainly Western society did not celebrate puberty with rites and rituals, but in some respects, the customs of Aboriginal peoples were not all that different. For many, menstruation and the separation/isolation allowed the girl to learn to be the kind of woman the culture needed. Following the rites correctly contributed to the health of the girl as an adult and determined the success of her life. The advice given by physicians was part of the conventions of puberty in Western society and designed to shape a girl's life to fit the needs of her society.

If First Nations societies often saw puberty as a time to separate the young woman from the group, so, too, did many physicians view puberty as a time of separation. Within the context of Western values, however, that separation was essentially negative, a taking away of choice in the name of protection. Physicians were convinced of the need to place certain restrictions on young women's activities. At times, they were quite vague about what they wanted done. In the early years of the century, they generalized about the need for fresh air, exercise (in moderation), a proper diet, plenty of rest and sleep, and the avoidance of excess such as late nights, too much partying, etc.[48] Such admonitions, if followed, would be healthy for anyone, although physicians did seem to direct them more specifically to young women than to young men. But often practitioners were very detailed about what they advised and why it applied to young women. Of particular concern was control over girls' educational experience.

Physicians did not see themselves as educational experts but as experts on the physiological makeup of women and as such they knew the limits of young women's physical energies better than educators. They used the logic of science to bolster their arguments and cited one another as experts in a way that brooked no denial. Underlying most of the medical assessments of education for girls was the belief that the body controlled if and when education should occur. It was a privileging of body over mind, an appeal to the immutability of nature. The problem with the education of girls as it existed (at the high school or university level) was that it coincided with a time when young women's bodies were undergoing tremendous changes that physicians saw as central to female development and, as we have seen, physically and psychologically upsetting to young women. It kept girls sedentary and indoors when they should be outdoors and more active. Education was simply another pressure when young women needed to be relieved of pressure. That being the case, education had to make adjustments.

One article in the 1900 *Canada Lancet* insisted that "all young women students would have better health could they be relieved of work during the menstrual cycle."[49] The implication was that girls needed to work at a different pace than boys because of their bodies. Curtailing their education, then, was the price girls paid for being female. Such a view contains several messages. First was the problematic nature of menstruation and the frailty of girls to endure it without making adjustments in their lives. Second was the inability of girls/young women to compete with men if they had to absent themselves for several days every month. Third, women's bodily needs suggested women's need to be educated in a different way from men. The proper development of the female reproduction system at puberty required up to five years or more and if, at the same time, girls were being educated then an "antagonism between brain growth and body growth" occurred, with dire consequences for both. The specific concern about education was that it demanded too much nutrition (blood) for the brain, leaving the rest of the body weakened.[50] Body had to have priority, for once body broke down it was not always possible to repair it. Physicians were very specific about the problems that education caused or could lead to. Some were immediate – exhaustion, "constipation, anaemia, irritable hypersensitive nerves and derangement of the menstrual function," menorrhagia, headaches, palpitations, emaciation, and dysmenorrhea. Others were lying in wait to cause future harm – invalidism, uterine and ovarian disease, and nerve prostration.[51] Still others were more general, pertaining to the wellbeing of the race itself. For example, A. Lapthorn Smith, professor of clinical gynaecology at Bishop's University, Montreal, blamed higher education for causing increasing numbers of young women to marry too late and give birth to fewer children. Smith worried that education raised expectations in women, which could only lead to dissatisfaction with marriage and eventual high divorce rates, in part because wives might be better educated than their husbands. Some educated women might even choose not to marry at all! Smith's antagonism to women's education was palpable. It was by far the most unrestrained attack found in the medical literature in the early decades of the century.[52] And it was class based. Smith's diatribe focused on girls whose parents could keep their daughters in school as opposed to working-class girls whose families needed the wages they earned.

Physicians were not against educating girls, but argued education should be different and take into account the demands of girls' bodies and their future role in society as wives and mothers. In the early part of the century, physicians specifically advised slowing down the educational process so that girls could receive more rest and exercise. Some even suggested a more extreme solution: take girls out of the public school for a period of time.[53] Puberty and the menstruation that accompanied it dictated a different education for girls and a more restricted one compared to boys.

The continued belief in the problematic nature of puberty and what it entailed meant that the early concern about education of girls never disappeared. It did lessen, however, in the decades following World War I. By that time, the issue of women's access to higher education had been debated and the decision made to open the doors of universities, although not all faculties, to women. High schools were emphasizing physical education, offsetting some of the earlier criticisms of the sedentary aspect of education. As well, increasing numbers of schools were teaching home economics and thus Smith's fears of women being trained to reject marriage and motherhood were addressed.[54] Physicians' interest in education had never been central to their concerns about puberty and by the 1920s was only one of many factors they believed hurt girls during those formative years. But the earlier themes still existed, even if in lesser form. Some aspects of education were problematic; in particular competitiveness and ambition were refashioned into dangers for young women's health. The authors of the 1930 textbook *Diseases of Women* criticized the "acquisitions of modern life" under which they placed "exhausting school duties." School should train the mind, but not at the expense of the body. And if the body suffered, the student (the girl) should be removed from school.[55] Others were more accommodating, willing to recognize girls' future involvement in the workforce and the need for them to be educated to meet those demands.[56] Such physicians still believed pubescent changes were a drain on the female system but recognized, as did the general medical literature, that most young women took the changes in stride. Puberty was normal but normal didn't always mean unproblematic.

Pubescent Sexuality

Most, if not all, of the changes that came with puberty – whether physical or psychological – were connected to the creation of a sexual being. With respect to girls, the medical literature in the early years of the century reflected a tension in attitudes – a desire to believe in the "passionless" version of pubescent girls and the need to control the expression of their sexuality. One turn-of-the-century gynaecology text argued that the social norms of restraint in the Western world had resulted in undeveloped genitals in girls compared to those in less inhibited societies. Such a view suggested that body and culture were in a symbiotic relationship in that culture could change the body to ensure the existence of the desired passionless girl. Believing such a notion would eliminate the tension between social concepts of sexuality and theories about the sexual nature of the body. As well, the text separated Western society from other, less "inhibited" cultures. Such a view seemed in tangent with perceptions of menstruation in warmer regions coming earlier than in cooler ones, limiting mental development and encouraging a younger sexual initiation. Needless to say, such girls were more often than not racially identified. Nevertheless, in acknowledging the existence of social restraints on sexuality, the text recognized (as did others) female sexuality and its strength. Certainly the international medical literature on masturbation in young women lent credence to girls as sexual beings and actors, but contrary to the argument of some historians, not to the degree that young men were.[57]

In their practices, physicians faced the possibility that some adolescents engaged in sexual congress. The case of a 17-year-old "young girl" was reported in the case files of the Montreal General Hospital. She arrived at the hospital on 16 April 1907 after telling her parents that she had been the "victim of forcible seduction." Apparently she had been out with friends, had taken a glass of port, felt drowsy, and couldn't remember anything after that until she woke up in her own bed the next day. She was eventually brought to the hospital, where an examination determined she was still a virgin.[58] While such a case could raise physicians' concern about false accusations of rape, it also pointed to a young woman's fear of and perhaps interest in sexual activity. Her fear and that of her parents also attested to the wide belief that male pubescent sexuality was not under control.

Compared to the early years, there was an acceptance and calmness in the recognition of adolescent sexuality in the 1920s, '30s, and '40s as long as young people did not act on their urges in an unacceptable way. Masturbation in either sex did not create as much concern as it had, although in Quebec disapproval continued among many physicians.[59] The medical literature emphasized that young men were more influenced and dominated by their sexual urges and at an earlier age than young women with Canada's leading expert on "teenagers" referring to young men's sexuality as "aggressive."[60] The textbook literature essentialized male sexuality, as have some historians.[61] A young man's sexuality was less complex than a young woman's; indeed, young men were considered very much on a par with one another vis-à-vis their sexual urges. They had them and were told to curb them. Gertrude Roswell's experience with one young man, the son of a church elder, conformed to the image of uncontrolled male sexuality. She recalled her date with him at university during which he poured her a heavy drink; when he wasn't looking she poured it onto a plant. He later took her outside and tried to attack her and she threw him onto the ground, earning the admiring response that she held her liquor well.[62]

Physicians considered young women's sexuality more complex than men's. In young women sexual desire and modesty were at war with one another. C.A. Baragar, the commissioner of mental health for Alberta in 1932, went further and suggested "sex instinct" and ambition were also in conflict. He admitted that some young women were ambitious, even more so than their brothers, but fortunately (in his eyes) their desire to have children and family pulled young women in the opposite direction.[63] Even when some commentators and physicians in the 1940s were worried about what appeared to many as the loosening of girls' morals during wartime, most pundits still believed that controlling their urges was not difficult for young women since almost all still agreed that pubescent girls' sexual feelings were not as strong as those of boys.[64] When girls did lose control, physicians often deemed them morally and/or intellectually defective.[65] As Joan Sangster has illustrated, perceived lack of sexual control could result in young women being incarcerated, an eventuality that often had a racial and class aspect.[66]

Pubescent sexuality intrigued practitioners both in the early years of the century and throughout the years leading to mid century. They viewed puberty as a time when both sexes became sexualized, but in gendered ways as female and male sexuality were fascinatingly out of step with one another. In the early years of the century, commentators saw women reaching puberty at an earlier age than men. Not only did women's bodies reach physical maturity before men, but mentally and sexually they did as well. Dr J.A. MacKenzie, in the 1902 *Maritime Medical News*, estimated that women reached maturity at age 18 whereas men did not reach it until the age of 25. He estimated that women took 4 years to develop, whereas men took 10 years.[67]

A similar disjuncture between female and male maturity was stressed even more in the postwar period, although in a different and more complex way.[68] Publicity over the work of Alfred Kinsey raised the issue to lay Canadians who seemed to be more intrigued by it than an examination of medical literature revealed physicians were. John J. O'Neill in a March 1947 issue of *Saturday Night* explained to Canadians, "While girls reach a more mature bodily form a few years earlier than boys, they do not, Dr Kinsey reported, reach sexual maturity until many years later, the boys at 14 and the girls at 28 years, while their peak of activity is at 35. This does not prevent reproduction at a younger age." Such sentiments seemed to have caught the imagination of other journalists in the late 1940s as well.[69] The scenario these statistics depict is quite fascinating. Girls matured faster and at an earlier age than boys except in the area of sexual urges. Thus boys matured mentally later, physically later, but sexually sooner. It is no wonder that boys were viewed as a sexual danger – you have a sexually needy individual in a boy's body, with a boy's maturity. Girls obviously needed to be with older boys at least until their twenties, at which point boys mentally reached the maturity to match that of girls their own age. In sexual matters, however, women needed much younger men. Of course this assumes that the need is for sexuality to be equal in both sexes for a couple to be well matched, which for the society of the time may have been a false assumption.

Sex Education

Perhaps because of their own lack of formal education in matters pertaining to sexuality, physicians tended to endorse sex education throughout the period. They did not see themselves as the prime educators – that role belonged to mothers and, to a lesser extent, fathers; understood, however, was that medicine would provide the source material. But to be successful, education had to begin early, at or just before puberty, when most physicians and others believed the sexual instinct emerged in a significant way. Both boys and girls needed sex education. Particularly central for girls was an understanding of menstruation.

The association of blood with injury in our society meant that reassurance of young women was essential before they began to menstruate. In 1900, William Gardner, professor of gynaecology at McGill University, pointed out that, unless properly informed, young girls did not always realize what was happening to them. He described the fright that they felt on first menstruating when ignorant of what it meant. He suggested that some saw the process as unclean and tried to stop it using cold water, while others did so because they felt it interfered with "the pursuit of pleasure." Mothers needed to instruct their daughters, but Gardner did not think many did so, either because they simply overlooked it or being uncomfortable with the subject deliberately avoided it. He sensitively pointed out that such neglect eliminated "a most important source of influence and a body of confidence between mother and daughter." If left on her own, the young girl would learn about her body from others in a way "she had better not have known."[70]

The reminiscences of English-Canadian women and others of the early decades of the century suggest that being told the facts of life was a hit-and-miss affair. Young people did not learn it in any formal way in school. Beth Richards recalled that "sex education non-existent! Was very ignorant of 'facts of life' throughout high school years – made aware of 'scientific facts' in biology class at university." When Joan Carr was growing up, it never occurred to her to discuss menstruation with her physician. One went to the doctor only "when something went wrong." Wilma Hallman recalled that when she was growing up the facts of life surrounding sexuality were not discussed in her home, although living on a farm meant she had some rudimentary idea by watching animals. What she did learn from her parents was what was "proper" and what was not. Any other information on sexuality came via school friends. Dr Marion Hilliard's older sister affectionately recalled her mother giving her two books to read on the facts of life – *Perfect Girlhood* and *Perfect Womanhood* – but she found the information rather vague. The chapter entitled "Hands Off" was particularly so since it left her wondering "Off ... what?" In his study of the Saguenay area of Quebec, Gérard Bouchard determined that young women knew little about sex and many entered marriage unaware of basic sexual information. Neither did other cultures in Canada necessarily prepare their young women any better.[71] For example, *What a Young Girl Ought to Know* from the Sex and Self Series was considered by many Canadians as a respectable way of learning about sexuality. The religious leaders of the Ukrainian community in Canada even had it translated so that they could teach young Ukrainian-Canadian girls the "proper" customs in their new country.[72] Ignorance was no longer a virtue. But theory was different from experience and if the experience of American immigrant working-class girls is true in Canada then their preparation for menarche was not very good with mothers seldom talking to their daughters about the facts of life and menstruation before they had to. As in Canada, they were expected to learn from friends, sisters, or other relatives.[73]

Faced with the hit-and-miss aspects of sex education in the early years of the century, doctors' support for it strengthened over time. Society, through parents, teachers, and health experts, needed to inform and protect young people. According to a 1922 article entitled "Sex Craze" in the *National Hygiene and Public Welfare*, sex education would overcome "the perverted opinion and bizarre knowledge" many had about sex. In a commentary designed to be read by parents, William Blatz told *Maclean's* of the need for both sexes to be taught the "ethics of sex." Parents shouldn't threaten their sons and daughters but explain to them that "social ostracism" would be the result of sexually inappropriate actions.[74] For him, social ostracism was not a threat but a reality that young people had to acknowledge.

The beliefs of some young women indicate that sex education of some sort was in order. Thérèse Renaud remembered, "At the time of my puberty I was taught that children were conceived by rubbing ... One can imagine what a state I was in, on the streetcar, during business hours! I was not the only one to believe this nonsense. A young girl friend thought that to sit down on a chair after a man was enough for fertilization." Another young woman believed that she couldn't get pregnant from sleeping with a man since she had had her appendix removed. Physicians thought that information on the facts of life could protect young women from their own ignorance and the blandishments of men who told young women they could engage in sex without anything happening. But the facts of life were not always easy to hear. When Dr Marion Hilliard addressed the women students of Victoria College, University of Toronto, on sex, one young woman fainted. Hilliard's response was vintage: "Well do you want to hear from me or from some man?"[75]

Despite increasing support for sex education, its nature did not improve much in the interwar period or beyond. In Quebec, Catholic authorities condemned the idea of sex education in schools being taught in a collective way.[76] As it existed in English-Canadian schools, sex education did not provide much information on anatomy or physiology, but rather emphasized morality through the teaching of normative behaviour. Other avenues of instruction were needed. Some suggested that nurses enter the classroom to explain menstruation to girls. In the December 1947 issue of *Canadian Nurse* there was a notation of a Walt Disney film entitled "The Story of Menstruation." Designed to instruct "teen-age" girls, the reviewer found it worthy of support.[77] Letting readers know that the film was available to educational institutions may have been a way for nurses and others to educate girls in a way that caused the teacher the least amount of embarrassment.

Other more organized sources were available – the Girl Guides, the Canadian Girls in Training, and, less formally, ads for feminine hygiene products. Many of the latter were tailored to help mothers tell their daughters the facts of life.[78] Written explanations were more available in the interwar period and after. One woman recalled that her mother handed her a booklet from the drug store and then walked away. Not all books were equally regarded by the parent and the child. Jennie Graham recalled her mother gave her a book called *Growing Up*, "which literally talked of birds and bees and was quite hazy in its description."[79] Some of the "expert" books, however, may have been more explicit than parents wanted or felt their children needed. One post – WWII manual, for example, preferred to use "medical" terms such as penis and vulva rather than euphemisms such as "private parts."[80]

Some women remembered how awkward their mothers were in telling them about the facts of life and how vague the information was. Dorothy Atkinson's mother taught her the facts of life but made it clear that Dorothy was not to do "it." Dorothy was never clear what "it" was but she surmised from the "finger stuff the boys would do" at school. Despite her mother's warnings about sex, her mother was positive about menstruation, even if scientific detail was lacking, with the result that Dorothy did not fear or have negative feelings about her monthly periods. Betsy Lawrence, born in 1918, knew nothing until she started bleeding one day at school. Only when she went home did her mother tell her what was happening. Faith Matthews recalled that her mother simply told her there would be a "showing," whatever that was. When her period finally came she was away from home and an older relative explained what it was she had to do. Another woman remembered beginning to spot at a friend's cottage and when she came home and informed mother, her mother told her the story of Adam and Eve and explained that menstruation was a curse. Mothers were not the only source of information. Some women remembered being educated about their bodies by their fathers in a sensitive way, while others mentioned learning from midwives, sisters, aunts, friends, and even from watching dogs in the streets.[81]

Several themes emerge out of such memories. First is that physicians were seldom consulted. William Victor Johnston in his *Memoirs of a Country Doctor* remembered little sexual discussion in his Lucknow, Ontario, practice, which he put it down to the reticence of the Scots.[82] It may also have reflected the reluctance of people to pay for a consultation – to discuss "sex." Second is the variety of ways that young women learned. Third, many learned about menstruation after the fact. The result for some was significant trauma. One young woman thought she had "soiled" herself, another that she had wet her pants.[83] Fourth was that so many did not learn in a supportive environment and the way they learned may have distorted their view of menstruation and their sexuality. Perhaps for this reason, women had their own terms for menstruation, among them the "curse" and "not working."[84]

Neither was sex education much better for boys, although they did seem to know more than their sisters. Some received sensitive training from mothers like L.M. Montgomery, who determined that her sons would get the sexual education she felt she had been denied as a youngster. Others just learned through observation. Recalling his farm childhood in Saskatchewan in the early decades of the century, Max Braithwaite commented that there was "no need to show us self-conscious little films of male frogs clutching females, and releasing their sperm on the emerging eggs. Raw sex was all about us, natural and constant." Charles Ritchie received a talk on sex while at boarding school in Toronto at the age of 14 in which he was assured, "While sexual desires could not be avoided, when it came to sexual satisfaction it was a different story."[85]

The amount of literature, both lay and medical, that focused on the emerging sexuality of pubescent girls (and boys) reflected fears of young people acting on their newfound sexual urges. The reminiscences of adults about their coming of age also noted the confusion of many about what was happening to their bodies. Certainly many were not well informed given some of the sources of information. Whatever sex education was offered and by whom never seemed suitable or enough. Perhaps it never is. As well, the education offered could not help but reflect societal values and fears. As Christabelle Sethna has argued, what existed "had less to do with teaching children about sexual anatomy, biology, physiology and psychology and much more to do with channelling Canadians toward compulsory heterosexuality, reproducing the patriarchal nuclear family, maintaining the hegemony of the Anglo-Saxon race, building a healthy, patriotic citizenry and protecting the nation state from harm."[86]

Conclusion

Compared to childhood, the medical literature on puberty was extensive. Puberty fascinated. In trying to understand female puberty practitioners tended to use the male body as the basis of comparison and by doing so, women's bodies became the other, somehow foreign, and at risk. In trying to determine what the average age of puberty was, physicians were establishing what it should be. They were creating the vision of what a healthy pubescent girl was – all girls should be this way. Not coincidentally, the normative experience was that of white, middle-class, Anglo-Celtic females. Not coincidental either was that the attributes of a healthy puberty were those attributes society deemed suitable for women to have. While practitioners presented puberty as socially influenced, they tended to emphasize its challenges as scientific fact, used to guide society about what girls needed and what they should be allowed to do.

3 "You can't be at your best when you're sitting in a swamp": Menstruation

In *Gynaecology for Nurses*, Canadians Archibald Donald Campbell, gynaecologist and obstetrician-in-chief, Montreal General Hospital, and Mabel A. Shannon, supervisor of the gynaecological ward, Montreal General Hospital, blamed women for not knowing or keeping track of their menstrual cycles since "accurate knowledge of the dates of uterine bleeding is of the utmost importance to both the patient and the physician."[1] But it appears that it was more important for physicians. They saw it as a central phenomenon that distinguished women from men and, in the patient files they kept, were careful to detail the menstrual history of women who consulted them. As we saw in the chapter on puberty, physicians deemed menstruation's beginning as the onset of womanhood, providing woman with the possibility of assuming her destiny as a mother. Because of what they saw as its mysterious force, physicians found it fascinating.

In this chapter, I examine how practitioners perceived how menstruation worked. They acknowledged variation among women's experiences, although many of the pronouncements made suggested that they had trouble integrating variation into their theories. While their understanding of menstruation was being refined over time – the scientific rhetoric deepened and the explanations became more complex – the rhetoric and explanations did not seem to influence the way in which physicians assessed menstruation and its symptoms largely because menstruation is culturally bound up, both in how it is experienced and and how it is perceived.[2] Menstruation, with its broad symptomatic nature, is prime for medicalization since it allows practitioners to draw a line between what is normal and what is not. As already seen, many physicians saw menstruation at puberty as problematic in girls' lives.

And in the early years of the century that attitude persisted to include women's experience of menstruation as well. Over time, however, the negativity lessened, aided, in part, by the introduction of sanitary napkins and tampons, which made dealing with menstruation easier for women. But for many women, physicians considered menstruation a potential source of problems throughout their menstrual lives. As the quote in the title of this chapter indicates, some practitioners had difficulty seeing menstruation as something as other than a problematic experience even when it was a normal occurrence for most women for many years of their lives.[3] But it wasn't always normal, Three 'medical' conditions are focused on here: amenorrhoea (delayed or suppressed menstruation), dysmenorrhoea (painful menstruation), and menorrhagia (profuse bleeding). Practitioners had difficulty defining each condition in any precise way and the lack of clarity made treatment fraught, although by mid century hormone therapy was becoming a favoured response.

The Female Cycle

Three continuing themes emerge throughout the first half of the century with respect to the female cycle. The first was the tension between the medical desire for regularity and the reality of its variability. The second was the use of analogies and speculation to understand what was unknown. Third was the willingness of some physicians to accept that they didn't know. Modern studies have indicated the monthly cycle can vary from 15 to 45 days, although the mean is 29 days with a degree of variation of 7 days. Even during a woman's life the cycle changes, with it becoming most stable in her late thirties and then becoming irregular as she approaches menopause.[4] Very early on some practitioners acknowledged that the cycle varied from woman to woman and that the variation was nothing to worry about. Most, however, preferred to see a pattern of common experience. In a 1902 article entitled "Landmarks in the Uterus," Byron Robinson declared the following: "*Menstruation* (condition): Reproductive, uterine crisis. Duration of each crisis 10 days (a) premenstrual phase 3 days; (b) intramenstrual phase 3 days; (c) post-menstrual phase 3 days while (d) the intermenstrual phase continues 20 days. Menstrual function persists 30 years." Two themes emerge here: menstruation as a "uterine crisis" and the unwillingness to recognize variability. Jennie Drennan, from St Thomas, Ontario, acknowledged variability, but not necessarily in an individual woman. She hypothesized that woman's body had changed over the centuries as a result of the environment and society in which women lived and the lives they led. She referred to the monthly cycle as a "pathological condition arising out of a non-adherence to natural law."[5]

The tension between regularity and variation continued in the later years, although its intensity lessened. Francis H.A. Marshall in his 1922 text on physiology noted that while as a "rule" women menstruated every 28 to 30 days, many did not. Significant is that he refers to a rule even while acknowledging the degree of variation from the rule. Like Drennan, some practitioners believed variability could exist among women but not in the same woman. For the individual, regularity was expected to be the norm. Yet even this was not dependable; the more physicians learned, the less they could generalize. But the question, of course, is why did they want there to be regularity? Irregularity made physicians' task more difficult for how were they to know whether there was something amiss if there was no standard bodily behaviour to go by? Consequently, many continued to act as if there was. A 1935 major midwifery text was an example of the desire for regularity. Not surprisingly, given its own focus, the author of the text saw menstruation in terms of a failed pregnancy. His description was all about the endometrium and what was happening to it, but the detail went far beyond what textbooks in the earlier period could provide:

> From the end of the first menstrual flow up to the 10th day of the menstrual cycle ... the endometrium is in the repair phase ... On the 14th day of the cycle ovulation occurs. From the 14th to the 28th day of the cycle extensive hypertrophic changes take place in the endometrium, until at the need of the period it closely resembles the decidua of pregnancy ... If pregnancy occurs the corpus luteum continues to grow and these decidual changes pass into the decidua of pregnancy. If not, on the 28th day and throughout the menstrual flow the corpus luteum degenerates, the superficial layers of the endometrium with its glands and stroma also degenerates and is cast off with the production of haemorrhage from capillaries and accompanied by the secretion of the uterine glands.[6]

Despite the technical references and specificity, the description overlooks the variability of the female cycle. It is of a norm that for many women did not exist and that physicians knew did not exist. Women, themselves, did not seem worried by lack of predictability in their menstrual cycle. Betsy Lawrence, born in 1918, claimed never to have had a regular period until she reached middle age. Another remembered that hot weather seemed to influence her cycle and that she did not often menstruate when it was hot, but she just accepted it and did not worry about it.[7] She may not have, but for physicians trying to make sense of whether a body was healthy or not irregular menstruation was an issue about which to worry.

Menstruation's connection to ovulation, a connection only recently accepted by the end of the nineteenth century, intrigued physicians.[8] But there was still little understanding of how the connection worked. One of the reasons Drennan perceived the human female cycle as "pathological" was because it generally did not occur in other mammals. Her appeal to animal analogy as a way of understanding women's bodies had long been a favoured device of many and continued to be so.[9] For example, Henry J. Garrigues in his gynaecological text told his student readers menstruation "is found only in woman and some monkeys."[10] What emerged from such analogies was that women more than men were closer to nature, closer to their more primitive ancestors, and, as such, linked to other species. Such a concept was applied to all women, but as noted in the previous chapter in separating women into groups vis-à-vis age of menarche, a hierarchy of women based on race and within race, class and behaviour, was created. While Drennan accurately estimated that ovulation occurred 12 to 14 days from the beginning of the previous menstruation, she also believed that fertility was most likely during spring and autumn, which reflected women's earlier (prehistory) life when she was much like other mammals who only ovulated at "distinct periods of the year." Because of the inability to do animal experiments (since most animals didn't menstruate), the theory of menstruation's connection with ovulation remained just that and led to some interesting, albeit acknowledged speculation. Thomas Watts Eden in his 1911 gynaecology text referred to a belief "that ovulation and menstruation are quite independent." Others focused on the cyclical nature of menstruation as the explanation, but an explanation of what? According to one 1912 text, the cyclical theory was "a statement of unexplained fact." One unnamed author recognized cultural influence in the popular idea that menstruation was a purification of some sort.[11] Whatever the theory, it reflected the desire of physicians to understand and the frustration of not being able to, the willingness to speculate, and how such efforts reflected the importance they gave to menstruation.

Neither did animal or speculative analogies disappear in the later years, although the animal ones did lessen and were not as negative. William Graves in his 1920 gynaecology text connected estrus in animals and menstruation in women in a physiological way. As for the aspect of sexual excitement that appears in animals, he concluded that humans had lost "the periodicity of sex impulse" – at least men had, although women still had "some remnant of the sexual rhythm characteristic of animals." Women were still placed closer to nature and nature's creatures. By the 1930s, however, that linkage was being denied. J.B. Collip from McGill, for example, pointed out that ovulation and estrus were "synchronized" in lower animals, but in the human female they weren't. The only reference to an exception was to the Inuit who some believed did not always menstruate during the winter, which suggested to F.W. Hanley of the University of Toronto "a primitive breeding season in the human race."[12] The racial hierarchy of women based on how their bodies worked was being maintained.

Other analogies helped in understanding as well. The irony is that many were not "female" ones. F.W. Marlow, associate professor of gynaecology, University of Toronto, and attending gynaecologist at Toronto General Hospital, for example, explained to nurses that the flow of blood was the consequence "of a break in the irrigation system of the uterus, or a loss of balance between supply and demand." Whether his analogy helped his nurse readers understand is unclear, though its negativity is. Winnipeg's Ross Mitchell viewed menstruation not as a phenomenon in and of itself but rather linked to the failure of a phenomenon – fertilization. In the 1940s and beyond, Harold Atlee made the same point, but with a different analogy. He referred in his lectures to menstruation being a normal physiological process, a "scaffolding" that was erected for pregnancy, but if it did not occur then it came down because it was not needed.[13] Medical science had the ability to muddy the waters of understanding. For example, with the use of sex hormones it was possible to simulate menstruation in a woman who had already experienced the menopause or in an "ovarectomized monkey." Consequently, H.W. Ham and C. Horner from the Department of Anatomy, University of Toronto, found the usual definition of menstruation – occurring regularly and between puberty and menopause – lacking because it could not encompass the two above situations. The understanding of menstruation was fluid and as Ham and Horner admitted, its cause unknown. Although they considered an estrogen "deprivation" theory the best explanation, proof of it was not conclusive.[14] A review of a book entitled *Menstrual Disorders* in the *Canadian Medical Association Journal* probably expressed the feelings of many: "Because of the complexity of nomenclature hitherto employed in the literature, both scientific and commercial, the subject of the sex hormones and the endocrine control of menstruation has been an extraordinarily confusing one for many medical practitioners."[15]

Not everyone needed to understand. A descriptive narrative would suffice. J. Bland-Sutton and Arthur E. Giles in their 1906 *The Diseases of Women* explained to their readers that "the female organism presents a tendency to an alternation of nutritive and reproductive activity. The alternation has a monthly rhythm; but to inquire why is as fruitful as to ask why the respiratory rhythm should be about four seconds, or the cardiac cycle something under one second." Others used metaphors as a descriptive device. David Tod Gilliam told his readers that during menstruation "the ripe fruit falls of its own accord, the green fruit holds tenaciously to its stem." Still others simply presented information as if eventually there would be a fuller understanding once physicians could put all the information together. J. Clifton Edgar mentioned that menstrual blood had an odour akin to marigolds. To the odour, Joseph DeLee added its alkaline reaction and a certain maroon colour. Others provided details on the variations of the actual length and quantity of the flow.[16]

In the 1920s Marlow was similarly sanguine about never being able to determine the answer as to why or how women menstruated and repeated the earlier attitude of Bland-Sutton and Giles in their 1906 text. Nevertheless, he detailed what physicians did know such as the changing size of the uterus over the life of a woman, determining that during the menstrual years it was average in size, that is, it was "the adult type."[17] Seeing women who could menstruate as having an "adult" sized uterus established women who were able to conceive as the norm. The desire for normative standards was also reflected in the medical interest in the amount of blood "lost," the length of the flow, and the number of years of menstrual activity.[18] The detail known was becoming more refined and complex. At the same time, physicians referred to earlier generations for an overview of understanding. Marshall in his physiology text referred to specialists writing in 1897 and 1901 to explain the purpose of menstruation and its evolution. A 1941 text quoted information that had emerged in 1920. Building blocks of knowledge existed and were used. At times, the knowledge was cultural. A text written by Henricus Stander of Cornell University described the nature of menstrual blood. The description would not be so interesting but for its unstated and, perhaps unrecognized, connection to First Nations' cultures that separated menstruating women from the rest of the community because of the perceived danger/power of menstrual blood. Referencing the work of other experts, Stander noted that "that contact with a menstruating woman would cause flowers to wither promptly."[19] What the toxic aspect of menstrual blood meant was unclear; what was important was knowing it and adding it to the corpus of medical information.

Symptoms of Menstruation

Given the confusion regarding menstruation's cause, the frustration over its variability, and the foreignness of a body being healthy while expelling blood, the medical view of the symptoms of menstruation were often negative, especially in the first two decades of the century. Anne Fausto-Sterling has written eloquently on the meanings of terms used by physicians: "The word *symptom* carries two rather different meanings. The first suggests a disease or an abnormality, a condition to be cured or rendered normal ... The second meaning of *symptom* is that of a sign or a signal."[20] Physicians in the early years of the century (and as we will see even after) didn't make distinctions between symptom as a problem to be cured or symptom as a sign of normalcy. They often had a purist view of how the body should work – it should be without pain, it should be stable in its functioning, and it should not alter how an individual felt in any significant way. But menstruation could and often did all three. It complicated the concept of body as a machine, which had long been a favourite metaphor. Unlike a machine, the female body broke down on a regular basis and then "repaired" itself. No wonder that physicians saw it as a challenge for both themselves to understand and women to experience.

Popular descriptive terms in the early decades of the century designated menstruation. Among them physicians mentioned "being unwell," "periods," "turns," "courses," "flowers," "terms," "sickness," "the reds," "menstrual flux," "troubles," "monthly illness," "the flow," "the catamenia," "the monthly purification," and "menses."[21] While many were neutral, others indicated that menstruation was or could be problematic. Physicians often noted that one of the most common characteristics of menstruation was pain and some were adamant that women could not be at their peak either mentally or physically during menstruation.[22] The negativity of attitudes was strong and shared with other cultures. Even though many First Nations celebrated the onset of menstruation at puberty, the taboos surrounding menstrual blood deemed it powerful and restrictive.[23] The latter taboos meant that women were isolated, had their actions limited, and told what food they could and could not eat. The restrictions in white society focused on the weaknesses of woman and not on any power/danger that she represented to the wider community. The constructed interpretation of menstruation was a cultural marker.

In the interwar years and beyond, physicians continued to be confident of menstruation's symptoms. Pain remained one of the most often mentioned. Concern about physical and mental abilities also persisted. Mentioned were upsetting dreams, irritability, headaches, neuroses, heaviness and weariness, dark lines around the eyes, a lowering of temperature, an exaggeration of other diseases, chilliness, decline in calcium content of the blood, lower blood pressure, diminished urine excretion, congestion of the nose, upset stomach to the point of vomiting, sore breasts, and swollen ankles.[24] W.T. Noonan mentioned "hysteria, depression, epileptiform attacks or melancholia," and suicidal tendencies, linking such symptoms to "highly educated" women, those "trained to a great fineness in business operations," and "of a neurotic temperament."[25] These were women who challenged the norms of behaviour and perhaps it is not surprising that some practitioners saw such women's bodies in rebellion against their gender-challenging activities. Many of these "symptoms" correspond to what practitioners now see as PMS (premenstrual syndrome).[26] The focus on educated women in this example reveals that physicians were sensitive to class differences between women and, as we have seen in previous chapters, whether the emphasis was on the problems and weaknesses of the working-class woman or the middle-class woman varied.

Not all was negative. Dr Percy Ryberg assured the readers of his advice manual that menstruation did not bother the majority of women to any great extent. Others recognized the importance it had for women as "one of the insignia of sex" with a psychological and physical benefit. In 1932, C.A. Baragar, Commissioner of Health for Alberta, warned against any "association of ideas of invalidism" with it. A 1933 obstetrics and gynaecology text insisted to its readers that the pain of menstruation was, in part, learned behaviour and that if young women were taught that menstruation was not an "illness" then the pain would not be as great.[27] The psychology of health was important. By the 1940s, popular writers were telling women that future research on hormones would most likely bring them relief from any discomfort. Science would aid women. Pharmaceutical companies through their advertising were certainly selling that line to physicians.[28]

Dealing with Menstruation

For physicians, menstruation was an added complication of body that men did not experience. And it was a complication they associated with health problems and disease. The very cyclicity was problematic in a world that esteemed planning and control. It was also a "barometer" of woman's health that physicians learned to "read."[29] As for women, they learned to "deal" with it. Dr Hespler recalled that "you never said you were unwell; you just dressed more carefully and put on some extra makeup and go into classes." But doing so did not remove the sense of unfairness for some – after all men did not menstruate.[30]

Over time, however, women from many cultures devised practical ways of absorbing the flow so as to protect their clothing and maintain privacy about their periods. Those of native women varied in terms of what was used to absorb or catch the blood flow. Southern Kwakiutl women, for example, used a "diaper" made of cedar bark to catch the blood and also the leaves of the thimble-berry if the flow persisted. Others used algae, and still others moss or a squirrel's nest.[31] In European-based society, working-class women and others used napkins made of cotton or other material that could be washed and reused.[32] For middle-class mothers and daughters, disposable napkins were an option that emphasized the issue of hygiene. The real shift occurred in the interwar period when commercial napkins were advertised and sold more broadly.[33] Nevertheless, many women continued to make their own using rags and it was dealing with those that caused the most ambivalent feelings about menstruation. In the 1930s, Ruth Howard found washing the rags "sickening," but her family could not afford to buy disposable napkins. One woman remembers going to camp and not knowing what to do with her stained pads and so she brought them home with her.[34] But even napkins could pose problems. Jane Rutherford remembers her mother advising her to burn her Kotex: "You did not want anyone to see them."[35] Such memories were strong and coloured the way in which some women looked at menstruation.

Physicians had little difficulty with women using commercial napkins. W.T. Noonan approved the new absorbent pads because they did not vary and thus created a measurement to determine how much the woman was bleeding and whether it was excessive or not.[36] Tampons were more controversial. The Catholic church feared that their use destroyed a woman's virginity. Emil Novak's 1944 gynaecology text expressed a similar concern. Six years later, it would appear that the experts were still debating the value of tampons. Arthur Hale Curtis and John William Huffman in their *A Textbook of Gynecology* informed their readers that it would be years before evaluations of tampons' safety could be done; "Meantime, let us be cautious, and open-minded. Intravaginal sanitary tampons may be very useful and at the same time essentially harmless if worn for a few hours on special occasions. Routine employment throughout menstruation cannot yet be accepted as innocuous." Dr Hespler recalled that she often had to remove a tampon from women who had forgotten it was there or had shoved another one into the vagina behind the older one.[37] Other practitioners were more positive. In the 1930s Dr Mackay remembered switching from Kotex to tampons and being happy to do so since she found the former chafed her. She recalled that Harold Atlee liked tampons because they stretched the vagina, which he believed was helpful when you began to have intercourse. Percy Ryberg did not endorse commercial tampons, but did explain to women how to make their own and warned them to use a napkin at the same time. The use of both would alleviate the need to carry sanitary napkins around.[38]

The advertisements for menstrual products provide entrees into the perceived lives of women, their concerns, and interests. The advertisements for napkins put forward a variety of arguments to entice women to buy the products, for example appealing to a young woman's sense of breaking down "hidebound traditions." Although some advertisements stressed the "hazards, risks, embarrassment ... even humiliation" of the menstrual period, they also offered women a solution with their product, which was more than had been possible before.[39] Such ads taught women to see their bodies as offensive in some ways but with a commercial solution to the problem. In the 1930s, specific advertisements for tampons (usually Tampax) appealed as well to freedom, the ability to swim and bathe whenever the woman wanted. Wearing Tampax allowed you to forget you were wearing it. Even students and girls in business used tampons, suggesting that the makers of Tampax were aware of the virginity issue and were dismissing it as insignificant by letting readers know that respectable young women used them. Soon after the United States joined the war, advertisements with a war theme began to appear in Canadian magazines. The theme of being able to remain active continued except that the activities were now related to the war: dancing at an army canteen after putting in a day's work or being able to work in a munitions plant without slowing down. With the anticipated and then actual end of the war, the theme of freedom of life and movement was again stressed.[40] Tampax ads appealed to physicians in a different way, assuring them that "TAMPAX provided ... complete INTERNAL protection ... freedom from perineal irritation ... prevention of objectionable odor."[41]

Menstrual products shifted the public image of a menstruating woman from one of fragility with special needs to a self-reliant, confident woman able to go about her business. Whereas the advertisers catered to how women wanted to perceive themselves, the medical image was more wary. Sanitary napkins did not negate the problems that physicians saw many women having with menstruation. Given the medical understanding of menstruation and the kinds of symptoms they delineated as coming with menstruation, it would have been difficult for them to have done so.

Problems with Menstruation

Some of the problems women faced were more severe than others. With the main ones – amenorrhoea, dysmenorrhoea, and menorrhagia – there were no standard diagnostic signs. Rather the signs were fluid, which meant that physicians had to decide whether there was a problem or not based on the individual woman's history. As critics have suggested, "[T]he lack of clear criteria enabling differentiation between 'normal' and 'abnormal' menstrual phenomena is of fundamental significance. Almost any presenting menstrual problem couched in an appropriate vocabulary of distress could *potentially* attract a diagnosis of menstrual disorder."[42]

Amenorrhoea

Amenorrhoea is the delay of menstruation past an acceptable age or the suppression of menstruation once it has begun. We have already noted that the age at which young girls began to menstruate varied depending on ethnicity, living situations, health, etc. When did a delay become problematic? Even today it is not clear and intervening too early to stimulate the onset of menarche can cause difficulties.[43] As for suppression of menstruation, an assessment of whether it is natural (as in the case of pregnancy) or not is required. If the latter, then some judgment needs to be made as to what accounts for the suppression and whether it needs a response. While in the interwar years and after, the understanding of amenorrhoea had not changed, there was a tendency to describe most functions of the body in medical terms, which often had the consequence of making normal conditions seem problematic. Amenorrhoea was the absence of menstruation and most of the literature on it discussed it as a problem or as a symptom of a problem. But as one text made clear it was also simply a descriptor and pointed out that "before puberty the absence of ovulation, which is then normal, causes amenorrhoea."[44] But how can the absence of ovulation that has never occurred "cause" something that could not be without it?

By the early years of the century physicians understood that menstruation came at variable ages, but they still needed to know at what point and why menstruation was delayed to an unnatural degree. Causes were many to the point that every woman appeared at risk. Underdevelopment of the reproductive system was almost always a permanent cause and could only be determined with a pelvic examination, which some physicians were reluctant to do on young unmarried women except when all else had failed to determine or eliminate the supposed cause. Ill health such as tubercular disease or anaemia could cause delay or suppression. Many mental diseases such as melancholia could result in amenorrhoea with the latter being a symptom of the former. Indeed the mind was able to control the body and so any fright or upset could result in cessation of menstruation.[45] Less specific causation such as "unsuitable environment" opened up the entirety of a woman's life to examination. W. Blair Bell of Liverpool, England, believed, for example, that lack of exercise, poor air, too much exertion, and even "the deprivation of masculine society" could result in delay of menstruation. Lifestyle change could also be problematic. One American physician writing in the *Canadian Practitioner and Medical Review* argued that the "new woman" with her modern outlook had caused a shift in the "natural process necessary for perfect health."[46] As in so many areas, physicians considered deviation from accepted gendered and social roles as causative factors in the development of ill health. In later years, poor health and poor living habits remained a focus of attention. In 1935, the authors of one text referred to the "rare but dangerous neurosis, anorrhexia nervosa" as a cause of amenorrhoea. In an attempt to be more precise in classification, Max M. Cantor and others writing from Edmonton summarized that there were three types of causation: organic, nervous, and endocrine. They noted that ill health or disease could cause amenorrhoea as could "emotional ... environmental changes and similar disorders." All these causes needed to be eliminated before the endocrine cause became the focus.[47] Incomplete development of the genital tract remained the most serious because it was most resistant to treatment. In 1941 Melville C. Watson of Toronto described three cases with "congenital absence of the vagina." The three patients were married and two could engage in sexual intercourse "because the urethral canal had responded to pressure and was dilated for a considerable part of its normal length." The two women were well aware that they did not menstruate, but were more concerned that they were sterile. The third woman was experiencing problems with sexual relations, which is why she consulted Watson, and the only other time she had looked to a physician for help was for her amenorrhoea.[48]

In the early years of the century, treatment varied, although it was not "medically" invasive. Some physicians advised marriage as a way of curing or providing an encouragement to development. Such a view was intriguing and signified a belief that in most cases the problem was not permanent given the conviction among many practitioners that women who could not bear children should not marry. If ill health was a cause, then treating the health problem would bring about menstruation or its return. Blair Bell suggested "thyroid and pituitary extracts in combination with ovarian extract" for amenorrhoea linked to anaemia.[49] Endocrine treatment came to be a major response to amenorrhoea. In 1930 A.D. Campbell and J.B. Collip, both from McGill University, reported using "extract of placenta" to bring about menstruation in young women who had not yet begun. Eleven years later, R.V. Chapple from Sudbury, Ontario, reported on one of his patients, age 16, brought to him by her mother. A detailed examination, both vaginal and rectal, ensued and a diagnosis of a slightly infantile condition made. Treatment consisted of estrogen, Emmenin, gonadotropic factor (gonadotropins are protein hormones that stimulate the gonads), and APL (a trademark preparation of human chorionic gonadotropin from human pregnancy urine or from serum of pregnant mares). The result was the onset of regular periods.[50] Bringing the young woman to the attention of the physician and giving her a rather invasive examination followed by powerful drug treatment without doubt focused her attention on the perceived failure of her body. The treatment also underlined seeing hormones as a key to sexual identity, the possible psychological impact of treatment on the patient, and the growing role of pharmaceutical companies in providing drugs (in this case hormone derivatives).

The latter became widespread. Some practitioners used diethylstilboestrol (synthetic estrogen compound), despite some concerns about its carcinogenic effects.[51] For Cantor and his colleagues, once they determined an endocrine cause treatment began with "large doses" of estrogens and progesterone. But like many, Cantor recognized that primary amenorrhoea was the most problematic to treat. Certainly hormone treatment was questionable in that case since all it did was to create an artificial bleeding. His voice was one of common sense when he concluded that in the absence of any "constitutional disease and of any desire for pregnancy" there is little point in treatment beyond "giving of thyroid and correcting any dietary failing." Emil Novak agreed, deeming estrogen therapy largely ineffective. The patient might be pleased because she seemed to be bleeding, but the bleeding did not represent the presence of ovulation and she would not get pregnant.[52]

Despite the adoption of drug therapy, old standbys remained such as advising marriage. One 1930 text on the diseases of women maintained that as long as "there is no organic lesion which in itself is a bar to marriage," marriage when the woman has not menstruated is "perfectly proper." The expectation of the authors was "under the influence of a happy married life," the amennorhoea would disappear.[53] Such an attitude is revealing. It suggests some conditions prohibited marriage and some did not; in this case, the woman should have the ability to conceive even if that was in the future. But it wasn't marriage per se that was necessary. Apparently the marriage had to be a happy one in order to overcome the functional disturbance of amenorrhoea.

Amenorrhoea was a serious condition. Without menstruating, the central process of being female was absent and being absent denied the woman her social role of motherhood. Physicians were agreed that intervention needed to occur but when and how? The when varied depending on the range of average or even extreme age of menstruation the physician believed in. As the case described by Chapple reveals, sometimes parents of young women put pressure on practitioners to do something to help their daughters reach womanhood. The how of treatment also varied depending on what the physician determined as causation. In the later years, hormone therapy became more popular even at the same time that advocating marriage maintained its presence.

Dysmenorrhoea

Many physicians in the early decades of the century mentioned the commonness of pain during menstruation. But when did pain require a medical response? In his text Thomas Watts Eden admitted that the dividing line between normal and abnormal pain was unclear – each woman had her own tolerance; he advised, however, that once the pain interfered with the ability of the woman to continue with her work or daily life then a physician had to accept that she was suffering from dysmenorrhoea.[54] The real question for practitioners was what caused the pain. Some referred to physical causes, whereas others looked to bad habits of dressing and late hours as contributory causes as well as any predisposition to neurasthenia.[55] One 1906 text separated causes into physical or neurotic, while a 1907 text distinguished between "mechanical" and "neuralgic." For his part, W. Blair Bell argued that painful menstruation was "probably one of the penalties women are paying for the advantages of evolution and civilization."[56] Others maintained that certain women were more prone to dysmenorrhoea than others: it occurred more in single women, but when it did occur after marriage, it seemed linked to the woman's sterility or at least with those women who had not yet given birth.[57] Such a view conforms to the broader medical perception of the female. As noted, practitioners often saw the female body as designed to bear children. Not doing so, then, went against the divine plan or at least the biologically driven one. A price was to be paid when a body did not or could not fulfill its destiny – in this case, the price being dysmenorrhoea.

Dysmenorrhoea crossed cultural barriers as did treatment. First Nations' medicine acknowledged menstrual pain and devised remedies. The Cree used skeleton weed or prairie pink in a tea form. The Dene, too, used a tea made from the inner layer of the birch tree or crowberry branches and berries. In the north, heated sand placed on the abdomen eased the pain of menstrual cramps.[58] Similarly, the response of doctors varied, albeit more so: the use of morphine or whiskey for the pain; advising marriage as a cure; various types of surgical procedures – dilation, divulsion, currettage, and removal of a diseased ovary. Some surgeries "improved" upon nature. In 1907, Mrs Susan Doane, age 38 and married only one year, entered the Royal Victoria Hospital, Montreal, and underwent surgery for an infantile uterus with dysmenorrhea. While the case record contains details of the surgery, whether it was successful is unclear.[59]

The pain of menstruation continued to be a significant focus in the interwar years and after. Some women had pain that was debilitating. Mrs Deborah Feist, age 23, entered the Victoria General Hospital, Halifax, on 23 November 1920 suffering from neurasthenia and her case record noted that she had always suffered from pain severe enough to send her to bed for the first two days of her menstrual cycle. There was no specific connection made between her pain and her perceived neurasthenia, however.[60] Feist was unusual only in the degree of pain she experienced. But since the measurement of pain was largely subjective, the estimates of women experiencing it ranged widely in the interwar years and after. The 1924 text by J.S. Fairbairn repeated the notion that the degree of incapacity of the patient was the only way of determining dysmenorrhoea. Harry Beckman in his *Treatment in General Practice* followed a rather inclusive definition claiming that "50 percent of women suffer from dysmenorrhoea, the severity of the cases varying from a mild physical and mental discomfort ... to severe attacks of pain that wrack the patient's back, head, legs, and lower abdomen for several days." He did admit, however, that dysmenorrhoea was a "symptom" and not a "disease." He offered the term "essential dysmenorrhea" to describe the condition of all women with pain. A 1935 text was equally vague in its definition. It recognized that most women experienced some discomfort, yet not all could be deemed suffering from dysmenorrhoea. Like Fairbairn the text agreed the definition should be individualized by how it affected a woman's life, but the effect did seem rather inclusive – "any degree of pain during menstruation sufficient to interfere with a woman's work or pleasure."[61]

One summary of which women suffered most from dysmenorrhoea occurred in 1939. It repeated some of the beliefs of the earlier period in that it was the unmarried, the nulliparus, the sedentary, and the younger woman who suffered. In the 1940s one text explained to nurse readers that dysmenorrhea seldom occurred "in the obese or plethoric" woman. Indeed it would seem that the "attractive woman" suffered more than one who was not in fashion.[62] It was as if "civilization" itself had caused the problem. Such a perception of cause was not singular. In the 1930s, some commentators had argued that the "hot house" girls of the modern period compared unfavourably with the women doing physical work on the farm.[63] Physical or disease causation was still mentioned, but TB, which had been listed in the earlier period, was no longer seen as significant due to better treatment modalities for the disease. Physicians also blamed bad environments – overly long hours; overly hard work; poor hygienic conditions; constipation from limited washroom facilities; too much standing; poor nutrition during the years of puberty; and the traditional bête noir of some, education of women – as elements of causation or aggravation of dysmenorrhoea. Most problematic as a cause, as in amenorrhoea, was the lack of development of the organs of reproduction. For some commentators, the female body itself, even when fully developed, seemed poorly designed.[64]

Since he took a relative approach to the definition of dysmenorrhoea, Fairbairn was not accepting of most of the theories that explained it. From his point of view, the trouble with causation theories was that they explained why all women might suffer but did not explain why some did not. As for the psychological theories put forward by Freud that it was "the expression of some repressed instinct of a sexual character, or of the reproductive function with a mimicry of the pains of labour," Fairbairn was only willing to accept that "temperamental and psychological factors play a very large part."[65] The psychological factor certainly appealed to many, but it was not a neutral perception; some deemed such women as "self-centred in their psychological outlook."[66]

Whether the cause be environmental, physiological, or psychological, the challenge for physicians and women was how to lessen or eradicate the pain. Women had their own ways of coping: drinking ginger ale, drinking a cup of hot water with a teaspoon of ginger in it, taking aspirin, or placing a hot water bottle on the abdomen.[67] Patent medicines were available. Lydia Pinkham's Vegetable Compound Tablets had a history that went back to the nineteenth century. Some women used "modern" products such as Midol, which advertised in the women's magazines with the lure of testimonies from users, assurances of its non-narcotic properties, and touting of its creation by "specialists." Most of all it promised the freedom to have fun.[68] Physicians' responses to dysmennorhoea were more interventionist simply because it was when women's remedies did not work that women turned to the medical profession for help. For less serious cases, commonsense advice was offered such as the use of baths, laxatives, exercise, or drinking watered essence of peppermint or two or three alcoholic drinks a day – the latter disapproved of by some. Sedatives or the use of pessaries also were advised.[69]

Physicians noted that childbirth often resulted in an end to the problem. Fairbairn mused about the psychological rather than the physical impact of childbirth, suggesting that "the fulfillment of the desire for maternity" could bring about the cure.[70] Evan Shute from the University of Western Ontario admitted that some women were helped by marriage and childbirth, but he was clear that most were not. Jennie Graham's physician acknowledged he didn't know everything about her dysmenorrhoea, but opined that when she became sexually active or after she had a child, her situation would become better. In the meantime, Graham recalled her doctor performed a d&c and when that didn't work, gave her a mixture of codeine and belladonna.[71] Other treatments were more invasive. Beckwith Whitehouse from the University of Birmingham reported in the December 1933 issue of *Canadian Medical Association Journal* that one young woman, age 27, had experienced "severe dysmenorrhoea" and had had a radium bromide inserted in her uterus to cause amenorrhea. During the two years when she did not menstruate, she at times had headaches and vomiting when the normal menstruation time would have been. To relieve those symptoms, doctors bled her. Eventually menstruation began again with no symptoms. At the Victoria General Hospital, Halifax, doctors at times used X-ray treatment. Harold Atlee in the 1930s was a strong believer in dilation of the cervix, but he also was willing to go further. He reported performing a presacral sympathectomy (excision or interruption of some part of the sympathetic nervous pathway) on six women. All had been given sedation and encouraged to adopt a "hygienic regime." Four had had dilatation of the cervix. None of these treatments had worked and so Atlee decided to proceed to the next step. Indeed, one young working woman "insisted" on the surgery that would most likely result in a cure. By the 1940s, however, some were beginning to insist that surgery of the kind Atlee did for dysmenorrhoea was rarely needed and physicians would be better off operating less and studying the nature of dysmenorrhoea more.[72]

Not surprisingly given all the attention being directed to hormone therapy for other conditions, physicians used it for dysmenorrhoea. Not only did they use it but some were engaged in studies of it. W.G. Cosbie, physician at the Toronto General Hospital and its historian, recalled:

Two junior members of Dr. Hendry's staff, working in conjunction with Professor G.F. Marrian of the Department of Biochemistry, established the beginnings of endocrine therapy at the General Hospital in 1934. J.B. Collip and his co-workers at McGill had isolated two gonadotropic hormones which they had given satisfactory trials in the treatment of dysmenorrhoea and functional uterine bleeding. On the basis of the work Dr. Melville Watson undertook a detailed study of 150 patients suffering from severe menstrual pain, using the preparation Emmenin. He found that approximately one-half of the patients responded favourably to the treatment, and that anatomical and psychic factors were responsible for lack of success in the remainder.[73]

The above gives a sense of the excitement within the clinical and research areas. Physicians debated the use of various hormonal mixes, but there was little doubt they saw great potential in them.[74] In the medical journals pharmaceutical companies plied their wares. The Leeming Miles Co., Montreal, advertised dexedrine sulfate tablets for menstrual cramps. One of their ingredients was dextro-amphetamine sulphate, a nervous system stimulant.[75] Practitioners saw pain as a symptom of abnormality, of ill health, and so the pressure was on to do something about it.

Menorrhagia

If dysmenorrhoea and its diagnosis were in large part based on the perception of degree of pain, menorrhagia – excess blood loss – was even more subjective. How could it be diagnosed since it really depended on the number of days of bleeding, the actual blood loss during those days, and most importantly on a woman's perception of whether there was a problem and what was normal for her? Not surprisingly, in the early years of the century, the perceived causes of menorrhagia were broad and unfocused. Some determined that excessive bleeding was "pathologic" in a young "virgin." J. Clifton Edgar reported that blood flow increased with "high living, rich diet" and potentially any stimulation of mind or body. He also linked it to climate and wealth. W. Blair Bell agreed that sexual stimulation led to a heavier flow as did prolonged nursing. He also linked acute mania with menorrhagia, at the same time being intrigued by the opposite, that is, the menstrual disorder causing the mania.[76] As with any disorder of menstruation, poor health also affected it. While the range of causes was rather overwhelming, it reflected the all-encompassing integration of body with mind and environment.

G.C. VanWart reported on one of his patients in 1907. She had begun menstruating in 1899 just before her seventeenth birthday. Her cycle was always irregular and profuse bleeding as well as pain kept her to her bed. His eventual diagnosis was that follicular ovarian cysts were causing the menorrhagia. For this patient, the degree of bleeding resulted in a significant interference in her life that required bed rest each month. Treatment was curettage and eventual removal of both ovaries in separate surgeries. Not all treatment was so invasive. Just as causes ranged widely so did treatment. For some it was removing the perceived cause – if it was poor diet, improve the diet; if it was too much sexual stimulation, lessen it. For some curettage was both a diagnostic tool and a curative one.[77]

The acknowledgment of the variation in the amount of flow among women continued, but with little discussion of how to determine when it became a problem in an individual woman. Evan Shute was one of the few physicians who admitted in writing that he was "making no effort to define what is meant by 'profuse bleeding.'" Such a term had to be determined by the patient. At the same time, he did try to give a sense of when to be concerned – a period lasting more than five days and when the first two days necessitated the use of five pads or the soaking of three. He admitted that some criticism might come from those who maintained such criteria would make menorrhagia common. His reply: it is.[78] Thus something that was common was made problematic.

Alton Goldbloom warned about this tendency and advised his colleagues if there did not seem to be any "ill effect" to give young women's bodies time to "adjust" themselves. When Gertrude Roswell began to menstruate in the 1940s her periods were painful and the flow "heavy." Her mother took her to see a woman physician who performed an internal exam, much to Roswell's mother's dismay. The only thing Roswell remembered as a result of the exam was not having to take gym classes for a period of time. Roswell was fortunate if not having gym classes was her physician's solution, for, compared to the earlier years, more radical treatment was available. In older women radiation near menopause to cause permanent amenorrhoea was used. A. Stanley Kirkland, radiologist at the General Public Hospital, St John, supported radiation even in young women, seeing excessive bleeding at menstruation as potentially resulting in "anaemia, loss of strength, loss of earning power, loss of fertility, invalidism and not infrequently death." According to him, other treatments had been tried such as drug therapy and surgery, the latter possibly "mutilating and dangerous, and short of a complete hysterectomy, none satisfactory."[79]

As with amenorrhoea and dysmenorrhoea, physicians adopted hormone treatment. In 1942 Elinor Black, from Winnipeg, Manitoba, reported on Mrs L.W., age 30, who began menstruating at the age of 15. Her cycle was always regular, but painful and profuse to the point of necessitating staying in bed for two days every month. No pelvic disease could be found. She had been treated for four years with APL, progesterone, and theelin (an estrogenic hormone) but with no effect, so on 17 November 1938 Black gave her 25 mg of testosterone propionate and repeated this every other day until she had received 125 mg. Her period became slightly reduced and so the treatment continued for a short period. When the patient experienced tightening in the throat, the therapy stopped, but her January period was "incapacitating" and so treatment resumed in February and continued for three months. Her period flow was reduced and dysmenorrhoea lessened. Black judged the male hormone treatment a success and the fact that the patient gave birth was proof of no ill effects.[80] Certainly hormone therapy had an aura of being modern, but caution was needed since long-term effects were unclear. In 1948, for example, J.L. MacArthur of Montreal took a conservative stance in warning his colleagues about estrogen treatment. He admitted that large doses controlled menorrhagia, but noted estrogen's carcinogenic potential.[81]

Menorrhagia was a condition similar to dysmenorrhoea in that both were open to interpretation. Amenorrhoea was not to the same extent. Physicians responded to menorrhagia because patients came to see them and their determination of causation reflected the values of the society, particularly in the early years, and what was happening in medicine in treatment in the later. As with dysmenorrhoea and amenorrhoea, physicians perceived the causes of menorrhagia as quite varied and consequently treatment could be as well. In all three disorders, diagnosis was a matter of perception, largely on the part of the patient and dependent on her ability to convince her physician that something was wrong. Physicians could not assess the degree of pain or flow – they had to accept and trust the descriptions of their patients. For amenorrhoea the diagnosis was clearer – the patient either had started to menstruate or had not or had started and subsequently stopped. But there was still the decision to be made how to assess the delay or stoppage. Once convinced of the problem, physicians had to determine causation, but possible causes for all three conditions were broad so that for the physician the challenge was to determine which cause fit the specific patient.

Conclusion

Several themes emerge from this examination of menstruation. The medical description of the female cycle became increasingly detailed, complex, and laden with scientific language. Underlying the descriptions throughout the period was a sense that menstruation posed a problem for most women and that the process of menstruation placed them at a disadvantage compared to men. The use of animal analogies, metaphors of a system too easily pushed out of balance, and the symptoms or signs of menstrual activity had within them a negativity about the functioning of women's bodies. A dichotomy, however, existed between the negativity of the medical literature and the advertisements of sanitary products that encouraged women to fear not – freedom, activity, cleanliness, and sweetness were all possible during menstruation. But problems did exist – amenorrhoea, dysmenorrhoea, and menorrhagia to name three. The similarities between the three different ailments were striking; in particular the difficulty in defining them and making an assessment of when a woman's experience goes from being at one end of being "normal" and crosses the line to being pathological.

4 Understanding Sexuality

In 1919, W.H.B. Stoddart, author of a text on mental disorders, pointed out that "many doctors, who presumably regard themselves as scientific men, consider the strictly scientific study of sexual matters to be improper."[1] His remark illuminates the tension felt by many practitioners about sexuality. As physicians and "scientists," they knew the power of sexual urges and they accepted them as part of the physiological make-up of humans, both men and women. But as citizens, as men, they also feared that power and the consequences if expressed in an inappropriate way. In looking at medical views of sexuality, it is impossible to separate the scientific from the social – each influenced the way in which sexuality was understood.

Since Michel Foucault's pioneering *History of Sexuality*, in which he posited the rise of the medical profession's involvement in the discourse on sexuality, historians have looked to doctors as shapers and reflectors of sexual sentiments held by the wider society and have argued that sexuality is, in part, a constructed force. While some non-Canadian historians have suggested that psychologists, social workers, and sociologists increased their importance in "constructing sexual ideology and practice," in Canada they certainly did not have the kind of influence that physicians maintained – the medical model held sway and others built on it rather than creating a new one.[2] Practitioners incorporated the subject of sexuality in what they defined as medical, even though their approach encompassed their personal and social opinions. Many Canadians gave weight to that rhetoric, both because it confirmed their own ideas and attitudes and because of physicians' status based on their knowledge of the body. Generally that picture of the body was a closed one, a comforting view of stability. At times, however, rifts appeared.

This chapter examines the medical perceptions of sexuality in Canada. The argument of the chapter revolves around the sources of doctors' knowledge: their medical education and their experience with patients, and attitudes shared with the rest of society. From those sources five points are stressed. First, to understand medical attitudes towards sexuality you need to understand the situation of physicians themselves. What did they think they knew? Second was their personal sense of vulnerability vis-à-vis sexuality when the patient was female. Third, by including a discussion of male sexuality, the gendered (relational) aspect of the sexual discourse is acknowledged. Fourth, in examining medical descriptions of female sexuality, it becomes clear that tension and ambivalence in beliefs and attitudes permeate the medical literature. Within the examination of sexuality in each sex, a study of the sexual problems many faced, and which physicians acknowledged, offsets the medical attempts in other discussions to create a normative model of gendered sexuality. Last, the urge to control sexuality was the underlying theme that physicians stressed and many women internalized, albeit in their own ways.

Medical Training and Knowledge

Two contextual factors in determining medical perceptions of sexuality were doctors' training and what they thought they knew about sexual issues. Early in the century, physicians wrote as if they had a responsibility to advise patients and others on sexual issues, despite the limited education on sexuality they received in medical schools.[3] Thus it is not surprising that the literature Canadian physicians were reading and in particular publishing contained mixed messages and reflected practitioners' personal ambivalence about sexuality. Certainly reticence concerning sexuality was easy to find. In a letter to the editor of the *Canadian Journal of Medicine and Surgery* in 1901, J. Hunter pointed out that while it was "fashionable" to speak of various physical ailments, "the strictest censorship must always be kept up lest any reference should ever be made to the sexual functions."[4]

In the years after WWI, some changes in attitudes did occur. Despite the continued lack of training of physicians on the subject of sexuality in the interwar years and even afterwards,[5] Canadian physicians were aware of and participated in the various discussions on sexuality in the medical literature (professional and popular) more than they had. Admitted more publicly was that the sexual instinct was a source of pleasure and its expression necessary for health.[6] Freud's influence was present, although not strongly endorsed or even overly controversial. Certainly few actually read Freud's work – rather his ideas were becoming part of the cultural fabric and often distorted. His ideas were ones to adopt, modify, or reject. Percy Ryberg was perhaps typical. In his popular advice manual, *Health, Sex and Birth Control*, he expressed concern about what he saw as rejection of sexual repression and the adoption by "pseudo-psychologists" of "free indulgence of what they call the 'libido.'" Sex did seem pervasive, as Ryberg made clear: "Take a look around at any newsstand and see how many magazines covers and advertisements are calculated to appeal to some form of sex instinct ... Advertisements continually harp on the theme 'would *he* like it?' or 'would *she* like it?' ... Even soap will provide you with 'the skin you love to touch'! ... Any visitor from Mars would think we were a race of people whose sole interest in life was sex."[7]

Canadian physicians were major participants in the discussion of sexuality despite their medical education having ignored the topic. They may not have been trained but at least they "understood" the body, the site of sexual pleasure, and they understood sexuality's power. As society in general and the specifics of urban life in particular placed temptations in the path of both men and women, Victorian morality seemed to be passing. The sexes were coming into closer proximity with one another as increasing numbers of women entered the work force. The disruption of war, the growing emancipation of women, and the economic problems that were delaying marriage all meant that sexual activity was increasingly occurring before marriage.[8] World War II amplified these trends.[9]

Women a Threat

Part of physicians' working context was their vulnerability. Late-nineteenth-century practitioners were sensitive to the problems facing a man (even a physician) physically examining a woman and warned one another about the dangers of false accusations by patients of sexual impropriety.[10] Such fears persisted into the new century. A 1902 editorial in the *Canadian Practitioner and Review* entitled "Blackmailer Attacks Physicians" described one couple who blackmailed physicians based on the woman's accusation of seduction. In 1911, while working at the University of Toronto, Ernest Jones, a protégé of Freud, was charged with seduction by a patient. Fortunately for Jones, the university president, Sir Robert Falconer, rejected the accusation and made it clear to the woman that she and her lesbian partner, a doctor herself, were open to legal action for making such a charge. The various interpretations that such a case could provide do not negate the existence of the original complaint and the fear that it could engender (whether true or false) in the medical community. The medical fraternity was a small one, and although in this case there was an attempt to keep the accusation contained, it is likely that some rumors about it or other accusations against physicians were widely discussed and became part of the lore of medical practice. In 1912 Barton Cooke Hirst, a major American figure in the obstetrical care of women, advised the student readers of his textbook about the dangers of being accused of assault by female patients. He noted that erotic females existed and during a regular vaginal examination with a speculum had been known to become orgasmic. Doctors' defence should be to "secure the services of an office nurse, who is ... a safeguard against a serious risk of attempts at blackmail." Hirst made his warning believable by admitting that four or five of his personal friends had been falsely accused.[11] Neither Hirst nor other commentators could conceive (or would admit) that some of their medical colleagues did in fact take advantage of their patients. In the script they wrote for one another, doctors were the victims.

Although lessening, the medical fear of false accusation of sexual impropriety with patients never totally disappeared. Former women students of Dr Harold Atlee, chief of obstetrics and gynaecology at Dalhousie Medical School, Halifax, recalled that during their training in the 1920s and 1930s, Atlee (like Hirst) made a point of telling his male students never to give a vaginal exam without a nurse being present.[12] Atlee wanted both physician and patient to be comfortable in their relationship. He understood that both were sexed beings and that neither one left their sexual identities outside the medical office. Dorothy Atkinson might have wished for a similar awareness on the part of her doctor. She was living in the Beaches area of Toronto in the 1940s when she went to her physician for a routine check-up. He was chatting with her while giving a vaginal exam, and with his finger still in her asked her how her husband felt about sex. Atkinson recalled, "I remember I was stunned ... frozen and I knew there was something wrong but it was me it wasn't him."[13] Her willingness to accept responsibility for her own discomfort reflects the status practitioners in Canada had reached by the 1940s. But her inner reaction revealed how other women might voice their concern about the impropriety of what they saw physicians doing in the examination room. Their unease and the fear of doctors of being falsely accused reflected how powerful both parties saw the sexual drive to be.

Normative Male Sexuality

Physicians, most of whom were male, had a sureness about what male sexuality was like. They had experienced it and their perception of it clear; it was and should be heterosexual. Indeed for adult men, marriage was deemed necessary for the full functioning of manhood. And despite suggestions by some historians that the issue of sexual control declined by the turn of the century, much of the literature in the early years continued to focus on the need for it largely because commentators envisioned the adult male's sexual drive as strong, bordering on uncontrolled and aggressive.[14] Men's role in sexual play was dominant and confirmed even by the actions of their sperm, which "exert[ed] no small amount of energy in their vigorous flagellate movements."[15] Lay and popular medical literature speculated on the reasons for the strong sexual urge in men. The belief by many men that sexual activity was necessary for their health was one. Less focused on health was the common belief in the wider society that sex was simply a natural male urge, existing in a much more uniform way in men than it did in women. And it was an urge that would last throughout most of their lives. Man was a sexual being and as pundits comforted themselves, only in advanced old age did lack of vigor become an issue.[16]

With some exceptions, in the years following WWI, physicians continued to view men's sexuality as central to their being, in the words of one practitioner an instinct "second only to that of self-preservation." It was a result of evolution, a reflection of being the active force in society, or as one 1940 text concluded, it was just nature.[17] But there were problems attached to a strong sexual nature. F.S. Parney of the Department of Pensions and National Health, Ottawa, warned that men had to get over "a false conception almost amounting to swagger in the case of many young men, that promiscuity is a sign of virility."[18] Like nature, men's sexual urges needed to be controlled. But for Dr George Melvin from Fredericton, New Brunswick, it was not man's responsibility alone. He used the advancements of women to make the point that woman "must needs take upon her shoulders the full equal responsibility with the masculine half of humanity for the abounding commonness of promiscuity."[19] He expressed a certain unease and hostility towards changes in women's lives – if they wanted to be equal so be it, but they had to accept the consequences and responsibilities that went with equality. While not saying that the sexual urges were the same in men and women, he was suggesting that they were significant in both. An article on sex hygiene in *Canadian Health* in 1930 reiterated an older view of control when it emphasized a woman "should be careful not to arouse the sexual desire of men by words or acts or suggestive clothing, for their sexual desire is easily aroused."[20] Such an article placed responsibility on the woman but, unlike Melvin's diatribe, painted the man at the mercy of his urges and did so in a way that infantilized him. Generally, however, that type of scenario was dying out in the postwar period. The belief was that men could and should have control over their bodies.[21] Interestingly, the belief that men could control and moderate their sexual urges seems to contradict the arguments of some American historians, who insist that sexual aggressiveness in men became a more accepted aspect of men's identity in the period after WWI.[22] Others argued that such a call for control was Victorian. If so, the Victorian era lasted a significantly longer time in Canada than it did elsewhere. But the difference may lie in the writers consulted. There is little doubt that the emphasis on control of sexuality declined if you look at the "liberal" writers on the topic, those foreshadowing the future.[23] But physicians were not necessarily "liberal" or if so not in the same way. The more liberal writers on sexuality often wrote in an abstract context; that is, they conceptualized what they might like sexuality to be. Physicians at times also did so, but even their abstract notions were grounded in the patients they saw – girls and women who had been raped, women bearing illegitimate children, men with VD. Such realities reinforced the older desire for control (not denial) of male passions.

"Problems" with Male Sexuality

Given the centrality of sexuality in the definition of manhood, a significant worry in the international literature early in the century was non-performance. Perceived causes of impotence were many: use of birth control, masturbation, opium and alcohol use, disease of the nervous system, injuries to the head or back, physical malformations, abstinence, old age, and excessive sexual relations.[24] In his 1906 text *Genito-Urinary Diseases and Syphilis*, Henry H. Morton tried to offset the hysteria over masturbation that was prevalent in the popular literature of the time and blamed that hysteria for the "psychical impotence" often found in nervous young men. Morton was more sympathetic than some about causation in that he did not focus on moral factors. He agreed that the excessive use of drugs could result in impotence but also noted that "workmen who are exposed to the exhalations of certain chemicals – such as arsenic, antimony, and lead - are affected in the same way."[25]

Concern about male performance persisted and even increased as Canadian practitioners joined the chorus throughout the interwar years and beyond. They described the problems linked to ejaculation: excessive nocturnal emissions, spermatorrhoea, and premature ejaculation.[26] Of even greater moment were men who did not have the required sexual feeling towards women and could not perform the act of sexual intercourse either for medical reasons, because of sexual exhaustion caused by their excesses in earlier years, or because of venereal disease.[27] Men's inability to perform was obvious. Some linked the inability to neurosis expressed in the inability of the man to transfer affection from his mother to his wife. Or in the words of Edwin Hirsch in the Canadian imprint of his 1948 text, inability to perform could simply be the result of "sexual fear, sexual ignorance or sexual stupidity."[28]

If impotence in men was at one end of the sexual spectrum, the misuse of sexuality was at the other. Through the medical texts they read as students and as practitioners, physicians learned details of what some considered the more sordid aspects of human sexual behaviour, in particular male behaviour.[29] Excessive masturbation, for example, could turn thoughts away from women.[30] In a 1905 text on legal medicine by Frank Winthrop Draper, the author informed his readers of men who sexually assaulted "little girls" to gratify their "lust." Others did so due to "the disgusting and altogether repulsive and horrible idea entertained by the ignorant and profligate that if a man afflicted with gonorrhea has connection with a healthy chaste virgin, he will be cured of his venereal disease." Neither was Draper the only physician who mentioned the rape of young girls or the misguided belief in the curative power of intercourse with a virgin.[31] Control was needed and, not surprisingly, physicians endorsed, as many women's organizations did, a single standard of purity based on that of women. Such a view tended to essentialize male sexuality (in need of control) as well as female sexuality (in control). Charles C. Norris in his 1913 text *Gonorrhea in Women* was not sanguine, however, about the ability of men to change. Nevertheless, men needed to be educated (warned) about the dangers of excessive sexuality and how it could diminish their energy. It was that threat that underlay many of the antimasturbatory treatises of the time. As an anonymous writer noted in the *Canadian Journal of Medicine and Surgery*, men must shift focus from "evil desires" to "healthful labor."[32] If not, their physical, mental, and moral health would be compromised and psychological conflict develop.

If the literature is to be believed, many men had difficulty channeling their urges into "proper" behaviour. As late as the 1940s physicians worried that old beliefs continued among some men; for example, that sex with a virgin could cure gonhorrhoea.[33] While most physicians did not believe that masturbation could cause disease as had once been the case, some still suggested that it could weaken the body, lessen muscular vigour, even leave a man unable to satisfy the sexual needs of his wife.[34] For others, the problem with masturbation was not the act itself but the conflict about it that often ensued, which could lessen men's virility.[35] Being virile was central to manhood and revolved around a heterosexual relationship. New in the years after WWI, however, was the medical discourse on homosexuality. For the medical literature the homosexual act was an indication of infantile sexuality, a view with Freudian overtones.[36] Some of the international literature suggested it was also dangerous behaviour and could lead to neurosis and insanity.[37] Voices of compassion did exist that tried to separate the biological (scientific) view of "inverts" from the social. In the 1940s Ryberg's was a voice of calm even as he disapproved. He believed homosexuality emerged when young men were thrown together with no chance of sexual outlet with a woman. Thus as an identity it could be contingent. If not, he comforted his readers that as a continuing phenomenon homosexuality was a product of genetics not environment; that is, homosexuals were born, not made. In 1950, S.R. Laycock, a psychologist with the Saskatoon Canadian Mental Hygiene Association using the work of Alfred Kinsey, noted that 37 percent of men had had some kind of overt homosexual experience. It was consequently not unusual or atypical. It did not necessarily determine identity, but he insisted it was not normal.[38] Lacking in the discourse was an acceptance of different "types" of sexual expression that existed in some other cultures. Rather, the medical commentators either condemned homosexuality outright or tried to explain its existence, while being negative about it.[39]

Normative Sexuality in Women

Compared to men, what was normal sexuality for women was less clear. As we have already seen, intriguing for physicians in the early decades of the century was the close association made between sexuality in women and menstruation, a phenomenon many saw as problematic and that they endeavoured to understand by comparing it to the rut in animals. One turn-of-the-century textbook appealed to a form of evolution that had "cooled" the "primeval sexual instincts" in women, but had offset that cooling by forming a sexual urge that, unlike oestrus in animals, lacked periodicity – that is, it functioned all year round.[40] Or as Dr Jennie Drennan argued, as a race became more artificial in the way it lived, it became more sexually inclined, to the point that the body would even change its way of functioning.[41] Such beliefs suggested, if not a sexuality equal to men's, one that did exist. In part, the acknowledgment of the sexual woman was linked to the age-old notion that sexual satisfaction in women stimulated conception, which some historians have argued ended at the end of the Enlightenment century, but which many physicians as represented in the largely international literature continued to believe or if not believe were unwilling to dismiss out of hand.[42] At the same time, there was a sense that women's sexuality was more varied than man's and less predictable.[43] All agreed, however, that women had more control over their sexual urges than men.

The international literature being read made clear that the natural site of arousal in women was the clitoris.[44] Not until the interwar years did some descriptions reflect Freud's emphasis on the vagina as the seat of sexual pleasure and even they were not dominant. The explicit description in some texts of the pleasure women experienced in heterosexual intercourse is perhaps surprising. In his 1912 obstetric text, Hirst told his student readers about the nature of the orgasm:

> These interesting experiments upon animals have been confirmed by observations which gynecologists occasionally have the opportunity of making upon erotic females during a specular examination. It is justifiable, therefore, to state that in the orgasm a woman's uterus becomes broader and shorter; that it descends into the small pelvis; that the cervix projects into the vagina, becomes broader, shorter, and softer, and that the os opens; these actions being intermittent, the uterus might be likened to an animal gasping for breath. It would appear that the intention of this action is to suck the seminal fluid into the uterine cavity.[45]

Three points emerge. First, Hirst did not question the morality of a physician watching an orgasm in his patient – it was "science." Second, one result of that "science" was to hypothesize women's active role in

the potential conception process. Third, the animal analogy continues. Women aroused are like animals aroused. The belief in the sexual
woman led some physicians to worry that without a normal sex life,
sexual energy could easily be diverted into nonhealthy channels and
cause physical problems. Thus single women (which included widows)
were at risk. One text, in what can only be seen as an antagonistic and
misogynous tone, described the single woman who, "As a result of her
unsatisfied physiological requirements ... either throws herself into
some desperate enterprise – suffragism or theosophy – the sophistry of
which suits well her mental attitude of vagueness and indefinite desire;
or she may drift into a condition of apathy and neurasthenia."[46]

By the interwar years, physicians were more accepting of female sexuality than their predecessors. Yet ambivalence remained. Doctors still
emphasized the differences between the two sexes – women's sexual
response was less than man's[47] – although those differences were no
longer seen by many as fundamental. But at times they were not sure.
Physician writers could both acknowledge sexual feelings in some
women and suggest that others did not share them. Toronto doctor
Frank Walker divided women into different groups depending on race
with each one having a different type of sexual response.[48] While most
physicians still acknowledged the clitoris as the centre of sexual feeling in women, not all did. Some adopted the Freudian view that the
mature sexual response was centred in the vagina.[49] Neither was there
consensus on sexuality after menopause.[50] What physicians did continue to agree on, although to a lesser extent than before, was that pleasure might aid in conception. Textbooks continued to follow the path
of their predecessors – orgasm wasn't necessary for conception, but it
wouldn't hurt. Physicians also acknowledged that it was a widespread
belief among women who, unable to conceive, often blamed their infertility on their lack of sexual satisfaction.[51] Such a belief gave primacy
to reproduction over sexuality, while at the same time acknowledging
woman's sexual nature.

What comes out in the medical literature is that physicians were
hedging their bets because they could not generalize female sexuality.
What all agreed on, however, was that female sexual feelings should
be expressed only within a marital relationship. Those unable to marry
would have to restrain themselves even though some doctors saw normative sexual activity as positive and healthy for women. At the same
time, physicians were aware that not all women fit the sexual norm
that physicians considered natural. Four sexual problems in particular

concerned practitioners: frigidity, the inability to experience and enjoy sexual intercourse; enjoying intercourse too much; masturbation, sometimes deemed normal, at other times not; and lesbianism, recognized but not accepted as normal.

Too Little or Too Much Sexual Drive

In the early years of the century, international literature dominated the discussion of frigidity. Sometimes the result of physical problems such as painful intercourse (dyspareunia) or the lack of technique on the part of the husband,[52] both causes provided hope for a cure. Frigidity caused by the underdevelopment of pelvic organs, especially the ovaries, which some considered the seat of sexual feeling, however, did not.[53] Such women were destined to have a life of nonsexual response. Some Canadian voices joined the international discussion by the 1930s and '40s, perhaps a reflection of the increased emphasis they placed on sexuality for pleasure within marriage. Non-Canadian commentators, however, continued to dominate by force of interest and numbers. Some advocated new treatments such the use of psychoanalysis or the female sex hormone, reflecting the idea that causation lay either in the psyche or the body.[54] Emotional frigidity was difficult to treat, although some texts remained optimistic that a loving husband could work wonders or that knowledge about how sexuality worked would break down the floodgates of sexual repression.[55] Others were not as hopeful, believing sexual repression could both originate in neuroses or result in them. Whichever it was would be difficult to determine and take significant time to treat.[56] When the cause of frigidity was physical, concern was tempered by limited optimism. On 10 January 1943 Mrs Emily Lauts, age 39, entered the Kitchener-Waterloo hospital for dilatation of her vagina. The case record noted that her hymen was unruptured and that her "parts" were "very small" and that after five months of marriage she had not had marital relations. On discharge the record claimed, "This has been a perfect cure"; "can fulfill marital duties." But at times little could be done, as in the case of Mrs H., who was suffering from maldevelopment of the uterus. Age 24, she had never menstruated, had never experienced sexual feelings, and "since she was married had rarely experienced sexual satisfaction."[57]

If the Canadian literature did not express much concern about frigidity in the early years of the century, it did so about the problems of excessive sexuality. Doctors related to their colleagues the experiences of patients who had become excited by "use of the current" or "close application to music." As already seen, women consumed with desire frightened practitioners but such women also fascinated.[58] So fearful was the image of the nymphomaniac that R.W. Garrett, professor of obstetrics and gynaecology, Queen's University, in his turn-of-the-century Canadian text, mentioned clitoridectomy and oophorectomy as cures.[59] Concern about prostitution was part of the worry about excessive female sexuality. Leading physicians in Canada such as Helen MacMurchy, who had undertaken an Ontario study of the "feebleminded," and C.K. Clarke, an expert in mental disorders, believed feeblemindedness and mental deficiency were attributes of most prostitutes. Feebleminded women simply did not have the mental strength to resist their sexual urges or to resist the pressure of men who wanted to take sexual advantage of them.[60] Then there were promiscuous girls who didn't charge for their services except for being willing to receive a gift on a date.[61]

The efforts to combat venereal disease after WWI kept prostitution to the fore of concern. Whatever drove women to prostitution, its morality (or more accurately its immorality) was central to all the discussions.[62] J.J. Heagerty, head of the Venereal Disease Control in Canada, reported on Canadian studies that indicated prostitutes were "recruited from girls who leave school before fourteen years of age." And as the earlier period did, Heagerty associated prostitutes with the feebleminded. Amanda Peate was an example. At age 16 she entered the Victoria General Hospital, Halifax, on 17 August 1921 suffering from syphilis. Her case record states that "Pat. admits having sexual intercourse about June seventh." On examining her the record adds, "Pat. is fair young female of very low type of intelligence." C.K. Clarke described one girl who had been examined at the Psychiatric Clinic, Toronto General Hospital. His descriptions focused on her working-class status, her mental age, and her inability to decipher moral from immoral behaviour:

> Jennie J. Age 19 ... left school between 15 and 16 ... To the ordinary observer nothing unusual would be noticeable; the trained investigator would soon discover her defects, mental and moral. And the Biet-Simon tests show that her mental age was less than twelve ... Like many of her class she earned small wages, did the simplest kind of work, and went from factory to factory with persistent regularity ... it was evident from her statements

and language that there was little about vice that she did not pick up ... Is a typical high grade moron. Has had syphilis for a year and a half. During her whole conversation was chewing gum and did not show the slightest hesitation in telling her story. This girl's good looks make it difficult to save her from herself, and society from her evil influence as a distributor of venereal disease.[63]

Clarke seems equally perturbed by her habit of gum chewing – perhaps not showing enough deference to him – and her lack of remorse about her activities, as the activities themselves. Physicians considered morally defective women especially problematic, women who actively engaged in looking for sexual excitement and in doing so went from a nonmoral stance to an engaged immoral one.

World War II brought the fear of sexual transgression to a peak. Modern adolescent girls were a problem as they went "soldier hunting in juke joints and dance halls."[64] Also worrisome were women in domestic employment or in personal service who, according to some, were "responsible for a rather large number of military and civilian infections." And wives of soldiers looking for "diversions" while their husbands were away were suspect.[65] Soldiers were at risk! In a study of the source of VD in the Royal Canadian Air Force, the contacts in order of significance were: "waitresses, office workers, factory workers, domestic help, prostitutes and housewives."[66] While some temperate voices were heard, they were in the minority. Percy Ryberg in his 1942 manual described prostitutes as ordinary women who had failed, women who had rejected or not been able to have "an honourable living" or "a fulfilled sex life with an understanding and loving husband." Perhaps the most sympathetic was Gordon Bates, the general director of the Health League of Canada. A few years after the war he pointed out that women were not the only source of VD, men were as well. In addition, "Where women are underpaid and under-privileged, prostitution will develop. Equal educational and economic obligations for women will ultimately destroy prostitution."[67] No matter what the reason for prostitution, the perceived sexuality of women was at its centre. Doctors' belief in the existence of the erotic female confounded the generalities of women's lesser sexual feelings compared to men and strengthened warnings about the examination of female patients and the necessity for doctors to protect themselves from false accusations of impropriety or rape.

Most discussions of rape, however, occurred in textbooks where authors were preparing their student and practitioner readers for court testimony as to whether a woman had been raped or not. Those discussions have some intriguing aspects. In discussing the forced sexual intercourse of a prostitute, Henry Chapman in his turn-of-the-century text acknowledged that this was still rape, but admitted that "the evidence would have to be very strong to convict." Even the rape of a respectable woman, he believed, was contingent on circumstances – how big the man was, how small the woman. Physicians directed their students in cases of rape to look for signs of the woman being at fault. One 1907 text even pointed out that the rape of men by women occurred because of the belief by some women that it could cure their venereal disease. Another put forward a more disturbing scenario – the rape of boys by women. According to John J. Reese, "This crime is rarely brought before the courts, but seems to be more common than has generally been supposed. Boys are occasionally induced or forced into sexual intercourse with adult women to gratify the erotic feelings of the latter without the danger of pregnancy." Interestingly, while the Canadian medical literature did not refer to this, the National Council of Women's publication *Woman's Century* did.[68]

The threat of the overly sexed woman continued to intrigue in subsequent decades.[69] Anxiety about false accusations against men remained and physicians directed their students to remember that women sometimes dreamed of rape as a way of escaping responsibility for their sexual desires. And *A Handbook of Medical Jurisprudence and Toxicology*, the most used book on medical jurisprudence in medical schools, continued to describe how difficult it really was for a man to rape a woman.[70] Certainly the price paid by women who acted beyond the sexual norm could be significant. A Newfoundland woman recalled, "It was a serious thing for a child to be conceived out of wedlock," and recited the story of a young woman who while pregnant remained upstairs "out of public view" and even after the birth of her illegitimate child remained upstairs, "afraid to come down, afraid of her father." Dr William Victor Johnston recounted a similar incident in his Lucknow, Ontario, practice.[71] Illegitimacy was confirmation of a sexual act outside of marriage and hence a source of shame. While some parents were supportive, society as a whole was not. It was left to others such as Aboriginals to welcome the birth of the child rather than bemoan the circumstances of its conception.[72]

Masturbation

As we have seen, one aspect of sexuality that garnered significant attention was masturbation. In the early decades of the twentieth century, most pundits saw masturbation as somehow not normal as a sexual act. Adults were to get their sexual satisfaction through heterosexual intercourse and any substitute for this was viewed as problematic, as not being healthy or complete, and being against nature.[73] The problem that complicated the issue was that masturbation was widespread and could occur in one who was "otherwise" a good citizen.[74] Some physicians maintained some of the Victorian attitudes towards masturbation. One of these was the belief that women did not masturbate to the same extent as men.[75] But despite the gendered perception of who masturbated, there was a sense that once started, it was difficult to stop. Masturbation became a "habit" and one that seemed to sap the willpower of individuals to stop. A turn-of-the-century textbook by H. MacNaughton-Jones told its student readers of one unmarried woman with the reputation of doing public work. Until she read about the dire consequences of masturbation she wasn't aware that it could result in so many problems. Even though she sought help, however, she was unable to resist the temptation. Her doctor's response was to treat her by giving her cocaine under which influence he "freely cauterized the clitoris and the surrounding sensitive area with the galvanocautery." What was particular disturbing about his description was that in relating the case he concluded that "it was not the effect of the cauterization that effected a cure, so much as the influence on the patient's mind of the assurance that it would do so, and the time afforded for her will-power to assert itself."[76] Certainly the use of the placebo has an honoured place in medical practice, but surely cauterization of the clitoris goes well beyond the placebo effect. Was the woman being punished for transgressing? Other treatment was even more invasive. One 1917 text suggested excision of the clitoris and nymphae.[77]

Physicians believed that masturbation in women could result in loss of health and physicians needed to know whether their patients masturbated in order to make a proper diagnosis and to determine treatment.[78] Henry J. Garrigues, however, pointed out that to ask a woman "point-blank whether she masturbates [was] rather rude and risky." He suggested that during a physical examination to inquire whether "she is bothered with heat in the genitals, and whether she scratches or touches them." As he pointed out, "[T]he guilty one understands the physician perfectly well."[79] If the discussion of masturbation wasn't enough for many Canadians to cope with, medical practitioners were convinced that they could "tell" if a person masturbated. In both sexes it could result in a tremor of the face when talking or widely dilated pupils. Sometimes the signs in women were only visible under examination as in the case of an "elongated or turgescent clitoris with pigmented labia."[80]

Even more significant, masturbation could result in psychological, emotional, and mental disturbances. It could make women unwomanly. Not needed to be said was that the very act of masturbation in a woman suggested self-centredness, self-absorption, and an interest in sex. As studies of insane asylums have revealed, masturbation was associated with nervous disturbance in both sexes. The reasons for believing that masturbation was connected in some way to nervous disorders was the belief in what was often termed "vital force"; this was the source of energy in an individual, which could be depleted through sexual activity. Since masturbation was a nonproductive activity in that it did not produce children, it was especially seen as wasteful and indeed was equated to "excessive indulgence in the sexual act."[81]

Controlling masturbation remained an issue in the post–WWI years, but physicians presented it using a different framework. As noted with male masturbation, increasingly many practitioners took the attitude that it was quite normal and harmless except if done to excess. Indeed, William R. Houston, the writer of the 1936 *The Art of Treatment*, suggested that not having masturbated was "one count in the evidence against a psychopath."[82] In married people, however, some physicians did not consider masturbation normal and certainly not mature adult behaviour.[83] Whether normal or not, physicians in their discussions did recognize that adults, even married ones, masturbated. While many of the discussions did not make gendered distinctions, occasionally references to sex-specific masturbation occurred. Some practitioners felt that women were more secretive about masturbating than men, suggesting that it was still seen as somehow more unusual in women. At the same time, it was a natural response in women at certain periods of "sex desire," which one study found to be particularly high in the spring or at the end of menstruation.[84] William P. Graves in his 1929 text argued that it was more common in women than in men due to some women's inability to get sexual gratification within marriage because of the "impotence or indifference on the part of the husband." Graves was one of very few commentators who referred to the general effect masturbation had on women's physiology and to the consequent "lengthening and attenuation of the labia minora" in an "asymetric" way. Following Graves, one 1942 medical jurisprudence text suggested that masturbation was particularly prevalent in the unmarried woman and that it led to "hypertrophy of the labia and clitoris" as well as destruction of the hymen.[85] Of course the reason for such a text referring to this was to raise a warning sign for defence counsels of accused rapists.

The association between masturbation and mental problems in the interwar period continued, although the emphasis was more on it being a symptom of mental disturbance rather than a cause.[86] Attitudes do not shift quickly and many practitioners trained in one perspective did not necessarily shift it in later years. In addition, psychoanalytic theories gave new support to the association by suggesting that masturbation, if engaged in by women, was a sign of infantile sexual development, that is, the inability to transfer sexuality from the clitoris to the vagina.[87] What was key was not the masturbation per se but the conflict such an inability of transfer caused or the guilt about the act of masturbating itself. Such conflict resulted in neuroses caused by the "morbid trends of mind associated with popular delusions about its dangers."[88] Physicians were clear that masturbation was a normal occurrence and people should not feel ashamed of or in conflict about it. In 1934, Baruch Silverman of the Mental Hygiene Institute in Montreal related a case involving a young woman:

A married woman, of 22, had had for two months feelings of depersonalization. She awakened feeling self-conscious. She did not "feel herself." Her surroundings appeared normal but she felt very small. Her body felt light. After concentrating on a subject she frequently began to wonder who she was and where she was. This woman, who had been married for 4 years, and had had a child who died at the age of 17 months, had experienced considerable difficulty over the question of contraception. Her husband had religious compunctions on this matter, and this resulted in a good deal of marital conflict which created a state of tension in the patient and made her resort to masturbation with accompanying severe conflict. This went on for about 18 months, when she finally determined to give up the habit, and shortly after developed this rather marked psychoneurotic state.[89]

Little in the telling of this tale suggested that Silverman saw masturbation in and of itself as bad. Even the fact that a married woman resorted to it was not commented on. It was resorted to for reasons that were reasonable to the woman. The problem was that she felt conflicted about it.

Lesbianism

A last area of specific concern about female sexuality gone awry was sexual inversion or lesbianism. While there is some debate in the historical literature about how instrumental the medical profession was in creating a homosexual identity, there is little doubt that a medical model of it emerged in the early years of the century.[90] But for most Canadian physicians, the issue was an abstract one and seldom faced in their practices. In the interwar period, however, the literature they were reading and writing addressed the issue. The authors of some texts used Freudian references in seeing lesbianism as the result of a woman's inability to make the shift from self-love to object-love.[91] Some Canadians, however, were surprisingly less dogmatic. In 1930 W.T.B. Mitchell wrote about one of his patients in Montreal. A young woman, age 23, had compulsive feelings about glass and pins and in consulting Mitchell had related to him a lesbian relationship she had had between the ages of 9 and 12 with a school friend. At age 12 she discussed it with her mother, who was "shocked," which increased the girl's fear. As Mitchell concluded, condemnation had shut down the young woman's sexual responses and channeled them into a neurosis. Percy Ryberg took the same tact with same-sex relationships in women as he did in men. He believed lesbianism abnormal if persisted in, but recognized, as did others in the international literature, that in some individuals it was contingent, a "natural reaction to surroundings" that offered no heterosexual relations. Neither was he willing to condemn all special relationships between women. While some may have been problematic, he insisted others were "very beautiful and of life-long duration."[92] Inversion was an act that challenged the stability of heterosexual relations and, as a result, much of the written commentary saw it as abnormal, although the more recent the literature the less morally judgmental it was as awareness of homosexuality and lesbianism increased.[93] Certainly the mainstream medical literature did not see it as a significant threat except to the individual herself.

For most physicians same-sex relations, frigidity, excessive sexuality, and adult masturbation to excess were outside the normative model for women's sexual response. While some of these "conditions" had physiological and/or psychological origins or consequences, all were to a greater or lesser extent socially constructed in their meaning. They represented something gone "wrong" in the lives of women who experienced them and, consequently, physicians believed they had an obligation to express concerns about them. Their existence and the lack of consensus among physicians about the nature of the normative sexual response in women complicated what physicians considered their mandate – to care and to cure – and made holding onto a normative model of female sexuality difficult.

Controlling Sexuality

While the acceptance of sexuality in women was clear and the willingness to discuss the subject increasing, physicians found some aspects of sexuality socially as well as medically problematic. Accepting sexual urges as a normal physiological response was one thing but, as we have seen, accepting the response in its various forms was quite different. Underlying all the discussion of sexuality was the belief in the need for and the ability of women (and men) to control their sexual feelings, not to deny them. Physicians' interest in the control of sexuality was a reflection of the broader norms of society. Being in control was something society esteemed, for being in control was what separated humans from animals. Uncontrolled sexuality had unwanted consequences such as disease and illegitimate children.

For many women self-restraint was part of their early experiences with sex. Becki Crawford, born in 1915, recalled in the interwar years that her most "daring" action was going into a man's apartment, even when her presence was "totally innocent." Eunice Jordan didn't marry until she was 31 and insisted that before marriage there was only kissing and hugging, although she did learn what French kissing was. She didn't think men knew that much more about sex than she did. Both Drs Mackay and Hespler recalled the emphasis on "moral" relations. Young men would come to the house; you would not meet them anywhere else. And perhaps on the third or fourth date you might be willing to kiss your date. For many, sexual experimentation was unusual. The costs were too high. Isme Southern, born in 1919, remembers a young girl who lived across the street from her who had become pregnant and, as a result of people whispering about her, she only came out at night for a walk.[94] These women's experiences or beliefs reveal the lack of resistance on the part of many women to the values of the day and the difficulties they faced when they did resist and were "caught."

For some women, however, the knowledge of sexual experimentation was more widespread and personal. Betsy Lawrence remembered some sexual experimentation among her friends. Dorothy Atkinson recalled being at a movie with a young man and having him touch her breast. She felt a "brand" there for weeks afterwards. Betty Mackenzie met her husband at Trinity College, Toronto, in the 1930s. They married several years after graduation; in the meantime there was some experimentation but "not all the way." Wilma Hallman did go "all the way." She was married in 1929, but before that had had sexual intercourse with her husband-to-be. Financial difficulties prevented them from marrying when they wanted to, but clearly the fear of losing respectability or even getting pregnant did not offset the need to "give in" to their sexual desires. Geraldine Mitchell lived openly in 1949 with the man she eventually married. She paid a price for doing so, however, in the alienation of her father. Her experiences were actually much broader than many women's for she had had relations with more than one man before her eventual marriage. Yet the incident she remembered most vividly was spending an evening with an Irishman in New York. They didn't have sex because he was married, but she thought it was the most exciting night of her life – he taught her to read James Joyce.[95] What all of these women had in common was the sense that they had made the decision. They were taking personal responsibility for their actions. That responsibility is confirmed by a study reported in *The Public Health Journal* as early as 1923. When asked the reasons for their first experience of "immorality" women placed "mutual agreement" first.[96]

Taking responsibility for your actions was a form of control – personal control. As historians have argued, in whatever form it existed, control of sexuality was closely linked to preserving the social order. The irony is that depending on their vantage point historians either emphasize the control aspect or the lessening of concern. But the two are not mutually exclusive. The nature of control shifted, but the goal of control did not. Joan Sangster and others have detailed the repercussions of young women who didn't exert control. Whether it was their parents or the state who imposed it, many reaped punishment to the point of incarceration. Working-class women were particularly vulnerable as were women from cultures that appeared different from the white European-based ones. Part of the constructed differences was sexual – seeing in specific groups of women a heightened sexuality not under control.[97] Despite the increased openness about sexuality and decline in the moral concerns about it over time, societal concerns remained. The form it took defined identity with social and, in the case of rape, legal repercussions.

Conclusion

While most Canadians may not have shared the medical literature's interests or concerns, what the literature did through its influence on the practitioners who read it was to set up a conceptualization of male and female sexuality that was full of tension. Binaries dominated – men were sexual aggressors, initiators, women were not; sexuality was central to a man's identity, not for a woman's. But the binaries were never as clear cut as historians have suggested. Physicians nuanced their views – yes, they felt that men's sexuality was more aggressive than women's, but not beyond the control of most men. Women's sexual drive was weaker than men's, but it did exist and its recognition increased over the period under study. In their discussions, they both essentialized their descriptions and discussed exceptions. They were attempting to create a normative model to guide them but the complexity of the subject posed difficulties. Nevertheless, they persevered, changed emphases with the passage of time, and learned to live with the contradictions between the realities they saw in both society and their practices and how they wanted the world of sexual expression to be. The medical literature made clear that the male sex drive was the standard to which women's sexuality was compared, even when it was clear that doctors had little desire for women's sexuality to approximate men's. At the same time, it was women's sexuality that fascinated.

5 Advice on Marriage and Motherhood

In 1903, the Ontario Medical Association meeting in Toronto announced that "[t]he medical profession should educate the public on unsuitable marriages, and the disaster to the children that may be born."[1] Seven years later Dr John McCullough, the Ontario Board of Health's chief medical officer, examined the issue of infant mortality and blamed it not on poverty or poor sanitary conditions but on the ignorance of mothers.[2] Both comments address the significance that many practitioners placed on marriage and motherhood and the need for education to meet the needs of both. Just as practitioners incorporated sexuality into the ever-widening definition of medical subject matter and exposed what in many respects were their personal or social views through the rhetoric of science, they did the same with marriage and motherhood.

Marriage is both private and public. Historians of the family have stressed the emergence by the early decades of the last century of a marital ideology in which there was a more equitable relationship between husbands and wives than previously.[3] But we should not overestimate the degree of change even in the ideal. As is evident in medical rhetoric, the roles of men and women in marriage were to be supportive of one another but, at the same time, distinct and unequal. Within physicians' view of normative marriage, a concept of gendered power was evident even as they recognized that it was not always fair to the woman. The norms of medicine itself bolstered that hierarchy in the medical consent forms practitioners used and the advice they proffered on how to treat a wife infected with VD by her husband. Where the gendered hierarchy lessened was in physicians' concept of healthy sex within marriage. Out of their concern for healthy marriages came the desire of many physicians to have some sort of marital control in place that recognized their expertise about who should and should not marry. The eugenic nature of such control was evident as were the ideological premises of what an ideal marriage meant.[4]

Motherhood, too, is both private and public. For physicians, becoming a mother was central to the specialty of obstetrics. Being a mother, however, was less obvious a medical concern. Nevertheless, physicians increasingly advised mothers (especially new mothers) on how to raise their children. Underlying the advice was the assumption that too many women, as McCullough pointed out, were ignorant of how to take care of their children. In looking at the feeding schedules emphasized it was obvious that physicians did not see being a mother as instinctual. The example of breast feeding also revealed a profession pressured by what new mothers wanted, what was easier, what was better for the child, and their own professional involvement. Not all were compatible.

Marriage

Marriage as the Norm

Practitioners (and most Canadians) deemed marriage the only legitimate venue for having children. Throughout the first half century, physicians were of a mind that children were the purpose of marriage and they were leery of a woman marrying if she could not have children. Only occasionally was there any suggestion in the medical literature that the central core of marriage was the husband/wife relationship. While Sir Comyns Berkeley and Victor Bonney in their 1942 *Textbook of Gynaecological Surgery* conceded that most men and some women defined marriage in terms of the spousal relationship, they saw such individuals as lacking. According to them, women who did so exhibited "male sexuality" and men who did so greatly underestimated the importance of paternity in men's lives.[5]

Assuming the woman could have children, physicians discussed the best age at which to marry. Early in the century some worried that too many were delaying marriage (despite statistics to the contrary).[6] One of Canada's leading gynaecologists and surgeons, Dr Lapthorn Smith, complained that young women instead of marrying at 18 or even younger, which he believed they had done in the past and which he felt was the optimum age, were delaying marriage until they were 26 or 28. As already noted, Smith blamed the expansion of education for this state of affairs and argued that nothing good would come of it.

Other physicians were not as apocalyptic but were made uneasy by what they perceived as the desire among the successful to delay marriage in order to enjoy a materialistic life.[7] At the same time, marriage should not occur at too early an age. Physiological reasons militated against it as did social attitudes that considered marriage in the early teens as "bordering on Oriental customs,"[8] the latter term a reference to the "yellow peril" that many Canadians believed existed. Age of marriage did not seem so important in the post-war years, perhaps because the trend to younger marriages was more evident and the increase that took place in the 1930s was understandable due to the economic situation.

Marriage at the right age brought benefits. Sexual activity was healthy for women, "the absorption of prostatic fluid" being " essential" to her "full physiological evolution."[9] It offset the stress of unmet sexual urges that in women could result in menstrual problems.[10] Not only did marriage help maintain health, some physicians saw it as a solution for certain ailments or diseases in both sexes. While the concept of marriage as a cure "for what ailed you" was not widespread, it had existed in the nineteenth century and continued into the twentieth. Practitioners and authors of texts referred to the medical belief that marriage was a cure for suppressed menstruation, possibly a cure for masturbation, and a preventative measure against insanity. Some physicians even advised young men to marry in order to cure their "gleet" (inflammation of the urethra).[11] The emphasis on marriage as a cure for or prevention of health problems remained strong. Becki Crawford remembered being assured by her doctor that her skin problems would clear up when she married. Other physicians considered it helpful in lessening amenorrhoea and some types of dysmennorhoea, and in preventing endometriosis. The social role of women impinged on the medical view. Woman's destiny was to marry and have children. A denial of that destiny could only be harmful; what was natural had to be healthy.[12]

The meaning of a marital relationship varies from society to society and within societies. In the early years of the century, Vilhjalmus Stefansson, in one of his journeys to the north, found that the obligation of a man living in the Mackenzie Delta and who married the only or the youngest daughter was to become part of her parents' family. If the husband at some point no longer wanted to accompany his wife's parents in their travels, he could leave his wife since she had to stay with her parents. In other communities in the far north explorers told of "marriage by capture." First Nations people also recognized the chance of violence in a relationship and, for example, on Baillie Island, near Point Barrow, had a custom of having a female child's navel string worn by her as an amulet so if her husband hit her he would develop a swollen finger.[13] In most First Nations' cultures, roles within marriage were very gendered but still evidencing a partnership based on family survival. The work of women was vital and in some cultures, such as the Netsilik Eskimo, taboos against men hunting were in place when women were doing particular kinds of work.[14] Marriage customs also varied according to class with the working class not always accepting the views of the middle-class or even those of some of their working-class counterparts.[15] While customs differed, almost all cultures viewed marriage (or some permanent relationship) as the bedrock of the family, the basic unit of society.

The marital relationship that physicians envisioned between men and women was a white middle-class one of ideological separation. The minutes of the 1904 Ontario Medical Association meeting in Toronto recorded what doctors envisioned in their own marriages: "the doctor should marry, but his wife should be kept out of his work."[16] While they did not see this as an unequal or unfair division, they were well aware from their practices that the inequality between the sexes could be visited physically on women – women contracting VD from their husbands, women paying the price of marital sex through the pain of and all too often death in childbirth. With the first there was the assumption that the "lower classes" were more prone to contracting gonorrhoea and thus it was more of a concern in childbearing among those women than women of the "upper classes."[17] The perceived class profile of VD did not waver in subsequent years. Milton J. Rosenau, a major figure in American public health, in his 1927 *Preventive Medicine and Hygiene* was clear that class mattered but he also added race to the mix: "It is estimated that the rates for colored race are more than double those for the white race." Canadian figures seldom mentioned race specifically, but they certainly emphasized class. A report from the Dalhousie Prenatal Clinic in the late 1930s estimated that 18.4 in 100 women tested positive for syphilis with the author reporting, "[O]f course, one would expect to find syphilis more prevalent in the women attending the clinic, because for the most part they are from the lower classes." One of the few comments on race came from J.J. Heagerty, head of the Venereal Disease Control in Canada, who reported on Canadian studies which indicated that prostitutes were "recruited from girls who leave school before fourteen years of age." Such girls had a low mentality and were compared to the "primitive and semi-civilized races" from countries such as Haiti or Siam.[18]

If VD was not a bad enough threat that came to women through marriage, James Winfred Bridges in his 1930 *Psychology Normal and Abnormal* told his student readers that "excess of ego instinct" on the part of men "constitutes what many women regard as the 'bondage of marriage.'" Samuel S. Peikoff recalled from his Rossburn, Manitoba, practice one maternity case in particular. The husband entered the room and said he wanted the doctor to focus on saving the life of his wife over that of the child. This was not an expression of husbandly love but of economic interest. According to Peikoff, the man smelled "like a brewery" and insisted he had lots of children but needed his wife: "She got cows to milk and bread to bake. She got to look after the keeds. I need her. She's a good woman." What Peikoff also noticed was that the wife appeared flattered by her husband's words.[19]

The medical system itself reflected the unequal aspect of marriage. Two examples were the consent forms needed for operations in certain jurisdictions and notifying a spouse that his/her partner had venereal disease. In the former the husband had to sign a consent form for an operation on his wife, the wife's consent alone not being sufficient. Especially crucial was surgery that would result in the wife's sterility, reflecting the idea that the husband's rights were also affected. Mrs Ginette Kendall entered the Royal Victoria Hospital, Montreal, on 25 August 1921. She was 38 years of age, had had two full pregnancies and two miscarriages, and was suffering from prolapse uteri and chronic cervicitis. Her case record stated, "[H]usband consulted, wanted more children, did not tie the tubes. It did seem as though it would have been better to ligate them out and fix uterus rather than suspend." Nonetheless, the physicians did a suspension. Angela Sidney of the Tagish and Tlingit tribes recalled that in 1929 when she underwent surgery the doctor told her husband, but not her, that the surgery would result in her not being able to have more children. The doctor's action in performing the surgery without her knowledge left her with an incredible feeling of loss. Whether this specific "sterilization" had a racial motivation as well is unclear. The history of medicine has certainly reflected a racial bias in such surgeries and when this specific procedure occurred the eugenic movement was gaining strength.[20] But if it was racially motivated, the gendered aspect of it also cannot be overlooked. As late as 1950, the Montreal General Hospital had an operation consent form that stated, "A wife, although 21 years of age, must have her husband's consent." The patient in whose record a copy was found was a married woman age 69.[21]

The second example revolves around the question of a physician's obligation to a wife whose husband he was treating for VD. Whether a physician owed responsibility to the innocent party was an agonizing question, but one that most doctors argued was solved, in legal terms, at least, by the concept of doctor/patient confidentiality. In 1910 S.M. Hay from the Toronto Western Hospital instructed what should occur when the wife had contracted a venereal disease from her husband: "In giving your instructions [to the wife on her own care] be careful to arouse no suspicion that might lead to domestic unhappiness. We should endeavor to lessen suffering in the home, as well as in the patient, not to cause it."[22] Thus the physician was to protect an innocent wife by keeping from her the knowledge that her husband had infected her. She was not given the option of protecting herself. What information a wife had the right to know remained an issue. In 1924 George Ross's solution was not to tell the wife but to treat such women without them being in any way the wiser. Some physicians in Quebec followed a similar approach, telling the woman not that she had VD contracted from her husband but that she had anaemia and "treating" her for that.[23] Physicians certainly were concerned about the infection of innocent individuals and did not ignore the potential dangers of marital sexuality as has been suggested in some historical interpretations,[24] but they also did not want to see marital breakdown and so tried to work out a way that the innocent wife could be protected. The underlying assumption was that the wife was the innocent party, that she would also be a patient of the physician, that she would have contracted venereal disease and not know it, and that she would come in to see her physician. There was no discussion of what to do if the woman did not come and consult the doctor on her own.

The Marital Sex Act

Where the push for mutuality within marriage was strongest was in the bedroom. In emphasizing the pleasure of the sexual union in a marital relationship, the international medical literature that dominated the sexual discourse saw men as sexually less aggressive than the "theory" of sexuality would suggest and women as more engaged sexual partners, although their agency was limited by the assumption that the man would be the initiator and director of the sexual act.

Nevertheless, the husband had to treat his wife with consideration with one turn-of-the-century text warning about sexual initiation if engaged in too "abruptly" when it was a woman's first time.[25] Physicians agreed good sex was confined to marriage. Assuming that women could make the transition from premarital purity to marital participation in sexual intercourse, the author of one 1907 obstetrics text considered the ideal would be simultaneous climax. That he believed it improved the chances of conception was a bonus.[26] But simultaneity of interest or result was not necessarily possible or even wished for in all cultures. Neither could mutuality be possible at all times. One area where physicians urged restraint was during a woman's pregnancy and for some time afterwards.[27] Such a withdrawal from sexual intercourse, they admitted, would be more difficult for the husband to accept than the pregnant wife. Nevertheless, similar prohibitions were culturally widespread. Franz Boas described the customs of the Inuit of Baffin Island to refrain from sexual intercourse for at least three months after birth.[28]

While many historians have suggested the liberalization of sexual attitudes in the post–World War I era, it was not without anxiety.[29] It went without saying that normal still meant within marriage, but not all marriages experienced sexual compatibility. In the memoirs of his post–WWI practice in Lucknow, Ontario, William Victor Johnston recalled one patient, Mrs D., who had just given birth to her fifth child in five years. Being able to go home after six days in hospital she asked to be kept in longer. When queried why she responded, "I want another two days away from my husband. He has had intercourse every night since we were married." Johnston asked, "[W]hy don't you say no sometimes?" While Johnston felt it a "reasonable question," Mrs D. did not, responding that her husband "would be angry. It is his right as a husband." As Johnston commented in his memoirs, "[W]hat a world of inner conflict and accommodation must have lain behind that statement!"[30]

To encourage sexual compatibility, the focus on mutuality of orgasm increased, at least in the literature being published.[31] Increasingly emphasized as well was the importance of the bridal night and the need for the husband to be considerate of his new wife. The assumption was that the man would be the initiator of the sexual act and that it was his responsibility to control his own emotions to make sure that his bride experienced pleasure.[32] Noted was that some women might need time to become accustomed to sexual relations, sometimes lasting until after the birth of the first child. Dr Percy Ryberg in his advice manual was prepared to envision a different scenario where the bride was the experienced partner. That being the case, he advised it was her responsibility to teach her new husband that the sexual act meant more than "the satisfaction of his animal impulses," and that a "responsibility rests upon her for the whole future of their married life; a responsibility that is almost as great as in the case of the man who marries a virgin."[33]

Whether experienced or not, some women were very pragmatic about the prospect of the wedding night and prepared for it. Irma Avery consulted with a friend and a doctor about sex before she married but admitted that neither one of them told her very much. Social worker Becki Crawford was 27 when she married. She had asked her physician for a checkup and while there enquired if was anything he could do to make the wedding night easier for her since she was a virgin. He said no, that her comfort was really up to her husband. Betty Mackenzie recalled consulting with her physician before her marriage in the 1940s to ensure that she was physically prepared. What she was interested in was stretching her vagina so that intercourse would not be a shock. Instead of doing it for her, her physician showed her how to do it herself. Mackenzie's story revealed her own interest in sexuality and her determination to control the wedding night, but also her physician's willingness to help her. But being "prepared" didn't necessarily guarantee a good wedding night. Even though she consulted a physician about birth control, Jane Rutherford still found her wedding night a "shock" just like the experts warned. Dorothy Atkinson on the other hand laughed on remembering her wedding night and thinking "is this all there is ... neither of us knowing very much."[34]

The wedding night was not the only concern of practitioners. They also stressed the importance of sexual technique throughout the marriage and emphasized the centrality of arousal for both partners. Medical texts and advice manuals were much more explicit in the post – WWI years than they had been earlier and contained detailed descriptions of the normal ways of making love. Readers of one obstetrics and gynaecology text were told, "The average woman prefers that her husband 'rewin' her and gain permission rather than take for granted the legal liberties granted by marriage."[35] Making love was more than having sexual intercourse. Physicians made it clear that sexual pleasure was owed to women and that it was men's responsibility to adjust their own sexual timing in order to provide it. In his manual Ryberg did place some responsibility on the woman to know her own body well enough so that she could enlighten her husband as to how to satisfy her. He pointed out, for example, that the left side of women's bodies were more susceptible to arousal than the right.[36]

Hygiene was also an issue. In his concern to have the wedding night go as well as possible, Ryberg advised against relations if the bride was menstruating. Edwin H. Hirsch pushed it further and suggested not engaging in intercourse just before, during, and after menstruation throughout marriage to protect the man against germs. Not going quite that far, a 1950 gynaecology text conceded it was still unhygienic to engage in sexual intercourse during a woman's menstrual cycle.[37] Men were not exempt from similar admonitions, but the ones directed at them never focused on the actual workings of their bodies as they did with women and menstruation. Neither did they have the tone of distaste that a menstruating body seemed to evoke. Rather they addressed more easily dealt with problems. Ryberg warned men that they needed to keep their underwear clean. He also noted, "A daily bath or shower may not be necessary, but the smell of male sweat and other body odours, especially the smell of feet, are not pleasant to a sensitive wife."[38]

Although the experiences of many women suggest that not all couples were living lives of sexual equity, some women did find mutuality with their husbands, although not always in the way that advice literature emphasized. Dorothy Atkinson recalled that her husband was not highly sexed: "We suited each other that way"; but he did know how to cuddle and after his death that is what she missed the most.[39] But it was not the quiet cuddling that the advice literature stressed. Without a satisfactory sex life there could not be a happy marriage. According to medical advice, both husband and wife were to enjoy the sexual act and for complete satisfaction orgasm was to be mutual. Some historians, however, have been somewhat ambivalent about the new ideal. They note that a more open attitude to sexuality posed problems for women since compared to men they were at more risk through possible pregnancies, birth control and abortion being illegal. Certainly it appears that male sexual urges were the controlling factor and the ideal was predicated on a male sexual model centred on orgasm.[40]

Desire for Marital Control

All societies have varying customs and taboos regarding marriage. Physicians were driven by their understanding of medicine to proffer opinions on what they hoped would lead to taboos or controls over marriage within their own society. By the early twentieth century, many Canadians were becoming concerned about the potential decline in the quality of the country's population, a consequence of several factors: immigrants coming to Canada who did not match the Anglo-Celtic base of the population, a perceived decline in morality, and the declining birth rate of the middle class and the higher birth rate of "others." Many concluded that marriage was too important to be left to the two parties concerned.[41] In 1907 Dr R.W. Bruce Smith, the provincial inspector of hospitals and public charities in Ontario, advocated "active measures" to stop the increase of degenerates. An editorial in the 1915 *Canadian Journal of Medicine and Surgery* concurred and suggested, "The final referee, in a modern utopia, will be the physician who examines both applicants thoroughly before marriage." Such attitudes persisted as the postwar years saw a heightening of eugenic beliefs. In 1934 Dr Morris Siegel published his *Constructive Eugenics and Rational Marriage* in which he made a plea for the restriction of marriage to those who were "fit."[42] Doctors wanted control; they believed that science provided them with the means to identify those who they believed should not marry. While at times physicians were not specific about whom the degenerates were, two groups stand out – those with VD and the feebleminded.

While both men and women could be the source of venereal infection, in discussion of marriage control physicians focused on the husbands as the "guilty" party.[43] This did not negate the wider belief that women were the source of VD, but rather reflected the separation of "good" women who were innocent brides and faithful wives from "bad" women who were sexually promiscuous. Due to the double standard of sexual morality, men were often "excused" sexual experience; given that women paid the price of such experience through pregnancy, it was generally believed that they were less likely than men to stray. Coupled with men's more active sexual history was the ignorance or denial on the part of some men of how infectious various venereal diseases were. Even more problematic were physicians who too often allowed patients with slight symptoms of gonorrhoea to marry and who gave advice to young men that marriage would improve their sexual hygiene. The result was a high rate of infection of wives. A report from the Toronto General Hospital noted that of 40 women who in 1917 came to the hospital and had had gonorrhoea, 28 of them had contracted it from their husbands.[44]

In such a scenario the required action was clear – the innocent wife and any future children needed to be protected from infection. The most popular protection proposed by physicians were marital health certificates, which could include blood tests to determine the existence or nonexistence of VD. John Joseph Cassidy, editor of the *Canadian Journal of Medicine and Surgery* supported such certificates, especially those that focused on men. Unfortunately, governments were not convinced about the value of legislating protection. In trying to understand their reluctance Cassidy pointed to self-interest: "[L]egislators, like most other men, have had venereal diseases."[45] The issue of marital health screening hit too close to home. Without marital certificates to fall back on, what were physicians to do? In his 1913 text Charles Norris took an unusual stance. If the man (or in rare cases the woman) had a venereal disease and still insisted on marrying, Norris advised student readers that the physician could break the bond of confidentiality and tell the prospective partner of her fiancé's condition. He believed that both professional and lay opinion would support him on this.[46] However, as with the case of married women, there is little evidence in the medical literature that his colleagues would agree.

In the interwar period and beyond, the push to control VD accelerated. Husbands remained the focus[47] and the solution for those concerned remained the prevention of marriage of those with VD. A judicial inquiry in Ontario by Justice F.E. Hodgins in 1919 supported the idea of a health certificate as a requirement for a marriage licence. While the province did not follow through, the Venereal Diseases Prevention Act did permit the Provincial Board of Health to stipulate that those who were being treated under the act could not marry or have sexual intercourse. How that was to be enforced was unclear.[48] What was clear was the medical support of marital health certificates. Aware of public hostility to such certificates, Toronto physician George W. Ross tried to assess the reasons for it, concluding that the public and politicians were reluctant to put "young and usually innocent women" through such an examination in order to identify the few who were infected. In addition, Ross noted that tests for gonorrhea were not foolproof. Nonetheless some jurisdictions were listening. By 1946 legislation in PEI, Manitoba, Alberta, Saskatchewan, and BC (still needing to be proclaimed) insisted on a premarital blood test for syphilis.[49] Such legislation sometimes had limitations. Dr H.S. Doyle, of the Division of Communicable Disease Control and VD Control of the Saskatchewan Department of Public Health, pointed out that the serological test for syphilis was intended to prevent marriage of the syphilitic person only if he/she was in an infectious stage and was planning to marry a noninfected person. If two syphilitic people wanted to marry that was acceptable; it was also acceptable if the woman or "girl," as Doyle put it, was already pregnant.[50] Such legislation was protective of an innocent party. Even if not yet infected, the "girl" who was already pregnant was no longer innocent. The spectre of illegitimacy, then, outweighed concern for her health or the health of the children she bore. Neither was eugenic consideration given to the health of the babies born of marriages between syphilitics. Knowing that VD often caused sterility, perhaps the hope was that such marriages would not produce children.

Those with VD were not the only ones physicians wanted to prevent marrying. The feebleminded were as well. Encompassing those considered mentally deficient and liable to become morally so, the fear was that the feebleminded could pass on their mental and moral deficiencies to their offspring. The actual numbers of people considered mentally challenged was not large. Nationally, the estimates were .3 percent of the population in 1900, but worrisome was the estimated increase to 3 percent by 1914.[51] Fredericton physician A.B. Atherton was quite typical in his focus on the women among them: "These must necessarily be a constant source of menace to us, because of the great risk of their bearing children of a like character."[52] The assumption underlying the focus on women was that while a man might have sexual congress with a feebleminded woman, the reverse was unlikely. And because women bore the children, physicians concluded there was a closer hereditary relationship between the mother and child than the father and child. The goal, then, was to stop the feebleminded, but especially the women, from marrying. In some jurisdictions restrictions on the marriage of feebleminded adults did exist. In the province of Ontario the marriage act forbade any clergyman to celebrate the marriage of persons whom he knew to be "idiots" or else pay a fine of 500 dollars.[53] But some physicians found the legislation unsatisfactory; it was not well enforced and it might not prevent the marriage of those not obviously idiots. Dr Gibson made the point explicit: what was needed "for the sake of future generations" were laws that would insist on a "reputable" physician providing confirmation of health of both parties before a marriage licence could be issued.[54]

The post – WWI years saw an expansion and development of the eugenics movement, which many physicians supported.[55] Marital health certificates were part of it. In the early 1920s C.K. Clarke reported that in a study of 767 cases of illegitimacy, immigrant mothers were over represented and, according to his findings, the majority of them were also mentally weak. In 1932 Dr R.M. Benvie, a member of the editorial board of the *Nova Scotia Medical Bulletin*, railed about the need to "check the increase of the unfit." Determining a physical disease may have been straightforward, but determining who was mentally unfit could be problematic – where was the line to be drawn? But Benvie didn't see the problem; for him deciding between the sound and the unsound was clear: "[T]he mentally alert are morally sound and vice versa, so that when one female produces more than one illegitimate, such a female is mentally defective."[56] Reproduction of such women had to be stopped.

VD and feeblemindedness were not the only barriers to marriage that physicians wanted to see implemented but they were the issues discussed most and they had a strong gender component. To a much lesser extent so did insanity and ill heath in prospective marital partners. For example, the authors of the 1910 *The Practice of Midwifery* believed that marriage should definitely be discouraged if the woman in particular had a hereditary predisposition to insanity or if she had ever had an attack of insanity. They assumed that the added pressures of pregnancy would bring about either the woman's first attack or a new attack of insanity.[57] And if pregnancy was not an option for that reason then it followed neither was marriage. In a similar way, doctors believed that certain physical ailments – alcoholism, epilepsy, heart problems, haemophilia, drug addiction, TB – prohibited women the option of marrying and having children because of their effect on a pregnant woman or the child she might eventually carry.[58] While the list of factors were not specifically gendered, the specific application was. Eugenic factors such as alcoholism and drug addiction could apply to both sexes, but the belief in the very close relationship between the mother and foetus emphasized such a woman was not a good marital choice. In addition, the physical and psychological pressures of pregnancy on women meant that the health problems that might prevent women from marrying were more numerous than those for men.

In the post-war period, similar concerns were raised. One article in the 1928 *Canada Lancet and Practitioner* urged, "Women contemplating marriage should even before becoming engaged see a good, competent obstetrician and be carefully examined as to their probability of being able to stand the strain of wifehood and child-bearing,"[59] suggesting a rather exclusive group who should marry. What had changed, however, was the increasing specificity of the concerns and the elimination of earlier ones due to advances in medicine. Some physicians argued that women with congestive heart failure should not marry, while those with "well established mitral stenosis, with *good* compensation and no history of failure" could marry as long as both the woman and her partner understood the risks represented by pregnancy.[60] The decision was theirs to make.

The concern about VD, feeblemindedness and to a much lesser extent insanity, and physical ailments existed for most of the period under review, but not all of it. Its peak was the interwar years, a time when eugenic thought was strongest. In the 1940s, the literature on all four and their relationship with who should not marry was simply not as visible as it had been. It does not mean that worry over who married declined, but that the solution endorsed – medical marriage certificates – no longer appeared in the literature. As we have seen, many provinces had introduced legislation that gave the state some form of control over who married. As well, the nature or purpose of marriage was shifting. No longer was it only for procreation (assuming it had ever been solely for that); the mutuality between the two partners was increasingly seen as an ingredient of a good marriage. There was also a sense that medical science could now meet some of the challenges that marital health certificates were designed to prevent.

Motherhood

Giving Advice to Mothers

A marriage between two healthy and moral people was assumed to lead to the birth of equally healthy and moral children. But the ideal picture of who married was not guaranteed. So physicians (and other Canadians) were faced with ensuring that children born were raised properly. The solution was advice to women on how to be good mothers. And the advice proffered was essentially reflective of the middle-class, white Anglo-Celtic ideology of motherhood.[61] In a modern industrial society, mothers were to accept a scientific model of motherhood, informed by the most up-to-date findings of scientific hygiene, childcare, and household management. Only if mothers were able to immerse themselves in such matters would their families receive the care they deserved.

In the early years of the century, mother was the front-line physician and medical advice books abounded with recipes that women could follow in order to care for their families. Child welfare clinics and classes in mother care also were available. The underlying assumption of both was that mothers who were taught to care for their children would decrease children's health problems. But as Rima Apple has pointed out, such education of mothers "made them responsible for the health and welfare of their families, but ... denied them control."[62] As a response to the tremendous loss of life in World War I and the influenza epidemic, the emphasis on training mothers intensified in the interwar period. No assumptions could be made about what women knew or didn't know. A good and a modern mother was a woman who listened to the experts.[63] The new thrust in childcare was the establishment of a schedule for the child and mother's responsibility to enforce that schedule. Underlying the medical focus on scheduling (regularity) in the child's life was the belief that the environment or training of the child could determine the child's future; that is, environment could help overcome any personal or family heredity or eccentricities. Of course, adherence to medical advice would ensure such an environment.

The ability of medical advice to reach women significantly increased. Women were being delivered by physicians in hospitals, surrounded by the trappings of medical science, and captive to the blandishments of doctors and nurses alike about how to care for their babies. The image of science and medicine was high and so advice from nurses and physicians had a certain amount of weight and cachet. In some hospitals nurses demonstrated the best way of bathing a child. Others opened motherhood clinics. In 1934 *Chatelaine* began a column in which Dr J.W.S. McCullough, chief inspector of health for Ontario, would "answer questions sent ... by mothers on the care of their babies, and other public health matters."[64] But we should not exaggerate the ability of all these forums to reach women. The Kingston General Hospital's *Annual Report* for 1936 revealed that only one woman in its outpatient roster attended mothercraft classes. Certainly the medical profession could give advice, but it was the mothers of the land who had to take and implement it. An ad for evaporated milk in the 1934 *Manitoba Medical Review* played on doctors' fears that women weren't listening to them but to other women.[65] The unstated message: advice from other women was not dependable.

Certainly not all women wanted or could follow the advice with its emphasis on middle-class mothers and providing the accoutrements of a middle-class home. At times, poorer women reacted against the advice, feeling shortchanged and frustrated. Some continued to turn to midwives or other women in the neighbourhood to help them, feeling that doctors' advice was too difficult to follow. Others simply did what seemed sensible. Nell Brinkley in a 1931 *Chatelaine* article on modern mothers acknowledged the "scientific attitude" that existed but did not feel "there are many girls who are extremists in hospital-like child culture." She described her own policy: "I know that though I am very careful of what my boy eats, of what he reads and of the impressions he absorbs, I do not do it by rote, but because that is the way that I think. I rocked him to sleep when he was very new sometimes because I wanted to. Now he goes to sleep by himself as easily as if he had never been rocked."[66]

The emphasis on training and following doctors' instructions (if indeed they were followed) took away from the spontaneity of mothering. What seemed to be natural responses were now deemed problematic. Dr Alton Goldbloom, one of Canada's most noted child doctors, carried on a detailed correspondence with Mrs H.V. Banford, from Kenogami, Quebec, between April 1924 and October 1925. It revealed the concern of a mother about her infant son and her need to have advice on a wide variety of issues concerning his well-being. Goldbloom was incredibly patient in meeting her requests for help. In one letter, dated 13 January 1925, he wrote a detailed response concerning the infant's habit of waking up at 10 p.m. He was very clear about what Mrs Banford had to do:

When he awakes and wishes to play, he must awake and play in the dark entirely by himself. He may have the necessary attention of changing his diaper if he is wet, but that only without a look in his direction or a word to him, so that he will quickly realize that the night is the time for sleeping and for nothing else. When he sees that his efforts at attracting your attention are productive of no results whatever, he will give them up. The restlessness, of course, may be due to teeth, but even this is not sufficient excuse for even slightly spoiling a baby.

"Spoiling a baby" was to be avoided. In a speech delivered in the 1930s to a symposium on child psychology Goldbloom made his message even clearer: "[W]hat we call behaviour problems in children, are in many instances only behaviour problems of the mothers."[67] The advice given to offset these problems separated mother and child. Mothers had to constantly monitor their children but not engage with them.[68] Mothers were to be the conduit of care not the origin of care. No longer were women to take their children to see a physician when they noticed that something was wrong; they were to take their children to the physician on a regular basis in order to see *if* anything was wrong.

The WWII years and postwar period continued many of these themes. With fathers either away in military service or busy with the increased demands of a war economy, childcare experts feared that mothers would become overly protective of their children, that they would transfer the attention usually paid to husbands to their children. Although women were being warned about the psychological damage that they could do to their children, physical care was not assumed. An ad for the Metropolitan Life Insurance Company endorsed a pamphlet by the Canadian Medical Association entitled "Food for Health in Peace and War." The advertisement, published in *Chatelaine*, told its women readers: "In language that you will understand, the book explains much of what years of study and research have taught doctors and scientists about food in relation to nourishment and health."[69] The patronizing phrase "in language that you will understand" perhaps gives the best insight into attitudes to motherhood. Women were uninformed and emotionally immature. They might raise the children, but they needed to be told how to do it.

Underlying the advice was an incredibly optimistic belief that nurturing was everything. It could shape the future by shaping the children. Such a belief was the flip side of the eugenic beliefs of the interwar years that we saw as the motivation for marital health certificates. But the latter simply were to prevent the minority deviants – the mentally and physically challenged or ill – from entering a relationship that could produce children. Those not deemed deviant were the focus of the advice literature by physicians, psychologists, and childcare advocates. The extent and range of the literature had expanded from the early years. If followed, there were consequences to the mother/child relationship. If not followed, there was potential blame of women and subsequent guilt in them. A more detailed examination of one example of advice – breast feeding – follows.

Breast feeding

After birth, the first task of a good mother was to breast feed her child.[70] Throughout the first half century, most commentators assumed the naturalness of breast feeding. A 1913 pamphlet entitled *A Little Talk About Baby*, published by the provincial Board of Health, Ontario, saw little mystery in nursing. Breasts secreted milk as easily as the salivary gland secreted saliva. In the interwar period Dr Helen MacMurchy chided women that any woman could nurse – they simply had to want to do it enough; that is, they had to exert their will.[71] The assumption of "naturalness," however, was a contested one. In 1918 Alan Brown, then attending physician at the Hospital for Sick Children, argued that increasing urbanization created a more artificial existence and, as a result, city women, unlike their country sisters, were not as prone to nurse their children. Yet in emphasizing modern woman's distance from the natural, Brown and other medical experts unconsciously emphasized breast feeding's relationship to the primitive, itself a deterrent in attracting the middle classes to nurse their children and a veiled slight against those who did. In 1938, Brown was still sending women mixed signals. He both berated women for not breast feeding and, at the same time, hardly made it seem attractive. In the 1938 *Canadian Public Health Journal* he wrote a commentary to explain why the quality of mothers' milk was variable and quoted an unnamed person:

> Milk production is milk production, whether in woman-kind or the lower animals. A Jersey cow if frightened or teased about her calf will give perhaps a quart of milk at the next milking time instead of the expected three gallons. Even a hog or a dog that drives her from the pasture, or a strange milker will affect the quantity of her milk. A woman is much more susceptible to nervous reactions. Milk production in all our minds is associated with green meadows, still nature and kind-faced old cows standing in quiet streams (not listening to a baseball game or a prize-fight over the radio).[72]

Brown's source clearly did not feel that pregnant women should be listening to baseball games or prize fights over the radio. Less clear was whether Brown agreed and thought they should join the cows in the stream.

Despite the mixed messages, there was consensus on the importance of breast milk for a newborn infant. What varied was the degree of that importance. In the early decades of the century the argument in favour of breast milk was that it saved babies' lives. One physician in the 1907 *Canada Lancet* made it clear that women should be made to nurse. A moral imperative surrounded the issue. A woman who did not nurse was, in the words of one turn-of-the-century textbook, "unworthy to become a mother."[73] The loss of life during the Great War only intensified the concern over infant deaths. Indeed, it put infant deaths in perspective – their death rate was higher than soldiers at the front.[74] Neither did the concern about infant deaths abate. Indeed, in the interwar years the rhetoric of breast feeding's value increased. H.W. Hill, dean of the faculty of public health, Western University, pointed out that two-thirds of infant deaths were the result of nutritional problems or infectious diseases and that artificial feeding often caused the former. Helen MacMurchy's 1923 booklet on motherhood contained 15 pages on breast feeding; the 1930 edition contained 22. She emphasized that women who did not nurse were failures as mothers, an attitude that the Montreal Department of Health booklet on infant care endorsed. Women who did not breast feed were "committing almost a crime."[75]

Breast milk was the "natural food of the infant," "essential" and "wholesome," and no substitute for it existed.[76] Especially important in breast milk was colostrum, the first secretion. Henry Jellett in his 1910 text was very specific about what colostrum did. It "acts as a mild purgative ... and so exerts a beneficial effect on the infant by clearing away the meconium [dark green material in the intestine of a full-term foetus]." The language of analysis is specific, technical, and "scientific." In 1912 George S. Strathy, assistant pathologist at the Hospital for Sick Children, also made the advocacy of breast milk a scientific stance, pointing to the relationship between antibodies in breast milk that provided the infant with some kind of immunity. The importance of breast milk could not be overestimated.[77] It was not just the infants who benefitted either. Throughout the early years of the century physicians agreed that nursing immediately after birth helped the involution, that is, the contraction, of the mother's uterus after childbirth. It brought a closeness between mother and child, and a feeling that the mother was doing all she could for the health of her infant.[78]

While most physicians publicly endorsed breast feeding, they did not support extended nursing. J. Clarence Wesbter in his 1903 text accused women who prolonged breast feeding of doing so as a form of birth control. Even worse, he noted that "in some countries – e.g. Japan – it is customary to nurse two or three years. The practice is an evil one, as it usually leads to deterioration of the mother's health. Anemia, loss of weight and strength, and neurasthenia frequently result."[79] Several messages are encoded in Webster's text. Preventing conception was not a concept that Webster endorsed. Linking prolonged nursing to Japanese women at a time when fear of the "yellow peril" was signif-icant in North America was a way of convincing white women that prolonged breast feeding was a foreign custom and one they should not emulate, especially when such nursing also was deemed by some physicians as going back to a more primitive time. Seeing an infant at the breast was one thing, but the image of a two- or three-year-old child at the breast was something else again. Whether Webster's unease was linked as well to some of the Freudian theories on child sexuality of the time is unclear. Certainly the specific link was not made. And if all of the above was not enough to dissuade supporters of extended breast feeding, Webster's prestige as a physician would carry the day in his specific listing of physical consequences that could ensue. Neither did these concerns go away. While acknowledging that extended nursing occurred, medical commentators did not support it, rejected it as a birth control measure, argued that it drained the energy of women, and continued to associate it with "uncivilized" peoples.[80] In addition, they pointed to studies that linked mastitis, the result of "stagnation of the milk of nursing mothers," to the development of breast cancer despite reports that women in Japan and Italy, where extended nursing was the norm, had lower rates of breast cancer mortality.[81]

The issue of prolonged breast feeding reflected physicians' willingness to engage in an aspect of childcare deemed natural. Indeed, they inundated women and one another with advice on all aspects of nursing. Each physician, within the broad limits of agreement, had his own opinion on how soon feeding should begin. Throughout the first half century, physicians who recognized the importance of colostrum tended to support early feeding.[82] For those not impressed by the importance of colostrum, early feeding was not significant. If the child was hungry, it could be given sugar mixed in boiled water, diluted cow's milk, or some form of supplementary feeding.[83] Once nursing began, however, physicians agreed on the importance of regular feedings but often disagreed when they should occur or at what age they should change.[84] The schedule could become quite complex. In 1906 Adam H. Wright described the system used at the Burnside Lying-In Hospital: "Let the babe nurse every six hours during the first day, every four hours during second day, and every two hours for twenty minutes during third day and thereafter, except at night, when he should nurse at half-past ten, half-past four, and in morning, half-past eight."[85] Physicians acknowledged that not every child could be kept to the recommended fixed schedule but they continued to suggest it was best for the child if it was. Neither did feeding schedules get any easier, particularly in the '20s.[86]

What was clear over time was that despite the value of breast feeding, fewer women were engaging in it for any period of time. At a minimum doctors advised four to six weeks of nursing even for women whose milk was of poor quality. The optimum time was between six and nine months depending on the circumstances of the mother.[87] But if six to nine months was the optimum period, many women were unable to achieve it. A 1916 study in Toronto of 633 women who nursed found that 76 percent breast fed for three months but only 46.7 percent for six months. Such statistics did not compare favourably with those of rural women, 70 to 90 percent of whom nursed for at least six months. A Montreal study in the late 1920s concluded that 52 percent of new mothers were no longer nursing at six months. In the '30s and '40s estimates seemed more positive with two-thirds of Canadian babies being on partial or complete breast feeding, but for how long was unclear.[88] Few estimates, however, were based on any authoritative studies. Despite the realization that many women were not nursing, let alone for the recommended six to nine months, physicians continued to advise it. And most agreed any breast feeding was better than none.[89]

Why did physicians believe women were not breast feeding as much as they should? Mentioned early on was mothers' ignorance and selfishness and the convenience of bottle feeding. Even those who nursed their babies could be faulted. Physicians pointed out that overfeeding led to infant vomiting with the result that the desire to wean the child developed sooner rather than later.[90] Physicians also subscribed to a vague form of environmentalism and blamed the strain of civilization. Dr A.B. Chandler of Montreal suggested that "modern life with its housing conditions ..., its fast pace and the training of the rising generation [was] not conducive to mothers nursing babies."[91] Part of the environment was poverty. Brown, the Canadian who spoke out most about breast feeding, recognized poverty as the reason many working-class women returned to work soon after birth. There was no medical solution in such cases, only "sociologic aid." Others were not so kind and only proffered advice that a nursing mother should not return to work, which was hardly practical advice for many women. On the other side of the class divide Brown referred to the "more highly organized and hence more easily disturbed nervous organization" of the upper classes, which created an inability to nurse.[92] The medical officer of Fort William, Ontario, believed that middle-class women in his community had adopted bottle feeding because of its convenience and apparent modernity.[93] The environmental factor also led some to perceptive insights as to why rural women breast fed more than urban women. Brown, in particular, understood the complex of factors that encouraged rural women to nurse – their work remained in the home so they were available for nursing, they lived in a culture where breast feeding was supported, and they lacked the ice on which to keep "properly modified cow's milk." As well, rural women generally did not have easy access to physicians who might have been willing to assist in accessing artificial feeding.[94] The list of factors indicated that women did not control many of them.

The availability of alternatives to breast feeding gave some women choice. In previous centuries, especially in western Europe, wet nursing had been popular among the affluent. In North America, however, it was not common. Nevertheless, in the early part of the century, occasional references to it occurred. But while references to wet nursing existed, they were becoming increasingly rare.[95] Physicians were becoming convinced that with the advent of "the best modern methods of substitute feeding" wet nursing had (or should have) become a thing of the past.[96] Substitute feeding usually consisted of some form of modified cow's milk. In the early years of the century, the difficulty was to ensure that the cow's milk used as well as the water diluting it were pure and safe to drink. In Montreal, pure milk stations were set up to encourage bottle feeding. Thus the message went out that cow's milk was an acceptable substitute for mother's milk. But it was not the poor who took this message to heart. Middle-class women learned the lesson. It even became part of class pride when physicians such as Helen MacMurchy suggested that bottle feeding was an alternative for the intelligent mother.[97]

Bottle feeding became much safer in the interwar period, partially as a result of the increasing pasteurization of milk. In addition, in the interwar years and beyond physicians became strong proponents of giving babies additional foods such as orange juice and cod liver oil and thus breast milk was no longer seen as the perfect food.[98] Alternatives to breast feeding were usually under a physician's control; thus physicians made money from bottle-fed babies whereas they did not benefit to the same extent from breast-fed babies. Often physicians created their own formula. Alan Brown's consisted of 18 different ingredients.[99] Advertisements for prepared artificial formulas directed at physicians flattered them as experts who would know what product to prescribe.[100] But as public health nurses could testify, often physicians did not know what to recommend or how to decide on which milk was best. Physicians had received little training about breast feeding in medical schools.[101] What had once been "natural" seemed of less use than the scientific feeding now available. In the 1940s, for example, what had been deemed obvious – putting the infant to one breast at each feeding – was being challenged.[102] Such challenges simply confused many and made formula feeding appear easier and less worrisome.

Irma Avery remembered a woman in hospital being told she was too old to nurse – she was 32. Even though Jane Rutherford nursed her own children, she did not remember being encouraged to do so by anyone, including hospital personnel. Neither were Betsy Mackenzie or Becki Crawford. The latter had friends whose doctor had left the decision of whether to breast feed or not up to them. Crawford found this strange feeling that the doctor should have "at least" encouraged the woman to try to breast feed.[103] Some hospitals adopted the mixed feeding regimen. Dr Warren recalled that when she interned at Women's College Hospital, Toronto, it followed a combination of artificial and natural feeding, as did the Royal Victoria Montreal Maternity Hospital.[104] At a time when mothers stayed in hospital ten days to two weeks after birth, the scheduling/feeding pattern had been set for the woman to continue when she returned to her home.

Given the mixed actions of physicians and hospitals in the interwar period and beyond, the accusatory tone of earlier decades towards women who did not breast feed lessened. Physicians recognized the busy lives women led and acknowledged the kind of inconvenience that breast feeding schedules placed on women. Nonetheless, one mid-1930s text seemed to combine both approaches. It argued that after six weeks of age artificial feeding of the child was usually quite successful and that "a more liberal attitude may be adopted to meet ... maternal demands for weaning." At that point the author mentions "excessive neuroticism," suggesting the decision to wean was selfish and reflected the inability of modern woman to do her duty.[105] Others believed that some women were simply better able to nurse than others. For example, the thin woman was thought to nurse better than the fat.[106] Underlying most of these attitudes and beliefs was the conviction that if properly advised most women could nurse and that so many did not, especially among the well to do, was a function of psychological, nervous, or selfish factors rather than physiological. Yet physicians seldom discussed how to overcome the psychological factors. Infant feeding had become medicalized and with the shift to bottle or artificial feeding unforeseen consequences emerged. For the lives of more traditional people, the increase in bottle feeding in later years had a significant impact on cultural norms. For example, Richard G. Condon, in his 1970s study of Holman, North West Territories, noted that bottle feeding had changed the adoption age of children to immediately after birth rather than at age two or three, which had been the traditional pattern. Such a shift was true throughout the Arctic.[107]

Conclusion

Underlying medical perceptions of marriage and motherhood was the conviction that they were subjects that were best under medical purview. At one level it reflected a holistic approach to health – anything that impinged on a person's life could affect their health and thus necessitate medical advice. Doctors perceived marriage as a union between a woman and a man with the goal of having children and as a result, they were strong supporters of placing limits on who could marry, excluding all those who were not mentally sound and physically healthy. Rhetoric was not enough to ensure controls over who should not marry, so many within the medical profession supported marital health certificates. Underlying the concern was fear of increased procreation of the unfit. Physicians, at times, had an idealized view of marriage, specifically marital sexuality. Physicians may have differentiated the "natural" sex urges between men and women; when they discussed marital sexuality, however, they envisioned a mutuality of desire even though that mutuality was not necessarily one they believed was innate to both sexes. A social creation – marriage – determined when and how a biological urge was expressed.

Marriage's purpose was the creation of a family. Family meant children and for women fulfillment of the central role in their lives – motherhood. The desire for motherhood may have been instinctual but being a good mother was not. Over time, physicians argued that women needed to be educated in topics such as scheduling. The interest physicians took in breast feeding can be seen from different vantage points. It reflects their concern about the health of new mothers and their babies. It speaks to the increasing scientific understanding of the composition of breast milk. It was both a recognition of the importance of women's bodies and what those bodies did and yet the sense of breast feeding's naturalness was circumscribed. Physicians saw nursing as needing to be limited in time and needing to be *taught* to women. Practitioners' attitudes to breast feeding reinforced their tendency to place women's bodies in close alignment with animals, with the primitive. They did not always agree with one another but were of one voice that women should listen to them.

6 "On the fringe of knowledge": Infertility

"The value of the uterus is to be estimated by its probable sterility or fertility."[1] These words, written in 1944 by James William Kennedy and Archibald Donald Campbell, respectively surgeon-in-chief to the Joseph Price Hospital, Philadelphia, and associate professor of obstetrics and gynaecology, McGill University, focus on two themes. First is the significance of infertility in the period under study. Second is that the problem of infertility was often directed at the woman. Not only did her body represent the problem but the problem affected her worth or the worth of her uterus, one of the major organs that differentiated her from man. A failure in its function resulted in a perceived uselessness and lessened the differentiation between the two sexes – in essence made the woman less womanly.

While physicians were aware of the problem of infertility, they were unable to do much about it in the early decades of the century and, consequently, there was little Canadian discussion of it.[2] Such discussion came with the interwar years when more accurate information on the female cycle became available and the ability to understand the actual process of conception emerged. At the same time, concern about infertility increased, not because of any perceived increase in it but because of the changing context of society – the loss of life during WWI and the decline in the birth rate. If those who could conceive were limiting the number of children they had, perhaps a new source of population could be found through overcoming the infertility of those wanting but unable to have children. But as the chapter's title summarizes, medicine had few answers.[3]

The chapter begins with a discussion of what physicians knew about the process of conception and what they understood about infertility, the changing definition of infertility, and the complexity of the term "infertility" itself. What follows is an analysis of the perceived causes of infertility in women and men and the gendered nature of those causes and how they changed over time. Last is an examination of the treatment of infertility and its emphasis on surgery and hormonal treatment. Clear is that over the first half century infertility became accepted as a medical "problem." As such, physicians had the power to create both the basis and limits of its discussion.

Knowledge of Conception and Infertility

The perceived causes of infertility and their treatment depended on how much doctors and others understood about conception. Because there was little accurate understanding of a woman's fertile period until the mid 1920s, much of the advice given was inaccurate and guaranteed to lessen a woman's chances of bearing a child. As more information became available, physicians refined their understanding of the optimum period for conception. By 1930, estimates were that ovulation occurred from the twelfth to the fourteenth day after menstruation and that conception could best occur between the tenth and eighteenth. A sense of urgency was sounded a decade later when doctors concluded that the spermatozoon could survive only three days or less after ejaculation. This was a far cry from the five weeks one physician had estimated earlier in the century. Considering that the ova, too, had a life of only three days, timing had to be exact. By the late 1940s physicians had a sense that this was possible, thus aiding many couples in their efforts to have children.[4] As we have already seen, one contentious belief was that orgasm in a woman was necessary for or at least helpful in conception.

Considering the importance they placed on having children, doctors considered infertility as something to be deplored. Nineteenth-century discussions were not very specific except in seeing infertility as a consequence of other health problems. Such a view was evident in the early part of the century as well. When patient records are examined, whether a woman had given birth or not was almost always mentioned; when a childless woman consulted a physician for some disorder that was cured and she subsequently gave birth to a child, the birth was reported with satisfaction, suggesting that this "lack" too had been part of the disease, at least from the point of view of the physician.

Interest in infertility increased over time. From a perusal of the medical examinations given at Queen's University it appears that not until January of 1919 did a question concerning sterility appear.

After that such questions appeared with regularity in 1924, 1929, 1931, 1932, 1936, and 1937. This growing sensitivity to infertility is confirmed by Dr M.C. Watson of Toronto who in 1930 noted that in the previous decade over 500 articles on infertility (sterility) had been published. Researchers at the Royal Victoria Hospital, Montreal, had engaged the topic of sterility from the late 1920s until WWII intervened. Subsequently research resumed and the hospital established a fertility clinic, which continued the work of a previous one set up in November 1935. In its first year, 81 patients attended with that number more than doubling the next year.[5]

If sterility was becoming a "fascinating subject,"[6] it was also a complex one. No one definition of infertility existed throughout the first half century and the length of time a couple had to be childless before doctors viewed it as a problem varied. Physicians in the nineteenth and early twentieth centuries tended to be generous in estimating three years or more of not being able to conceive and bear a child before labelling a couple infertile. Others, however, were narrowing the limits. In his 1905 text Henry J. Garrigues acknowledged the three-year norm but argued that one year for those wanting children should be time enough. Still others suggested 18 months.[7] Whatever consensus had existed was lost in the post–World War I period, in part because there developed an understanding that different women had different needs depending on the urgency with which they wanted children, as well as their faith in medical ability to help them and their willingness to seek this help. Mrs Mary Donohue, for example, was 30 years of age when she entered the Royal Victoria Hospital, Montreal, in 1921. She had been married for only 16 months but perhaps because of her age wanted to begin her family immediately. J.S. Fairbairn recognized the pressure of age in his 1924 text. While he felt that two years of marriage should occur before sterility was discussed, he felt with young women, more time could be given before intervention occurred; with older women, those over 35, the period should be lessened.[8] Although some continued to adhere to the three-year guideline, many in the 1930s adopted twelve months and in the 1940s two years, but there was no uniformity.[9] The varying time used to define when a couple was experiencing an infertility problem reveals the way in which medical science constructs a definition and can change it at will.

There was even less consensus about the terminology used to describe infertility. By and large, doctors used the term sterility rather than infertility. While some physicians used "sterility" to describe a situation where an egg was never fertilized,[10] most did not, which allowed them to include the phenomena of habitual abortion, still-births, etc. But these generalizations do not really express the variations that existed throughout the 50-year period. Some doctors referred to the inability to conceive as sterility, absolute sterility, complete sterility, or primary sterility. Others referred to the inability to bring forth a living child as secondary sterility or relative sterility. Then there was what some referred to as acquired sterility, the situation where the woman might have given birth to one or two children but was unable to conceive again.[11] For statistical purposes, however, acquired sterility was not considered because it would have been impossible to determine whether or not one-child families were a result of choice or infertility.

The power that physicians had in defining sterility and its variations and the timing when conception could occur should not be underestimated. First, the labelling of women or men as sterile could be devastating to them. Second, childlessness, which is a social situation, became through the designation of "sterility" a defined medical condition. Third, by using the term sterility rather than infertility, practitioners were suggesting a fixed condition (infertility can be temporary and in many cases overcome). By preferring the more absolute term, physicians were able to take more credit for themselves than warranted when so-called "sterile" couples conceived after treatment. Fourth, the inclination to define and to place time constraints on fertility was part of physicians' desire to have certainty in their profession. It allowed them to measure and thus gave an aura of objectivity and preciseness to what it was they were doing. It is difficult to imagine what else they could have done; nonetheless, being aware of the sometimes arbitrary nature of the process does remind us of the socially constructed aspect of much of medicine's measurements and definitions.

Defined by childless couples, infertility did not affect more than 10 to 15 percent of the population.[12] But such figures include those who deliberately remained childless and so are the optimum percentage. When physicians specifically addressed sterility, the rates appeared relatively constant as well. One early-twentieth-century text estimated that one in eight couples was sterile. The Canadian authors of a 1946 textbook for nurses agreed, at least quoting the same figure for "gynecological patients ... personally concerned with the problem of childless marriages." Medical interest in infertility, then, was not linked to its increase in the population. Neither have recent estimates changed the figures.[13] As for what couples were sterile, physicians saw no class distinction,[14] despite, as will be seen below, their perceptions of many causes being class linked.

If physicians were interested in determining the percentage of couples that were infertile, they were also interested in apportioning blame – to either the woman or the man. But even while doctors continued to do this, they recognized that it was really a fruitless exercise. Encompassed under the discussions of infertility was the concept of selective sterility, "when two individuals of opposite sexes are unable to procreate, although each may be potent in this respect with another partner."[15] Doctors had long been intrigued by this; with different partners, individuals supposedly sterile were no longer so. As Dr W. Blair Bell speculated in 1917, though the cause of this was unknown, he felt that some aspects of "natural selection ... lie behind this so-called incompatibility." The conclusion: it was for the best that these mismatched couples remained childless, a matter of nature knowing best. Dr Pelton Tew in 1939 was not quite so deterministic. He simply noted that there was no one cause but rather "4.79 factors for each childless couple" and they were seldom associated with one partner only. Selective or sterile mating recognized the frequent impossibility of determining "blame." There was a sense by mid century that eventually determinations would be possible, but as medical knowledge existed at the time they were not.[16]

The Gendered Nature of Infertility

Emerging in the medical literature of the first half of the twentieth century was the perception of many physicians that sterility originated largely in women. As Henry Garrigues noted, "[H]er sexual tract being so much longer and more complicated, it is more apt to harbor conditions which prevent fecundation." There was little doubt that women's reproductive system *was* more complex than men's and the whole specialty of gynaecology with its emphasis on what could go wrong in women's bodies was brought to bear on what caused sterility in them. Nowhere is this more evident than in the 1946 *Essentials of Obstetrics and Gynecology*, by William Albert Scott, professor of obstetrics and gynaecology, University of Toronto, and H. Brookfield Van Wyck, assistant professor of obstetrics and gynaecology, University of Toronto, in which the authors list five joint causes, three gender specific in men, and five in women, with each of the five broken down into 11 different subsections.[17]

Although numerous, perceived causes of infertility in women can be categorized under three general headings – volitional, iatrogenic, and physiological. The first had its greatest acceptability in the early years of the century when there was much about women's lives that doctors blamed for women's inability to conceive or carry a child to term, from their sexual practices to the food they ate, the education they received, and even their individual personalities. Clear is the lessening in the judgmental quality of the discussions over time. The second major grouping focused on how medical treatment in one field led to problems in another, in this specific case how poor obstetrical practices could cause future sterility in women. Iatrogenic causes were virtually absent in the discussions of male sterility. The last grouping of factors was related to the physiological nature of the body, in the case of women its problematic nature.

Volitional Factors

Volitional factors encompassed lifestyle factors, many of which we have examined. For example, practitioners extolled the idea of female sexual restraint and while attitudes changed with time, throughout the first half of the century they perceived the female sexual drive as somehow more dangerous for women. It is not surprising, then, that they linked sexual excess and sterility. While less morally judgmental than in the early years of the century, doctors in the interwar period and later still pointed to sexual excess and other problematic sexual habits or even lack of sexual enjoyment as factors leading to sterility or to problems that could cause sterility.[18] How sexual excess and sterility in women were connected, however, remained unclear.

One medical link between sexuality and sterility was obvious – the dangers of contracting VD. In 1915 Dr Helen MacMurchy made the danger facing women plain: "Every year in this country thousands of pure women are infected in the relations of marriage, and in many instances their conceptional capacity destroyed." Gonorrhoea was of particular concern with physicians estimating it as causing the majority of infertility problems, in particular for the phenomenon of one-child sterility. Even as late as 1951 and well after the introduction of sulphonamide drugs and penicillin to treat gonorrhoea, it was pointed out that the disease could still cause "sterilizing lesions ... inflammatory lesions in the cervix and occlusion of the fallopian tubes of the wife."[19] The other major venereal disease, syphilis, posed a different problem. It did not cause sterility per se but it often did result in miscarriages and stillbirths with the same result – childless homes. One 1900 estimate was that 30 to 40 percent of syphilitic women aborted and in 1923 doctors estimated that syphilis destroyed 75 percent of the children of syphilitic parents either before they were born or within a year of birth.[20]

Linked also to sexuality were birth control and abortion, two top-ics we will analyse in more detail in the next chapter. Birth control was very much a moral issue in the early twentieth century and doc-tors strongly believed that it was unnatural and that anything unnatu-ral was bound to be detrimental to health; some made explicit a linkage between the use of birth control and sterility. By the 1940s, even after the moral argument against birth control had lessened, physicians still connected specific types of birth control, such as the stem pessary, as problematic for future fertility.[21] Abortion was even more problem-atic. Physicians perceived nontherapeutic abortion to be a cause of ill health and gynaecological disorders, some of which could cause infertility. Self-induced abortions were particularly worrisome. In 1930 Dr Dafoe estimated that 40 percent of the incomplete abortion cases on the Toronto General Hospital wards were self-induced. Equal concern was expressed during the war years that followed.[22] While much of the ill health of women that physicians saw as a result of abortions *could* have resulted in sterility, at least according to the understanding of the period, doctors also addressed the *expressed* link between self-induced abortions and subsequent sterility.[23]

While moral and sexual decisions that resulted in infertility were one aspect of the volitional "choices" that women made, more benign life-style factors were another. We have seen this emerging in discus-sions of higher education of women, their increasing involvement in the labour force, and even in the clothes they wore and the food they ate or didn't eat. In the early years, practitioners opposed higher education for women, arguing that it could undermine the proper development of woman's reproductive system. They were even less comfortable about the increasing participation of women in paid employment. Such con-cerns increased during WWI as more women entered industrial work in areas previously not open to them. There was a sense that because of women's reproductive responsibility they were particularly suscep-tible to industrial poison, especially the fumes of lead, mercury, arsenic, and phosphorous. In this case, the dangers of work were connected directly to female sterility. This was also acknowledged in the 1930s.

With thousands of women flocking to war industries in World War II concern emerged once again about the effect this work would have on their childbearing capabilities and how the exposure to poisonous substances would affect their health.[24] Other than pointing out the problem, however, physicians could do little to follow up their concerns.

Improper fashion and diet could also lead to infertility. As we have seen, of special note was any tight clothing around the waist and abdomen. As one American doctor explained in the 1902 *Canadian Practitioner and Medical Review*, "Tight lacing ... predisposes to pelvic disorders by interfering with circulation and exciting uterine displacements."[25] As we will see below, uterine displacements were a possible cause of sterility considered by physicians. Although the hostility towards women's fashions as a cause of disease declined as fashions changed and allowed the body more freedom, the concern about them never totally disappeared. As for diet, physicians in 1917 reported that nutrition affected "in a marked degree" fertility in animals and the same was true for women. In later decades the lack of vitamin E was added to an insufficient diet as a contributing cause to sterility and infertility.[26] In the 1930s and afterwards doctors expressed anxiety about the idealization of the "boyish figure" and the use of "extraordinary physical exercises and mechanical appliances to prevent the normal development of the hips and bust."[27] If they were too thin it affected their fertility and yet there was an awareness throughout the entire half century that infertility was also linked to obesity.[28] So women had to maintain what physicians considered a normal weight.

Lifestyle factors provided a greater latitude for intervention on the part of physicians and an almost endless scope of causes to blame for sterility. Nowhere can this be seen more than in the occasional blame that physicians placed on the very personality or nature of certain women. Dr Charles Shepard in the 1902 *Canadian Practitioner and Medical Review* was concerned about the emergence at the turn of the century of the "new woman" who because of her "new ideas and practices" had retarded the growth of her natural menstrual processes and had descended into ill health. The life chosen was a selfish one. The theme continued to permeate the literature on women. Dr W. Pelton Tew made this clear in 1939 when he explained, "Human energy is expended in two ways, for individuation and genesis";[29] women had to decide between their own needs and those of the species. The opinion of many practitioners was clear – delaying marriage was not an option.[30] Dr Jessie McGeachy was even more vehement at mid century about the blame the individual woman had to accept:

> In assessing a case of sterility from the emotional standpoint, it is important to judge the personality type ... For example, is she vain and egocentric, able to give love and attention only to herself in the way of clothes and personal adornments and elaborate housing equipment? If this is so, she has not developed beyond the narcissistic stage of childhood and she is emotionally unable to love anyone else but herself. Does she desire a child, not with the aim of being a good parent, but to be one of a group of women with social prestige because they can gossip about formulas and training? Is it too visionary to venture the suggestion that this type of egocentricity and emotional maldevelopment may be accompanied by altered physiology such as faulty ovulation?[31]

The attack on middle-class women and those with social pretensions was clear. McGeachy was reacting to the downside of modernity and women's role in it, and the fear both raised about the future. Volitional factors that could lead to problems conceiving or carrying a healthy child to term reflected physicians' social beliefs. Woman's life was to revolve around her role as mother. Anything that drew her attention elsewhere could be interpreted as medically problematic. And certainly some of the decisions women made were – sexual excess could lead to VD, too much energy expended in school or work *might* weaken an individual's health especially if it coincided with a poor diet. Underlying most if not all the factors, however, was a sense of woman putting herself first. Certainly the Freudian language of McGeachy made that abundantly clear.

Iatrogenic Causes

While all of the above factors are ones which the individual woman had some control over, the medical literature acknowledged that often women were not responsible for the problems that influenced fertility; their doctors were. The sometimes excessive intervention in treatment that many physicians followed had dire consequences for their patients. Of particular concern was the increasing intervention that the rise of gynaecology brought with it. In a few instances doctors explicitly connected specific treatment with infection causing sterility and admitted that surgery resorted to in order to cure sterility at times actually caused it.[32] Equally problematic were childbirth practices, which many saw as becoming increasingly interventionist and which gynaecologists blamed for many of the gynaecological problems of women. Certainly until 1950 many doctors deemed childbirth, or the medical practices surrounding it, a cause of or contributor to disease, ill health, and fertility problems. Of note in these discussions was concern over the increase in Caesarian sections and their relationship to subsequent sterility.[33]

Like Caesarian section, X-ray and radium treatments became tools in the hands of practitioners in the twentieth century. Effective in combatting various conditions, their connection to sterility was not always appreciated. In the early decades, radiologists consistently emphasized that only those trained in the field should attempt to use the new technology. Their need to repeat this, however, suggests that it did not always occur. In 1928 the use of "weak therapeutic doses of x-ray for sterility" was mentioned in the literature, a situation of some concern. In the 1931 *Canadian Medical Association Journal*, Dr L.J. Carter expressed reservations about X-raying women who could still bear children for he worried about the effect it would have on the children they bore. In 1943, D. Kearns made it clear that radium therapy could cause sterility.[34] Doctors could be part of the problem rather than part of the solution.

Physiological Causes

While some of the physician-induced responsibility was very specific, when examining physiological causes of infertility the view becomes less clear only because so many factors could impinge on the ability of a woman to conceive. Sooner or later doctors seemed to focus on every aspect of a woman's health experience in an attempt to explain her infertility – TB, rheumatism, cholera, enteric fever, cancer, scarlatina, myxoedema, anemia. Even depression was connected to it as a study done at the Toronto Psychiatric Hospital in the late 1920s revealed.[35] The various organs of generation were the main focus. Disease of the ovaries was a problem, but then any disease or disorder of the reproductive system had to be taken into account. As one 1935 text explained, "Sterility in woman may be divided into two classes: 1. Cases in which some defect of a sexual organ can be discovered. 2. Cases in which the sexual organs appear to be normal."[36] Essentially the world of gynaecological disorders was linked to potential sterility in women. Because it is clearly impossible to write a survey of all the perceived medical

causes of sterility in women over a 50-year period only the more prominent ones will be touched upon as well as those that indicate certain
trends within the profession itself.

A major issue in preventing conception was blockage of the fallopian tubes. For some, it appeared that nature had somehow gone astray
in creating them. As Dr R.E. Cutts exclaimed in 1900, "The fallopian
tube is, no doubt, the weakest part of the entire system. The small-
ness, length and tortuosity of its canal all favor its occlusion with the
slightest pathological change."[37] In 1920, I.C. Rubin introduced a test
for the patency or nonblockage of the tubes "by allowing carbon diox-
ide gas under pressure to escape into the abdominal cavity by means
of a cannula introduced into the uterine cavity." Escape proved the
patency of the tubes. No escape suggested blockage.[38] This test was
taken up quickly as an easy diagnostic procedure that had less impact
on the woman than previous exploratory surgery to determine the condition of the tubes. The excitement of the Rubin test was that it could
lead to cure through confirming the cause of the sterility and thus suggesting treatment – that is, removal of the blockage through surgery.

For other factors the situation was not as bright. Malformations of
any of the reproductive organs were clearly recognized as problematic,
but seldom was there a straightforward solution. Physicians comforted
themselves that malformations were not common and other than noting
that the physical examination should look for such malformations they
did not spend a great deal of time on them.[39] One "malformation" –
uterine displacements – led a chequered history and did attract the
attention of practitioners. From the turn of the century to the late 1930s
and beyond, most doctors had a sense that uterine displacements were
linked to sterility even though some challenges to such an idea were
made. One text in 1906 maintained that "anteflexion [uterus pointing
forward], which is by far the commonest so-called displacement associated with sterility," was in fact a condition of most women who had not
borne a child, indeed it could be said it was a sign of never having had a
child. But such a challenge was rare, although more seemed to emerge
in the later years.[40] As for retroflection, the strength of the linkage was
reflected in the words of Rubin: "Retroversion of the uterus per se is
not necessarily deterrent to fertility. If the husband is vigorous and fertile the anatomical abnormality is no barrier to insemination. When the
husband is relatively infertile, uterine retroversion may play an unfa-
vorable role in the deposition of the semen by reason of the external
os of the cervix not dipping into the seminal lake."[41] Thus it was not a

primary cause but it certainly did not maximize the ability to conceive. During the discussions of the various uterine displacements, there was the underlying sense that women's bodies should conform to a norm and that deviation from that norm was problematic, indeed had to be.

From a reading of the first half century of literature it would appear that any health problem could potentially lead to sterility. There was a recognition that abdominal growths, especially fibromyomata, interfered with conception. One strange note with respect to this was sounded in 1950 in the *Manitoba Medical Review*. In an article on "Psychosomatic Considerations in Gynecology" the author reported that one expert maintained that women with "satisfactory sexual lives" seldom had fibromata, while those experiencing "chronic psychosexual disturbances" were susceptible to them.[42] Intriguing also was the discussion of endometriosis that emerged in the 1930s. It was seen as a cause of sterility, and Drs Fallon, Bronson, and Moran in *Modern Medicine of Canada* claimed it developed "more readily in childless or sexually dormant women."[43] As in lifestyle factors, somehow the patient was being held responsible. Similar were "abnormal secretions" within the woman that, although not harmful to her, were harmful to the sperm. At times, such secretions almost seemed volitional, with references phrased in a way that the secretions appeared hostile to the sperm.[44] But the hostility allowed physicians to focus attention on the female secretions rather than the "weakness" of the sperm in not being able to survive female secretions.

Primary in physiological problems was endocrinal imbalance. In 1915 one article in the *Canadian Medical Association Journal* linked deficiency in production of thyroid secretion and deficient function of the anterior lobe of the pituitary gland to sterility. Physicians in the same journal in 1934 and 1939 agreed and pointed out how disturbances of the endocrine system (pituitary, thyroid, and sex glands) were significant and in the 1939 article claimed that nearly 60 percent of primary sterility was connected to these disturbances. Others concurred and as we will see below this led to significant hormonal treatment.[45]

As is clear from the above discussion, physicians focused on a great number of factors that they believed could cause sterility in women. When once a factor was established it seemed to persist throughout the period, although its popularity as a cause might ebb and flow and the attitudes towards it might shift. New factors were added to older ones as time passed. Many of these were beyond women's control such as those caused by disease or which existed for congenital reasons. The listing of factors that related to infertility was so long that the conclusion reached by anyone immersing themselves in the literature is that the female body simply did not function well.

Infertility in Men

When physicians looked at male involvement in infertility quite a different pattern emerges. As Cheryl Krasnick Warsh has argued, for most of the nineteenth century, physicians had generally believed that as long as a man was not impotent he could impregnate his wife. That belief did not last. By the end of the century and the early years of the new century, practitioners were emphasizing that impotence and sterility in men were two separate conditions.[46] As a result, physicians began estimating the percentage of childless marriages that were due to the sterility of the male partner. There was no consistency about the estimates but one trend was visible – physicians perceived male sterility as more important as time passed in that the lowest estimates (and to a lesser extent higher) gradually moved upward. For example, in the first 20 years of the century, physician estimates of male sterility ranged widely from a low of 7 percent to a high of 40 percent. In the 1920s and '30s estimates generally ranged from a low of 20 percent to a high of 50 percent. The 1940s saw a similar increase in the lower estimate of 25 percent and maintained the high at 50 percent.[47]

The recognition of male sterility, however, was not accompanied by any change in attitude. Doctors for the first half of the twentieth century continued to make the same points – that the male partner had to be examined and too much emphasis was being placed on the woman to her detriment. That they had emphasized the same points over again suggests that while physicians recognized male sterility, many had difficulty in transferring that intellectual recognition to medical practice. They simply could not accept the idea that male sterility might be as significant an issue as female sterility.[48] And they were not alone. In trying to explain the overwhelming emphasis on female sterility among their male patients, some practitioners concluded that men were rather ignorant of the possibility of their own sterility as long as they were not impotent. And if aware, they were loathe to admit it. As one Winnipeg physician put it in 1934, "The faith of the average man in his own procreative ability and his willingness to place the blame of an unproductive union on his wife are remarkable."[49] That some physicians themselves continued to focus on women more than men suggested the ability of physicians to ignore the "scientific" information available to them. They seemed to prefer to work within a wider worldview of men and women and the responsibility of each in reproduction.

When they did examine infertility in men, physicians worked within some of the same categories they did with women. Volitional factors that encompassed excessive sexual activity were explicitly linked to male sterility in the early years of the century. In 1903, Dr J. Ross explained that, while not a prime cause, "debauchery" on the part of the man was a factor in sterility. Three years later in their *A System of Gynaecology*, Thomas Allbutt, W.S. Playfair, and Thomas Watts Eden mentioned too-frequent intercourse in marriage as a cause of male sterility. But whether inside or outside marriage, sexual excesses remained a concern.[50] If outside marriage, the fear was it could lead to venereal disease in men and consequent sterility. Of particular concern was gonorrhoea. In men, it could cause a "devastating chronic infection of the prostate and obstructions of the passageways for spermatozoa in the male genital tract."[51] Linked as well to sterility in men were masturbation and birth control.[52]

Physicians also looked to other lifestyle factors. Less condemnatory was a sense that modern society was not conducive to reproduction. It removed both sexes from the realm of nature resulting in them having difficulty "mating." As part of that perspective one 1911 textbook expressed concern about the sedentary lives more men were leading. It was only decades later, however, that this kind of theme was picked up in discussions of infertility per se and focused on the professional man.[53] Other factors seemed to attract less attention. Interestingly, physicians did not focus directly on the kinds of work hazards to which many working-class men were exposed as they had with women. They had some sense of the dangers of chronic poisoning from arsenic, antimony, lead, mercury, and other occupational hazards but provided little detail.[54] And most concern was expressed after the early years of the century, perhaps a reflection of doctors' increasing sensitivity to an environmental impact on health and their social responsibility to raise it within a medical framework. Of more interest after 1930 was diet perhaps because the Depression concentrated attention on the problems of inadequate nutrition. Errors in diet were seen to result in fewer spermatozoa, and ones of immaturity and less vitality. The two aspects of diet on which doctors specifically focused were the ones they had connected to sterility in women as well – obesity and the lack of vitamin E.[55] Specifically linked to men was the attention paid to alcohol and its effect on the spermatozoon, a concern expressed over the entire half century.[56]

The focus on volitional factors as a cause of male sterility provided the medical profession with hope of cure since adjustment of decisions made did not appear to be out of the realm of possibility. With respect to venereal disease, damage may have been so extensive as to eliminate the possibility of cure but generally, if caught in time, the damage could be contained. Focusing on lifestyle also permitted an expansion of medical expertise into areas that may not have always been considered medical. Poor employment conditions and inadequate diet became medicalized, although physicians were never too specific in their attempts to counteract them other than through noting their existence.

More problematic for the individual in being able to do anything to help himself were, for want of a better term, physiological causes. As has been already pointed out impotency was a consideration. In the nineteenth and early twentieth centuries, doctors often saw it as the result of immoral acts, but both physical and psychological causes of impotence were acknowledged in a straightforward manner, particularly in the period after World War I.[57] At various times doctors remarked on specific diseases such as tuberculosis, diabetes, mumps, orchitis (inflammation of the testes), or epididymitis (another form of inflammation of a specific part of the testes), and others as factors in male sterility. Developmental problems leading to sterility were also significant.[58] Interestingly, considering the emphasis placed on endocrinal causes in women, doctors did not focus on this as a significant cause of male sterility and when they did it was only near mid century.[59] In some cases doctors viewed the physiological process of aging as a problem in the production of adequate sperm in men, although this was certainly not stressed perhaps because there was little physicians could do about it and when mentioned only seemed to apply to very elderly men.[60] Only rarely did physicians mention sperm problems being the result of specific medical practice such as treatment of other conditions through X-ray.[61] Unlike the case of women, iatrogenic causation did not loom large in male sterility. But as with the case of female infertility, over time the list of causes became longer as new ones were added with each generation. Prioritizing causes was rare, which meant that the inconsequential was lumped with the consequential – each patient was different and what was inconsequential for one could be consequential for another.

Treatment

Determining causation was the first step in helping patients who wanted solutions to their infertility. As causation varied so did treatment. At the turn of the twentieth century, the anthropologist Franz Boas described the custom among the Southern Kwakiutl of eating certain foods to increase the chance of a woman conceiving. Among some Inuit there were reports of spousal exchange as a remedy for infertility.[62] Much of the advice given to men and women over the years in Western society was of a type that they could follow and control. Individual men and women could change their lifestyle. If alcohol and tobacco were used, it should stop. If sexual excess was the problem for either partner, then the individual should show some restraint. If douching was causing a problem for the woman she was to cease. Both men and women were to live healthier lives – get plenty of sleep, exercise regularly, and eat well. For some people this was going to be easier said than done. For much of the first half of the twentieth century, many working-class Canadians did not have access to adequate food. Equally problematic, as we have seen, were the environmental hazards associated with some industrial work situations. There was no suggestion in the medical literature that laws protecting workers should be passed. There was no suggestion that individuals should change their work situation, which, in any case, would have been difficult for many workers to do. In any of the discussions about work-related poisons, the only direct reference to action was usually to suggest that perhaps women should not be involved in such jobs. All these indicate that individuals themselves could partially take the "solution" or resolution to the problem of their sterility into their own hands. The importance of such advice lies not in its efficacy or its feasibility but in the fact that it appeared to allow individuals to take charge rather than becoming totally dependent on medical treatment. This was not to last.

Medical therapy for sterility varied and, while some therapies were directed at men, such as the use of electric current in the early part of the century,[63] most focused on women. There was mention of the benefits of divulsion and dilatation, although some voices in the 1920s rejected such procedures, seeing them as conducive to sterility rather than an aid in curing it. Nevertheless, some practitioners were still raising its potential in the 1940s and 1950s.[64] Other therapies in use were pessaries for retroverted uteri or curettage, although the safety and efficacy of both was questioned by the 1930s.[65] Since the causes of

sterility seemed to be as numerous as perceived pathological conditions of the reproductive system, whatever the current treatment for
the condition was should, in theory, have been a potential cure for the
sterility.

New diagnostic tests did allow, in some cases, a better awareness of
the problem and where to concentrate treatment efforts. From early in
the century, but especially from the mid 1920s onward, there was more
emphasis on testing male sperm for quantity and quality. The ability of
the sperm to survive within the generative tract could be determined
from a postcoital examination and was more commonly used from
the early 1930s onward. Becki Crawford recalled that in 1942 she consulted a physician when she could not get pregnant and her physician
arranged for her husband's sperm count to be tested.[66] As some physicians pointed out, however, it was not always easy to get semen to
test either through a condom specimen (which seemed to be the norm)
or through a masturbation specimen in the doctor's office. Many men
found being tested a threat to their virility. In a 1948 article in the *McGill
Medical Journal* Rubin made the problem clear:

> The husband should not be told that he is sterile unless and until several
> examinations of his semen have shown absence of spermatozoa and testi-
> cular biopsy demonstrates absence of spermatogenesis. Much depends on
> the psychiatric judgement of such a male. If the husband is sized up as
> normal otherwise and it is assumed that he can take it, he should be told
> the facts. If despite careful appraisal of his psychic make-up one finds that
> his ego is deeply affected, it is well to modify ones [sic] opinion and allow
> for the possibility of nature with or without treatment, to bring back sper-
> matogenic function.[67]

As noted above, Rubin's test for tubal patency became available in the
1920s. The *Annual Reports* of the Royal Victoria Hospital, Montreal,
reveal that in 1930, 47 operations were performed on fallopian tubes, of
which 23 were Rubin's test. The next year there were 30 operations, 27
being Rubin's test.[68] Noteworthy is that Rubin claimed for his test not
only diagnostic capabilities but also curative ones at 10 percent.[69] Other
than repeating what Rubin himself claimed there seemed to be little
supporting evidence for this in the literature. The idea behind determining fallopian tube blockage was the possibility of its surgical correction/
removal through, among other means, a salpingostomy (forming an
opening or fistula into a uterine tube). However the success rate of such

surgery was low and its consequences in high rates of miscarriage and ectopic pregnancies so worrisome that some warned against it.[70]

Better understanding of the female cycle allowed physicians to give their patients more accurate advice on the most advantageous time to engage in sexual activity. After the mid 1920s physicians had a good sense of the range of days when intercourse would be optimum for conception, though the desire to refine it continued. As the authors of one 1948 article reported, "Knowledge of the exact time of ovulation is of special importance for relatively infertile women since conception is favored by intercourse on the day ova escape. The exact date of ovulation was determined by injecting patient's urine into rats." In the late 1940s daily oral temperature readings were advised to better determine ovular and anovular cycles.[71] While certainly not an invasive technique such as Rubin's test, what the taking of daily temperature readings did was to remind the woman every day of her childlessness even as it gave her hope of conceiving.

Surgery was occasionally mentioned as a possibility for a man's sterility, but most of the emphasis was on the woman. In part connected to the rise of gynaecology as a specialty and particularly the equation of gynaecology with surgery, the surgical solution was a favoured treatment second only to endocrine therapy. The types of surgery, of course, varied and there is no space to go into specific detail. Rather it is more appropriate to evaluate physicians' attitudes towards such intervention. In the September 1900 issue of *The Canada Lancet*, R.E. Cutts of Minneapolis told his readers about a case of one woman who had little apparently wrong with her but could not conceive. She had slight dysmenorrhoea and "a slightly enlarged uterus." She was advised to have a divulsion (separating and pulling apart) and curettage and when that was not successful "at her request exploratory abdominal section" occurred. During that surgery blocked tubes were discovered. Such a description in a medical journal sent out at least two messages. The first was that exploratory surgery was justified even when there was no obvious reasons for it. The second was the finding of a problem when none apparently had existed. The moral of such a case was that exploratory surgery was acceptable for non–ill health reasons and that female sterility was becoming medicalized. Cutts concluded from his experience that "conservative surgery of the ovaries and tubes" could be used to offset sterility. Lapthorn Smith described a case of sterility in a woman who was referred to him. He discovered "a long conical cervix, and the uterus was retroverted, but easily replaced. The cervix was amputated, the uterus curetted and the round ligaments were shortened ... So far she had not become pregnant, although many other Alexander cases [shortening of ligaments] have done so."[72] Of course the other cases probably did not include the removal of the cervix, an organ that was necessary for conception. Interesting as well was Smith's "correction" of the retroversion that many practitioners viewed as problematic for conception.

While some were willing to operate for sterility, F.A. Cleland, in the 1909 *Dominion Medical Monthly and Ontario Medical Journal*, argued surgery was unwarranted unless it was done "on account of the woman's ill-health alone." In that case if sterility was overcome it was all to the better. His concern about operating for sterility was that the procedures were often too dangerous and too extreme to justify as a solution for sterility. Even more to the point, surgery for sterility was not particularly effective. Others, too, continued to warn that abdominal surgery was likely not to be successful and could be harmful.[73]

Perhaps the warning was needed since surgery seemed to be increasing in popularity. In 1924 Dr Polak from the United States remonstrated in the *Canadian Medical Association Journal* that "more unnecessary operations have been done for the relief of backache, than for any one symptom, except that of sterility." Five years later Dr William Graves pointed out that surgery was significant therapy for sterility but too often performed "in a haphazard manner, success being more or less accidental." In 1935 the authors of one text told their readers that when nothing could be found wrong with the husband, the wife should be investigated and warned if an abdominal operation was necessary that no guarantees were possible about its success in overcoming her sterility."[74]

Most surgery was done because of some kind of "abnormal" situation within the reproductive system that physicians believed they could alleviate using traditional gynaecological procedures, for example through suspension of a retroverted uterus. But sterility was a frustrating condition in which many factors could come together and for which there was no aid. In such cases practitioners tried more adventuresome treatment. The oldest of these in the Canadian literature was artificial insemination. It was detailed in the 1870 *Canada Lancet*. Doctors in the early decades of the twentieth century, however, saw problems with it. E.C. Dudley described it as "revolting" and useless. Physicians in the 1920s and 1930s were more optimistic, although their unease had not totally disappeared.[75] In 1921 the Ontario Supreme Court found a case of donor insemination adulterous.[76] Nevertheless, the Rev Alfred Tyrer in the 1943 edition of his book *Sex, Marriage and Birth Control* described its use for sterile couples, using either the husband's sperm when it was suitable or if not that of a donor. His matter-of-fact attitude is fascinating. He claimed that up to 1941 nearly 10,000 such procedures had been successful in the United States. How many, if any, were done in Canada is unknown. Seven years later, in their text Arthur Hale Curtis and John William Huffman suggested to student readers that donor insemination was fraught with "undetermined legal problems, religious restrictions, and delicate personal reactions; [yet] even those of us who have a distaste for donor insemination should accord consideration to the advantage of the theoretically better heredity in a donor conception baby in contrast with an illegitimate or foundling infant."[77] Such a view goes back to the age-old belief of moral traits being hereditary. The desire was not for a baby but for a certain kind of baby. Besides artificial insemination, reports of other treatment methods occurred. Around 1930 ovarian grafting took place, taking ovarian tissue from one woman and surgically attaching it in another. Mention was made of the future when complete ovarian transplants could occur with the complications in law that this would entail.[78] But few references were made to these procedures after that date.

The discovery of hormone therapy made it the new hope in infertility treatment. As early as 1915 there was mention of lutein (a fat-soluble hydrocarbon pigment) therapy in the case of sterility and early miscarriages and later of different extracts including thyroid, pituitary, and ovarian, although there was not always the sense that physicians understood why these seemed to work.[79] Some doctors also questioned how successful and safe such extracts were. In 1930, one Toronto physician referred to the "scientifically unjustifiable prescribing of literally tons of internal gland extracts" while another pointed out in 1937 the "close relationship that exists between the oestrogenic hormones and the carcinogenic factor."[80] Despite such concerns, endocrine therapy continued to be a favoured way of treating not only sterility per se (in both men and women), but also conditions that would result in sterility, for example, amenorrhoea. To give a sense of the degree of development in this field one Montreal expert pointed out that at least 27 oestrogenic hormones were available in 1940 but that only six were standardized and only six had any "appreciable oestrogenic potency."[81] Reporting the successful treatment of male sterility with thyroid and APL (a trademark for a preparation to treat underdevelopment of the gonads), one group of physicians noted the case of a man who had been deemed sterile but whose wife became pregnant, the reaction to which was, "[W]e cannot attach too much importance to this unless we carefully consider the moral habits of the wife."[82] If such an attitude was common, then many marital relationships could have been put in jeopardy through the injudicious pronouncements of physicians. Testosterone was being used, but it was unclear to what effect. Some suggested that it actually decreased sperm count. All one physician could conclude in 1940 was that its value was unlikely and dosage needed to be supervised closely.[83] Diethylstilboestrol, a new synthetic estrogen, caused some excitement, but its danger was not always appreciated. One physician in 1947 pointed out that in hormone therapy "stilboestrol is almost consistently used in over-doses, with the result that toxic effects are commonly experienced."[84]

Doctors who wrote about sterility at times acknowledged that treatment was often experimental and not very successful. Patients needed to be given careful explanations, and indeed permitted to make the decision about the therapy, especially in cases when sterility was the only complaint. These careful voices were few and far between. As one physician in 1935 concluded, "The wombs of childless women have been subjected to so much assault in the guise of treatment."[85]

Infertility treatment changed greatly over time. By the 1950s there was a sense that sterility could be overcome, although doctors also recognized that much more information was needed before a new age of therapy was successful.[86] For women and men who desperately wanted children the situation at mid century was both frustrating and discouraging. Mrs M.H. of British Columbia related her experience to the editor of *Chatelaine* in 1947. Her husband had been tested and found to be fine; but, she wrote:

> With me the story has been different, a succession of doctors, each with a different theory; operations, "adjustments," injections, pills, medicines, electrical treatments, and so on. Each one has told me there is nothing wrong except the one defect each one found and supposedly corrected. I have had more pain and mental fatigue so far than would perhaps accompany a normal birth. But I would like to have some of the most recent discoveries in medicine tried on me – such as tests for excess acidity, X-rays to find abscesses, and even artificial insemination. Surely something can be done for us women who seem to be perfectly healthy and yet produce no offspring.[87]

Mrs M.H.'s letter revealed not only the diversity of treatment she had undergone, but also her awareness of what other procedures were possible.

Conclusion

A survey of attitudes towards and treatment of infertility in Canada between 1900 and 1950 reveals an overwhelming emphasis in the literature on female as opposed to male infertility. Despite the very early recognition of male sterility, the tendency of doctors was to focus on the problems of women, even as physicians increased their estimates of male responsibility for childless marriages. One explanation was the emphasis that Canadian society placed on motherhood, leading doctors and others to focus on women in their search for infertility treatment. The rise of gynaecology also played a part since here was a specialty already in place whose focus was the reproductive system of women. As Emil Novak stated in 1944, "It is of interest to note that the subject of sterility has become almost entirely a gynaecological problem." Urology simply did not play the same role and was not as developed or as focused as gynaecology.[88] Lastly, most doctors during this period were male and themselves recognized the difficulty that men in general had with the concept of male sterility. Throughout the discussions on infertility, little mention was made of the morality of intervention, the societal need for intervention, or the possibility of questioning the underlying assumptions of the right of couples to have children. Doctors worked in a technological world; they were fascinated by the developments in medicine and the possible applications these developments could have.

Although practitioners recognized some social factors involved in sterility such as work-related hazards and diet they spent very little time in agitating for any change. There was no evidence in the literature that the various medical organizations were trying to pressure governments or employers to make work sites less hazardous for workers. It would seem they left preventive work to their public health colleagues. Entranced by medical advances, they did not always consider the side effects of what they were doing or as some of their colleagues pointed out that in some cases their treatment of patients may have caused the sterility they later tried to treat. Doctors, however, were not alone in their belief in the efficacy of medical technology and treatment to overcome almost any health problem. Patients, too, believed in a technological fix. Although there is little sense of men and women coming to physicians for infertility in the early years of the century, by the interwar period this seemed to have changed, although at this point we only have the opinions of doctors to base this on. The voices of women and men, the childless couples, are not often heard in the medical literature. They were not being heard in the popular lay literature either. This is not surprising considering the position of medicine in our society. As Barbara Ehrenreich has astutely observed, medicine "stands between biology and social policy, between the 'mysterious' world of the laboratory and everyday life. It makes public interpretations of biological theory; it dispenses the medical fruits of scientific advances."[89] What is also lacking in the medical literature is any sense of the success rate of the various treatments partially because of the complexity of factors involved in infertility and the myriad of treatments for each available but it does raise the question of how informed were the choices that couples were making during this period. To what extent were they given adequate and accurate information about the causes of infertility, the efficacy of the various treatments available, and the potential side effects of treatment?

7 Controlling Fertility: Birth Control and Abortion

Not all women were interested in becoming mothers in the way that the ideology of motherhood suggested. Some wanted control over the number of children they had and when they had them. Others, a minority, made the decision not to have children at all, perhaps for health or personal reasons. For all such women there were few options. The Criminal Code, section 179 (c) of 1892, was unequivocal. It was an indictable offence "to offer to sell, advertise, publish an advertisement of or have for sale or disposal any medicine, drug or article intended or represented as a means of preventing conception or causing abortion."[1] While various amendments occurred over time, the thrust of the legislation did not. Birth control and abortion remained criminal offences in Canada for the half century under review.

In the latter decades of the twentieth century, scholars engaged in a historical investigation and debate of birth control and abortion.[2] Michel Foucault argued that contraceptives were "disciplinary technologies" that could both socialize and discipline our reproductive behaviour. Others viewed that interpretation as only part of the story, offset by contraceptives' ability to offer resistance to and liberation from the controls of race, gender, and class. The early feminist literature deemed birth control and abortion women's issues and was critical of any attempt to limit women's access to them, focusing on the medical profession as a major obstacle.[3] More recent literature has acknowledged that birth control and abortion "rights" for some women (such as Black or First Nation women) were and are very much an attack on their fecundity and the future of their peoples.

This chapter begins with an examination of fertility control within the context of the law, the decline and rise of birth rates, and the social attitudes of Canadians towards both. The public hostility in the early years of the century towards birth control was significant; with the inter-war period, however, advocates were increasingly engaged in a public discourse. No such discourse occurred about abortion. For the full half century, Canadians were hostile to abortion and seldom engaged in any kind of public debate about its value. Despite the various levels of pub-lic hostility to fertility control, Canadians in their private lives resorted to a plethora of methods to control the size of their families and physi-cians learned about many of them through contact with their patients. Medical attitudes about birth control and abortion were similar to those in the wider society in that physicians generally shared the negative social perceptions towards both in the early years and towards abor-tion in the later. While professional issues, including those of medical training, influenced attitudes towards both, they seemed to enter the medical literature more with abortion than with birth control because of the significance in ending a potential life as opposed to preventing a potential life. Abortion also faced practitioners with the medical reper-cussions of botched abortions, which were often more extreme than the results of various birth control attempts. Abortion's threat to women's health raised the dilemma for physicians of how to respond to women who approached them to perform the procedure, responses that were inevitably tied to their view of who aborted and why they did so.

Less fraught in the medical literature was the assessment of the vari-ous fertility control practices, an area in which their medical expertise dominated, albeit oftentimes embedded with social and moral over-tones. While much of the historical literature has emphasized medi-cine's opposition to fertility control, practitioners' hostility to birth control and even abortion was more nuanced than has been suggested. Support for birth control increased over time, a reflection of it having entered public discussion among Canadians. The only medical dis-course on abortion was when a woman's life or health was at risk, but within that discourse latitude existed in how dangers to life and health were interpreted.

The General Context for Fertility Control

Throughout the first half century and until 1969 birth control and abor-tion were illegal in Canada. The law did not mean that physicians could not advise their patients about birth control or even abortion, but they had to take care and ensure that there were sufficient medical reasons for doing so. The application of the law on abortion also encouraged an engagement by physicians with which some were uncomfortable. Abortion law focused on the abortionist, not the woman who was aborted or who self-aborted. In cases where the woman was dying from an abortion her dying declaration was used as evidence for the prosecution against her abortionist. Doctors were often present at or even the instigators of the dying declaration and would testify in court as to what they had heard. From hospital records, it is clear that medical staff asking their patients about the details of attempted abortions was not unusual and, more often than not, the cases investigated involved single or poor women rather than married or private patients.[4] Abortion's illegality, then, prompted physicians to seemingly work against their patients, the women who had aborted, and align themselves with the State.

Despite the law discouraging fertility control, Canada's birth rate began to decline by the latter decades of the nineteenth century and continued to do so until the 1940s when the rate increased. Not all groups in the country experienced the same pattern, however. The Inuit of northern Quebec saw their fertility decline in the 1930s, increase in the early 1940s, but unlike that of other Canadian women it remained stationary between 1946 and 1956. But whatever the pattern, both the decline and increase in fertility has intrigued historians. The decline in particular suggested some form of fertility control.[5] Public discourse on the decline in the birth rate revolved around birth control not abortion. The latter simply was not a topic for public discussion. In the early decades of the century, the discourse was minimal and largely negative. For many commentators, birth control signalled decline in morality and a sign of a woman's selfishness.[6] Such public negativity on the part of many Canadians continued even as the amount of literature on it increased. The Rev Mabel McCoy Irwin through the National Council of Women made her misgivings known. She worried that birth control would lessen men's commitment to fathering, lessen their respect for women, and allow men to be guided by their more sensual nature. For women birth control led to marital prostitution; it would "free" women sexually and therein lay its threat. Gender identity and relationships were very much formed by the potential of a woman who engaged in sexual intercourse to become pregnant. Take that away and the sexual conventions of society could break down. For Catholics, opposition to birth control was reinforced by the 1930 papal encyclical "Casti connubi," which forbade artificial contraception.[7]

Not all the discourse was negative. Availability of information on birth control increased. Canadians became familiar with the work and writings of birth control advocates like Margaret Sanger in the United States, Marie Stopes in Great Britain, and Georgina Sackville in Canada. Widely distributed was Rev Alfred Tyrer's 1936 *Sex, Marriage and Birth Control* and other birth control literature advertised through Eaton's catalogues.[8] Attitudes were changing. By the 1920s when the high maternal mortality rates became a focus of anxiety, some women used the argument that spacing of births would help preserve their health.[9] The Depression years emphasized the financial burden to many of having large families. As for the morality of birth control, some argued that birth control would lessen the need of many women to resort to abortion. Supporters also reassured Canadians that birth control was not a rejection of the maternal role but an embrace of it.[10] As a result, a birth control movement emerged with clinics that provided contraceptives.[11] In 1936 Dorothea Palmer, employed as a nurse by the Parents' Information Bureau, was arrested for disseminating birth control and after a lengthy trial, acquitted under the "public good" clause of the Criminal Act on birth control.[12] By the 1940s, birth control did not seem to engage public discussion as it once had. The country was at war in the early years of the decade and this captured the attention of public and the press. As well, the lines of the debate had been drawn. For those who felt birth control should be rejected on moral and religious grounds the maintenance of the law was encouraging. For those who felt birth control should be available to those in need, the expansion of birth control clinics, the not-guilty decision in the Palmer trial, and the increased availability of literature on birth control were comforting.

No comparable discussion of abortion existed in the public literature of the time. The Rev James Simpson was typical of opponents in the early part of the century in seeing abortion as "absolute murder."[13] Abortion opponents did not distinguish between foetus and child; they were one and the same. As with birth control, abortion was also caught up in the issue of sexuality and the fear of many that it allowed a couple to "sin" without punishment or consequences. Unlike birth control, however, public opposition to abortion remained strong throughout the interwar years and beyond. Neither did many birth control advocates disagree. Georgina Sackville in her birth control tract could see abortion only as murder. There was little or no discussion of the rights of the mother perhaps because the general feeling was that unwed women had to pay the price of their sexual immorality and married women did not need to worry about abortion or if they did want to limit the size of their families they and their husbands should practice sexual abstinence. Underlying the moral opposition was a class and ethnic component, abortion seen as the last resort of the less respectable.[14]

Methods of Fertility Control

Both the decline and increase of the birth rate reflected the ability of Canadians to control their fertility. In the early years of the twentieth century, many Canadians sought out information on birth control wherever they could – from friends, neighbours, family members, physicians, and the popular press. This was true even in a so-called traditional society such as Quebec, which historically had not been associated with significant use of birth control. Among the methods used in Quebec were marriage delay, sexual self-control, a form of rhythm method, condoms, and coitus interruptus (withdrawal). These and other methods were used throughout Canada. One Alberta woman recalled that it was her husband who decided that she would never go through another pregnancy because of the danger to her health. Unfortunately his understanding of physiology was rather lacking in that he assured his wife, "If you don't enjoy at that time, if you don't want it, then you won't get pregnant." While this may suggest some concern on his part and willingness to engage in the discussion, the solution devised was not particularly efficacious or considerate of his wife's sexual needs.[15] Other methods demanded more specific involvement on the part of the woman: prolonged breastfeeding; homemade pessaries of cocoa butter, boric acid, and tannic acid; botanical concoctions used by and learned from Native women made of "squaw" vine as well as cedar, cherry, or yarrow. The 1901 Eaton's catalogue advertised the "Every Woman Marvel Whiling Spray," a vaginal douche that some women used as a birth control device.[16] Certainly physicians were aware of the various methods being used. In their private and hospital practices, practitioners came to know of women's use of the vaginal douche, a sponge or cotton wool within the vagina to absorb the semen, and "womb caps," as well as pomade pots, candle-extinguishers, and small india-rubber balls in the vagina used as sperm barriers.[17] The variety of birth control methods had different appeals. Some were based on common sense, others on methods that seemed to have worked in the past, and still others on the most up-to-date understanding of the female monthly cycle – unfortunately more often than not, incorrect. None were technologically sophisticated and their use revealed the determination of many women to control the number of children they gave birth to and when. Each demanded something of the user or users: strong control over natural desires, keeping track of bodily processes, or a co-operative relationship between sexual partners. Many demanded forethought.

All these methods continued to be used in subsequent decades in one form or another. Condoms, long available, were cheaper to buy. Individual physicians were giving more accurate advice on the rhythm method. Cervical stems, intrauterine rings, and pessaries were accessible.[18] A study of the birth control clinic in Toronto during 1933–4 indicated that even before coming to the clinic women had used a wide variety of birth control methods, among them coitus interruptus, douching, condoms, suppositories, the vaginal pessary, and cervical pessary. Diaphragms, jellies, and condoms became the prime means of contraception advocated by various birth control clinics. Sterilizations also became seen as a permanent form of birth control during the '30s because of their eugenic connection. Eaton's catalogues continued to advertise items that women adapted as birth control devices and Ortho-Gynol jelly was also advertised.[19] Gérard Bouchard has traced the increased use of birth control by men in the Saguenay region of Quebec. In addition, more physicians were giving advice on the rhythm method and more hysterectomies being performed with priests remaining sceptical of the reasons for them but nevertheless agreeing to them. Other measures tried were abstinence, prolonged nursing, coitus interruptus, and urination after sex. Access to birth control across Canada, however, was still class based. Middle-class women seemed to be aware of condoms and vaginal suppositories, both of which were available in drug stores, but if working-class women were aware of them, they often were too expensive.[20]

Abortion methods were equally varied and accessible. By the turn of the century, medical books provided enough information on various methods for the enterprising abortionist or woman in distress to find useful. Advertisements in the popular press of patent medicines for "delayed" menstruation were blatant and visible for all to see and had been even before the turn of the century. Instruments such as covered knitting needles, known to many women as potential abortion "tools," were readily available. Neither were abortionists difficult to find, at least in cities. The medical literature listed other methods that women or their abortionists used: violence or severe exertion; taking emetics (agents causing vomiting); cathartics (agents causing bowel evacuation); ergot; emmenagogues (agents stimulating menstruation); concoctions made from plants; fasting; taking mustard baths; or drinking copious quantities of gin.[21] Some methods were more popular than others and some remained popular longer. Heavy exertion remained a tactic that was in the control of the woman and did not necessitate any help from others. The emmenagogues had appeal, perhaps because they appeared effective and their use allowed women to construct their situation as amenorrhoea rather than pregnancy. Drugs were not regulated to the degree they are today so access was easy. One physician writing in the 1922 *Canadian Medical Association Journal* worried about that accessibility and suggested that specific items be available only through prescription.[22] Given that many of the abortion drugs were available for legitimate purposes, controlling their use was difficult.

Much of the information physicians had about attempted means of abortion came from their women patients. Worrying about the apparent increase in abortions, W.A. Dafoe, a fellow in obstetrics and gynaecology at the University of Toronto, noted that women patients at the Toronto General Hospital were asked about the various abortifacients they had tried. The list was considerable: "quinine, castor oil, ergot, ... salts, lead pills, and the patent preparations such as pennyroyal and Beecham's pills," as well as "many others."[23] While physicians often learned from their patients what the latest abortion method was, not all women could remember what they had taken or were willing to say. Mrs Ruggoso took "all manner of drugs"; Eleanor Whelan, "some medicine"; and others resorted to "pills."[24] The means of abortion were sometimes cultural in their specificity. Finnish women apparently used hot saunas, alternating with submersion in cold water. One Alberta woman recalled that Metis women knew more about family limitation than she did: "They used a black bag from the bladder of a bear. They dry it, then mix it with some liquid, and then they'd lose the baby." Cree women used sweet flag. The women of Cape Smythe in the Arctic kneaded the abdomen of the women to dislodge the foetus.[25] In some First Nations communities in which the Catholic Church dominated, the traditional use of abortion declined. In others, there is evidence that native women shared their knowledge with missionary and medical staff.[26]

Two of the most favoured means throughout the half-century were the insertion of foreign bodies into the vagina and uterus and douching. The foreign bodies introduced were many: tents, catheters, knitting needles, sticks, scissors, crochet hooks, douche nozzles, stove-pipe wire, hair pins, slippery elm bark, coat hangers, pencils, and uterine sounds. Such items may not have been designed for abortion, but the appeal of all these devices was that they could be used by the woman herself and were available in most homes. One Canadian researcher in 1930 reported that of 71 self-induced abortions studied, 47 had been brought about by the insertion of foreign objects into the vagina.[27] Douching, which was often used by women for hygienic purposes, in the hands of desperate individuals became the means for abortion. And women were eclectic in what they used to douche. W.A. Dafoe noted the use of lysol, potassium manganate, vinegar, mustard, carbolic acid and mercury bicholoride, and sodium thiosulphate.[28] Whatever the means a woman first used to abort, if it failed to bring about the desired outcome she often resorted to others, an understandable response once the decision to abort had been made. If nothing else, the combination of methods points to determination and desperation. Miss Cynthia Moore, 25 years old, entered the Montreal General Hospital on 6 August 1935. Her case file noted:

> When the patient missed her period in June she went to a doctor who gave her pills to start them but they didn't work. She knew that she was pregnant however even though there were no other signs. At the end of June she noticed morning sickness. In the middle of July she took Quinine tablets but they didn't work. On Friday she got desperate & took a piece of wire – pointed on one end & about the thickness of a large knitting needle. It had been around the kitchen & was used to clean a gas stove. She washed it off & introduced it into the vagina & thence up to the womb ... going about 2 inches into the uterus.

Four days later, bleeding and suffering from pain, she entered the Western Hospital and from there transferred to the Montreal General Hospital where she aborted her foetus.[29]

Medical Attitudes towards Birth Control

When physicians attempted to explain Canadians' desire to control their fertility, their discussion revolved around birth control. The editor of the *Canadian Journal of Medicine and Surgery* in 1905 raised the economic plight of many modern couples (most likely middle class) who did not feel that they could cope with a large family and the demands that went with it. While acknowledging financial reasons, others simply blamed middle-class women for shirking their duty. An editorialist in the 1903 *Montreal Medical Journal* argued that women had been tainted by Eve and as Eve had been tempted by the fruit of knowledge so, too, were modern women being tempted by "false ambition."[30] In *The Public Health Journal* Sir Thomas Oliver, professor of medicine at the University of Durham, acknowledged that there were physical dangers associated with birthing but, in the next breath, he argued that for affluent women the physical dangers were really quite minimal. They had no excuse not to procreate. Such a view negated the real dangers of childbirth for all women and also ironically contradicted a theme within the childbirth literature that it was the more protected, the more civilized woman who was having more difficulty in giving birth.[31] Seldom were supportive voices raised. One somewhat sympathetic voice was that of Frederick Fenton, associate in obstetrics at the University of Toronto, who suggested that women were avoiding childbirth because they feared its pain. If physicians could reassure women and offer them "even a moderate degree of relief" then the decline in the birth rate might be offset.[32]

Hostile attitudes continued to be found throughout the medical literature. An editorial in the 1922 *National Hygiene and Public Welfare* dismissed the notion that birth control preserved women's health and argued that there was evidence that women who bore children were healthier than those who did not. Such a view harkened back to nineteenth-century arguments that whatever was natural was healthy and that bearing children was natural. The editorial concluded the reasons behind some women requesting birth control were "indolence and love of social pleasures."[33] The May 1931 issue of *The Nova Scotia Medical Bulletin* referred to a policy of that journal (since at least 1926) not to publish articles advocating birth control because the editors of the journal felt that it would lead to sexual immorality. Shortly after (in July 1931), the journal published an article condemning artificial birth control. The anonymous author asserted that there was no difference between taking life and preventing life, that once you allowed the prevention of life by mechanical means, ending it by such means would follow. Life would no longer be held sacred. Another took to task those who said the medical profession supported birth control, a stance the author did not believe given "the splendid attributes of the average and normal man in our profession."[34]

Dr Lacoste, medical officer of health for Tecumseh, Ontario, opposed birth control in general and saw sterilization as an indirect form. Such opposition did not mean he was without eugenic concerns but he felt that those who were increasing in numbers would find their numbers limited through "providence" in the form of earthquakes and wars. As proof, he pointed to the high murder rate in Detroit to allay the fears of his colleagues, the assumption being that the unfit would kill each other. The racist subtext of this would be identifiable to many since Detroit was noted for having a significant black population. What Lacoste thought society should do rather than focus on birth control was to rid itself of activities that led to "mental and moral perversion," namely the yellow press and moving pictures. Other practitioners were more "optimistic" about what birth control could do to stem the tide of racial suicide. Yes, the "better" classes used birth control, but if birth control could be expanded so that the lower classes, too, resorted to it, then at least balance between the groups could be maintained.[35]

For Catholic physicians, birth control was never going to be acceptable. They would find themselves in the position of those testifying in the Palmer trial such as Dr Joseph De Haitre, a Montreal obstetrician. He argued that the birth control devices used by the Parents' Information Bureau were unsafe. Under cross-examination, however, he had to admit he was not familiar with many of the methods advocated and that his opposition was based in his religious beliefs. Dr Ernest Couture argued that humans should not control the organs of their own bodies and any attempt to change them would result in dysfunction of the system.[36] For a physician to take such a stance was strange given the kind of medical intervention occurring every day. Physicians removed parts of various bodily organs or the organ altogether with little debate. They provided all sorts of medicinal aids to control the functioning of bodily systems. Clearly it was not the control of organs that was the issue, but the specific organ being controlled and who controlled it. Other physicians opposed birth control simply because their patient roster was largely Catholic or they were connected with Catholic institutions.[37]

Personal or religious morality may have directed attitudes but so did fear – the fear of race suicide. The discussion about racial suicide and its connection to birth control, however, was limited in the early years of the century, not because of unconcern about the former, but the distaste of discussing the latter. Nevertheless, having children was a public issue of national importance. The irony was, of course, that the burden was a personal one since the state did not provide much help to parents raising their children. Never queried was whether couples forced to have children through the nonuse of birth control would make good parents. Instead the worry was that the wrong "type" of people were reproducing, a concern that stemmed from the declining birth rate of the middle classes. For Dr Wickett those not using birth control included the "the outcast, the feeble minded and the criminal." Wickett also worried about English-Canadians being outnumbered by French-Canadians, clearly for her an outcome to be dreaded. What we might view as a private choice, then, had public consequences. And an editorial in the 1903 *Montreal Medical Journal* knew whom to blame – woman.[38]

As the eugenic movement increased in strength after World War I many physicians adopted its views. An editorial in the 1923 *Canadian Medical Association Journal* asserted that birth control was being used by those who could afford to have children and not being used by those who could not. The latter were seen as unfortunate, not simply because such parents could not afford to give their children the necessities of life, but also because of a belief that poverty was linked to some sort of moral inadequacy.[39] Dr George Chisholm, a psychiatrist and psychologist from the University of Toronto, testified at the Palmer trial that a crisis of biological proportions faced Canadians as a consequence of those with low intelligence giving birth to many children who in turn had low intelligence.[40] The Darwinian faith in survival of the fittest did not seem to apply here. Indeed the fear was that the fit would not survive because they practised birth control. A reverse racial suicide was needed, that is, birth control to limit the birth of the unfit. Concern obviously existed that the more affluent (assumed to be more intelligent and hardworking as evidenced by their affluence) were limiting the size of their families and that the poor would eventually overrun society. This concern, however, could sometimes work to favour the large families of the poor even though the argument was not intended to. For example, in *The Hospital, Medical and Nursing World* of 1926 an editorial expressed the view that popular wisdom assumed that the first child would be the best and the brightest since "the conservation of the desirable germ plasm is more certainly achieved in the first conception." Yet the editorial went on to suggest that there was evidence to prove that the last born not only measured up to the first offspring but "quite frequently" evidenced higher "moral and intellectual faculties." For the author, this meant that the better families should continue to have children. But surely the argument could be used to say that those families with large numbers of children, even if poor, were improving the stock if their later children were an improvement on their earlier ones.[41] Such an argument, however, would not have been posited by those concerned about the eugenic consequences of the declining birth rate. The belief in heredity would limit the ability of children born to the "lower" classes from going beyond a certain level and also the coterminous belief in environment would reinforce that ceiling. The irony is that an examination of the birth rates suggest that the decline was across class. Even assuming that historians are correct and that control of birth began first among the more affluent classes, by the 1920s the decline was such that it could only have occurred if the vast majority of couples were practising some form of fertility control. In his 1936 book *The Art of Treatment*, William R. Houston explained that the appeal of birth control was its modernness. Nonetheless he warned this modernity hid real dangers. Traditionally communities could protect themselves against "sex perversions," not consciously but through "the unconscious racial instinct against whatever menaces the transmission of the sacred flame of life."[42] Against modern science in the form of birth control, this unconscious instinct had little strength. Underlying such fears was a status anxiety of those with status in the society being overwhelmed by their "inferiors." Unless something changed, the nation, a race, or a species could be at risk. By the 1940s the eugenic argument lessened in intensity but it never disappeared. An article published in the 1940 *Canadian Doctor* asked whether a high fertility rate necessarily resulted in "good Canadians." In this case, the author used the example Quebec to reveal the dangers of a high birth rate – high infant mortality rates and high rates of TB. For this physician, these health risks were far more "deplorable" than the "hidden horrors" of a low birth rate.[43]

The medical discussion of birth control and its connection to eugenics was an important one in that it constituted an underlying context for general reactions to the issue of birth control. It reflected broader interests and concerns on the part of many physicians and revealed the way in which gender, race, class, and moral issues could become intertwined. But not only were they intertwined, they influenced attitudes on issues that were medical. We cannot expect physicians to leave their gender, racial, class, and moral views outside the medical office. Indeed, what emerges from the brief look at eugenic interest in and concerns about birth control is how often physicians framed their arguments about race, gender, class, and morality in ways that refer to health – their accepted and recognized area of expertise. Their arguments might not always refer to the health of the patient, but rather to the health of a class, a racial grouping, the state or even the species. If you will, such physicians had not only medicalized birth control but also the well-being of social and political groupings.

Faced with women who needed and wanted birth control, physician discourse on birth control became more positive. Over time, there developed a sense of fait accompli about birth control. In the mid 1920s, Dr Roberts, medical officer of health, Hamilton, Ontario, reported that birth control was becoming a fact of life, a situation about which he was unafraid. E.W. Montgomery, the minister of health and public welfare for Manitoba in 1929 and himself a physician, acknowledged that the "delicate subject of birth-control" might need to be considered to protect the health of women.[44] Physicians were concerned about prevention and, for some, birth control used for preventative purposes was unproblematic. Support also came from those who denied "ill-results to health" as a result of birth control.[45] While one historian of birth control has argued that those physicians supporting birth control did so on medical grounds, it is clear that medical supporters often resorted to a myriad of reasons, not just medical ones. Dr Herbert Bruce recalled the Palmer trial and the "powerful" arguments that the defence and its witnesses put forward, a mixture of medical, social, and economic reasons arguments that Bruce clearly supported.[46] By the 1940s advertisers were promoting their products through the medical press. The ease of use, the low cost, and effectiveness were all appeals that advertisers used to convince physicians to adopt their particular brand of contraceptive. Dr Mackay remembered that when she was practising in Sydney, Nova Scotia, she was measuring her women patients for the diaphragm and when other women heard about it they came to her. Percy Ryberg in his manual on birth control took pragmatism further. He was quite willing to point out, for example, that a "girl" who was going to engage in extramarital endeavours needed to protect herself and he proceeded to explain how. He did not endorse the sexual activity but he recognized that it did occur. His view of birth control within marriage reflected his and others' belief that a marriage was about the spousal relationship rather than solely on the begetting of children.[47]

Given the change in some medical attitudes, it stood to reason that medical students should learn about the safest and most effective means of preventing conception. Nevertheless for most of the period under review (if not all of it), medical training in birth control was largely nonexistent. In the 1930s, the University of Toronto's medical school became the first to offer contraceptive instruction to its students.

Elsewhere training in birth control was hit and miss. Even in the 1940s training of physicians in birth control remained minimal. Dr Richards remembered her years as a student when one lecturer was discussing the conditions that would be contra-indicative to pregnancy. The lecturer made it clear that "[u]nder these conditions tell her not to get pregnant – and tell her *how not* to get pregnant." As Richards describes it, this left her wondering "what I was expected to tell her." Certainly, she remembered no contraceptive information being taught to students.[48] Such experiences reflected the reluctance of organized medicine to openly challenge the law on birth control even for medical reasons.

The change in attitude and the support many practitioners gave to birth control reflected the changing mores of the society and in particular that of their patients. While this shift is not surprising it needs to be acknowledged because it was done within a context in which birth control remained illegal. William Scott and H. Brookfield Van Wyck pointed out that as far as the legality was concerned, physicians did not have to worry too much. The law allowed birth control for medical reasons and social and economic reasons for contraception could easily be converted to medical ones by physicians. They still needed to be careful, however, in recommending birth control, especially with respect to the moral and religious scruples of their patients.[49]

Medical Attitudes about Abortion

While the medical discussion of abortion shared a more intense version of the early hostility directed at birth control, there was little lessening of that hostility with time. In addition certain aspects of the birth control debate were replayed in the abortion discourse. Religion played a role in restraining a physician's options just as it did for birth control.[50] For all physicians, personal morality was a factor, as many shared the wider societal abhorrence for abortion. Given such attitudes, the perceived frequency of abortion appalled physicians.

Physicians in the early years of the century considered abortion "prevalent"[51] in society, and such views only intensified. Hamilton's O.A. Cannon speculated in a 1922 article that the greatest cause of early miscarriage was criminal abortion. Such perceptions would have had a powerful resonance with Canadians who had just seen the tremendous loss of life occurring as a result of the Great War. Loss of life – the child and potentially the mother's – from abortion seemed a waste and unacceptable. Increased estimates of criminal abortion emerged in the 1930s as economic conditions placed pressure on unmarried and married women alike. One study of abortion deaths (self-induced with septic conditions) estimated a rate of 11 per 100,000 live births in 1933 increasing to 15 in 1937.[52] As well, the statistics suggested higher rates in cities where access to temptations and abortionists seemed more prevalent than in rural areas.[53] While physicians in the 1940s remained concerned about what they perceived as the increase in self-induced abortions, there seemed to be less engagement with the issue than had been true in previous decades. The authors of one mid century American text noted, for example, that abortionists were becoming more proficient with the result that fewer cases of "infected instrumental abortion" were seen despite "increased sexual promiscuity resultant from a changing moral code and altered social and economic conditions."[54]

The area in which the medical discourse of abortion differed significantly from birth control was the role professionalism played: the difference between an abortion performed by a reputable physician and that by a criminal abortionist; the mentoring of colleagues; the conflation of morality and professionalism; the profession's alignment with the state; and abortion's connection to the maternal mortality rates. Unlike birth control, abortion was a medical procedure and considered part of a practitioner's knowledge requirement because of its potential therapeutic nature (see section on Medical Behaviour). For physicians, criminal abortion led to death because the abortionist could not or would not take the care that physicians were allowed to take for therapeutic abortions.

Professional mentoring in the early decades specifically included warning younger practitioners not to discuss the issue of abortion with their patients.[55] Saving life, not taking it, was the raison d'être of medical practice. In addition, physicians had long tried to separate themselves in the public mind from other practitioners – nurses, midwives, irregular doctors, etc. One way of doing so was to tar these "others" with performing illegal/immoral abortions. "Real" physicians did not do this and when such cases did come before the public, they brought dishonour to the profession. While the profession as a whole distanced itself from them, some practitioners tried to understand the motivation behind their colleagues' actions, concluding that money was central. But the consequences were not worth the financial gains. Abortion "lowered" a physician in his own eyes and abortion's clientele was "not a desirable one." Physicians needed to be the gatekeepers of moral-ity.[56] They also needed to protect themselves. An editorial in *The Canada Lancet* warned physicians that the single working girl who found her-self pregnant was particularly problematic. Such women "have no home, as a rule, and live in rooms or in boarding-houses. If anything goes wrong they have no means of securing proper care; and things are very liable to take an adverse course." If such women self-aborted and then needed medical attention afterwards, doctors warned one another not to treat them in these boarding homes. Rather "they should be placed at once under conditions where they cannot implicate their medical attendants."[57]

Similar concerns continued. Taking the moral stance protected the reputation of the physician and maintained his prestige among his col-leagues who were always watching what he was doing. The issue was so important that the 1934 examination in medical jurisprudence at Queen's University had the following question: "How would you safe-guard your reputation if called to a woman whom you found having a miscarriage?" The vulnerability of physicians is seldom acknowledged by historians. The usual scenario is of a powerful medical practitioner and the much less powerful patient. It is important to note that, at times, physicians did not see the situation in the same light. The moral stance taken was also a professional one and it aligned practitioners with the interests of the state. In 1944 at McGill University the following exam question was posed to medical students: "You have been called to see a young woman unknown to you and find that she is unmarried and is suffering from the effects of a criminal abortion. Discuss the more common situations in such cases and outline briefly, the proper action in each case with respect to (a) your duty as a physician, and (b) your duty to the state." Not all physicians were willing to accept the align-ment with the state over the needs of the patient. One doctor who had treated a young woman dying from a criminal abortion testified at the inquest into her death. He had refused to call the police so they could interview her and as reported in the *Saturday Night*, he "considered his a personal duty to the patient ... In other words any facts disclosed by the patient to the physician must of necessity be deemed secret." Velma Messinger remembered that when she had her first child, her physician asked her if she had ever miscarried. She admitted that she had had an abortion performed by a physician. Her new physician's response was to say that he would not put that on her chart and her husband need not know. This was a physician who worked for a Catholic hospital and who obviously aligned himself with Velma and what he saw as her need for privacy.[58]

Linked to professional status was the medical perception that criminal abortion deaths inflated the maternal death rate. A Manitoba study for the years 1928 to 1932 estimated that abortions accounted for 17.1 percent of puerperal deaths and that almost half of those abortion-related deaths were due to criminal abortion.[59] Some physicians argued that including such deaths in maternal mortality rates was unfair since if these pregnancies had not been interfered with they might well not have resulted in death. Physicians were having difficulty accepting that maternal mortality rates were high in Canada compared to other Western nations and saw abortion deaths, especially criminal abortion ones, as a way to explain them that did not cast aspersions on themselves and the quality of care given to women. The medical concern about abortion deaths artificially inflating the maternal mortality rate remained a major issue for physicians.[60]

Why Women Abort

The frequency of abortion forced physicians to come to terms with why women resorted to criminal abortion. At times, they displayed a real sympathy for the plight in which some women found themselves, at others they were quite dismissive and judgmental. It depended on which women they were discussing and the time in which they were writing. In the early decades of the century the stereotype of the woman who aborted was of a single woman of "easy" virtue who made the decision to abort easily. Such were the designing women about whom young physicians were warned. The repugnance felt by some was typified by D.W. Cathell in his turn-of-the-century text. In his estimate not worthy of sympathy were "unmarried negresses, ladies of easy virtue, and other low females (and sometimes even the wealthy, young and beautiful: in silk, satin, velvet and gold), who fear they are pregnant."[61] His association of black women with easy virtue was reflected in the wider American society for whom he was writing. More often than not such racial specificity occurred in medical textbooks, rather than the articles that appeared in Canadian medical journals. Other physicians, while rejecting the decision to abort, did attempt to distinguish between groups of women and their reasons. About the only woman for whom some physicians had sympathy was the young single woman, otherwise respectable, who had been seduced by a lover. Not only the woman's life would be altered by the birth of an illegitimate child but the lives of her family members as well.[62] The distinction between the "innocent" single woman and the designing single woman did not survive the second decade of the century in the published medical literature. The morality of abortion as an act was the focus, not so much the morality of the woman. She became disconnected from context. When differentiation between single women was made, class was the underlying factor.[63] Those who were poor and members of minority groups did not always have access to safe abortions because they lacked both · funds and a position of negotiation with those who could provide them, with a safe abortion. Middle-class single women had more access to personal physicians and to money to ensure a safer abortion than did their working-class sisters. Neither would they have come to the attention of hospital authorities or not as much. In addition, the image of a middle-class girl being seduced could still evoke sympathy.[64]

Although the working-class single woman was at more risk than her middle-class sister, she was not always without agency. Martha McNamara, a single 22-year-old waitress from Newfoundland, entered the Victoria General Hospital, Halifax, on 9 January 1931. In September of 1930 she had missed her period and so in early October she took some pills to encourage menstruation. She began to bleed in mid October and assumed that this was her regular period since the timing was right. She stopped bleeding and then began again 2 days later. On Monday January 5 she obtained more pills from her physician and took a large dose (7–8) for the next three days. She began to bleed again and entered the hospital whose record notes, "Patient admits having had opportunity to become pregnant." Part of a foetus was found in the vagina and removed.[65] Several themes emerge from this record. The fact that Martha was young and single and from outside the province suggests a person away from family and friends with few people to whom she could turn for help. Her narrative of what was wrong with her, namely irregular menstruation, indicates the ability of individuals to reshape what was happening to them. Of course, this may have been a story she concocted for her physician in order to get abortifacients, fearing that if he suspected she was pregnant little help would be forthcoming. The fact that her physician gave her the pills without testing her for pregnancy, however, is suggestive of complicity. The narrative suggests some agency on her part – she went to a physician for a problem that she had diagnosed, she presented him with the diagnosis, and she expected help. When she first took the pills she was very early in her pregnancy. When she returned to her physician for more pills, however, she was approximately four and one half months pregnant and there could have been little doubt about her condition; still there was no suggestion that the physician was suspicious. Perhaps he did not have to be; he knew very well what the pills were for. In either case, it reveals a physician willing to accept a lay diagnosis; he gave power to the patient or connived with her in the fiction of missed periods and gave her something to bring about an abortion. What this record also indicated is that Martha McNamara was able to exert some agency in fashioning her medical history. We know about McNamara's agency only because her attempt failed and she ended in an institution that was obligated to keep records. Women who aborted successfully did not leave documentation to the same extent. Thus our sense of who aborts and why and the situation of their lives comes from the "failures," those women who cannot afford the "better" abortionists, who cannot pressure their own physicians into helping them and who as a result of desperation resorted to any means and anyone to help them and who paid the price often in terms of ill health or death. These were women who could not ensure privacy in their lives.

While the unmarried woman was the stereotype of the woman seeking an abortion, physicians did not deny that married women sought out the procedure. In the early years of the century physicians warned one another to watch for the married women, those "cases where there is no previous guilt," that is, where extramarital sex had not occurred. What is intriguing is that although physicians could allude to women who had been unfaithful, they seldom focused their rhetoric on them, as if the idea of a married woman succumbing to infidelity was more than they could acknowledge. Instead, they focused on the married women who wanted to abort a legitimate child. Such women, they felt, were the majority of married women who aborted and the women about whom they were most concerned – aborting a legitimate child was a challenge to. the stability of the family[66] and none of the reasons put forward by women were acceptable: already having the number of children they wanted or could afford to support; being a newlywed; fear that their health could not stand another pregnancy or birth; their youngest child was still nursing; or being early in the pregnancy.[67]

The awareness of married women seeking abortions intensified after the first two decades of the century. The *Canadian Medical Association Journal* for December 1933 described a Hamilton woman who seven and a half months pregnant came to the Hamilton General Hospital on

20 December 1932; it was her ninth pregnancy. Five of her pregnancies had resulted in the birth of healthy babies, the eldest now being fifteen and the youngest two. A sixth baby had died at birth and two pregnancies had ended through self-induced abortions. Such a woman could not be accused of avoiding her womanly responsibilities. Dr Richards vividly remembered the horror of her first autopsy in 1942 when she was in medical school, of a woman who had died of septic abortion:

> She was the mother of seven children, in her early fifties. Thinking she was pregnant and unable to face another pregnancy she had gone to an abortionist who had used a device called "slippery elm" perforating the uterus and setting up purulent peritonitis (pre-antibiotic days). To compound the tragedy she was not pregnant.

Women interviewed confirmed this woman's sentiment. Several were married and had aborted because they had already given birth to the number of children they or their husbands wanted.[68]

One of the reasons hinted at for women's reluctance to continue to bear children early in the century was economic, but as the century progressed more weight was given to this consideration. While physicians and others in the health field recognized the economic argument, particularly in the 1930s when the Depression gave the argument more urgency, most physicians had little to offer women in dire economic straits.[69] Nevertheless, there was a sense by some that underlying women's economic concerns was a deeper pragmatism that overcame any moral scruples. H.S. Wasman in the 1947 *University of Toronto Medical Journal* addressed that pragmatism in words that conjure up Carol Gilligan's gender separation between men and women. Wasman wrote:

> Anthropological research has shown that most primitives had no compunction in terminating pregnancy by abortion just as there was little feeling against infanticide. Of course, primitives we will always have with us. Then, too, we must remember that many women in some matters at least, are realists, less concerned with principles than with results, hence, little impressed by the illegality of something they may desire. One must admit that today a considerable percentage of women do not hesitate to employ abortifacients or if they do hesitate, manage to overcome any doubt or vacillation with such success that abortion today is "big business." Again, abortion per se, appears to cause no mental trauma of importance – of course that is debatable.[70]

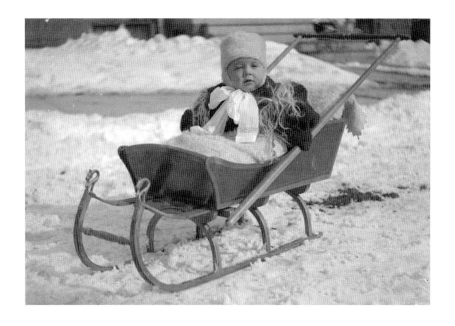

Child on a pull sleigh, ca. 191?; For the period 1900 to 1950, women's role was to have children. It was central to practitioners' understanding and assessment of women's physiology, psychology, and intellectual abilities. A.W. Barton fonds, C 121-1-0-8-6, 10019333.jpg, Archives of Ontario.

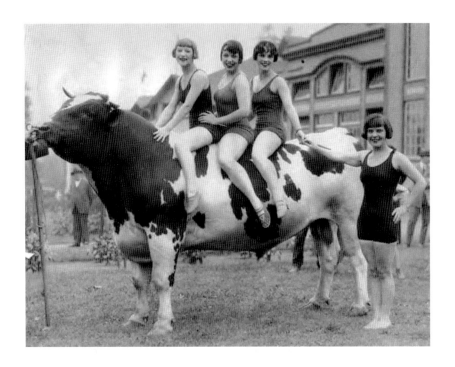

These young women represented much of what many physicians and other Canadians feared about modernity. Their bobbed hair, their swimsuits showing unclothed arms and legs in a public setting, not to mention being astride a bull challenged traditional decorum, restraint, and modesty. City of Vancouver Archives, CVA 180-296, 1927. Pacific National Exhibition, Dominion Photo.

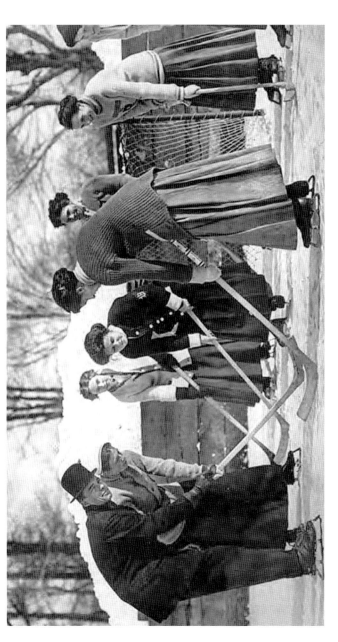

Varsity Ladies Hockey, ca. 1910. Physicians supported physical activity for women as a health issue. What they had difficulty condoning was the competitiveness of sport. The degree of competitiveness in the 1910 photograph was significantly curtailed by the clothes worn. B1990-004/001(11), Digital Image No. 2001-77-48MS, University of Toronto Archives and Records Management Services.

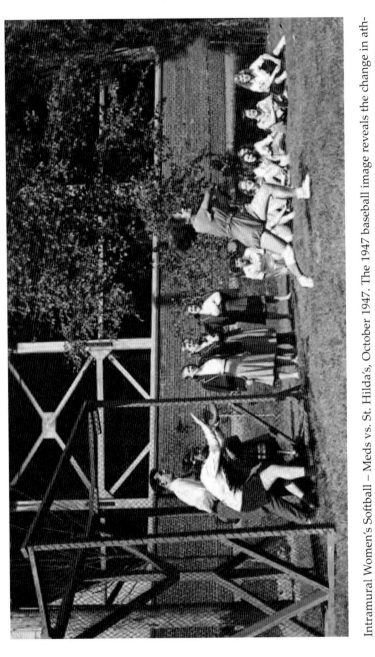

Intramural Women's Softball – Meds vs. St. Hilda's, October 1947. The 1947 baseball image reveals the change in athletic fashion to allow for concerted physical exertion. B2003-0001/011-4, Walter F. Mackenzie, University of Toronto Archives and Records Management Services. Coloured.

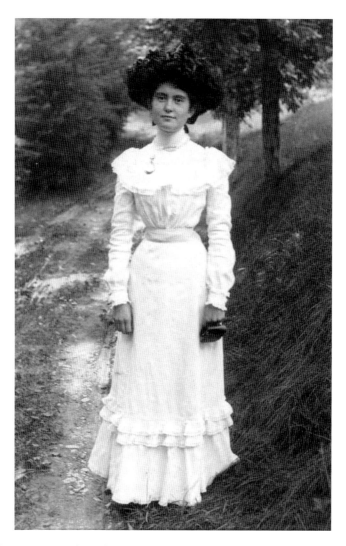

Ethel Brewster posed outdoors, circa 1898–1920. Many Canadians associated modernity with changes in women's lives that challenged the traditional sphere of women. Fashion trends over time provide a visual reminder of the "revolution" in the image of women. Here was reflected the turn-of-the-century covered body. Marsden Kemp fonds, photographs of people in eastern Ontario, C130-5-0-0-211, 10013496.jpg, Archives of Ontario.

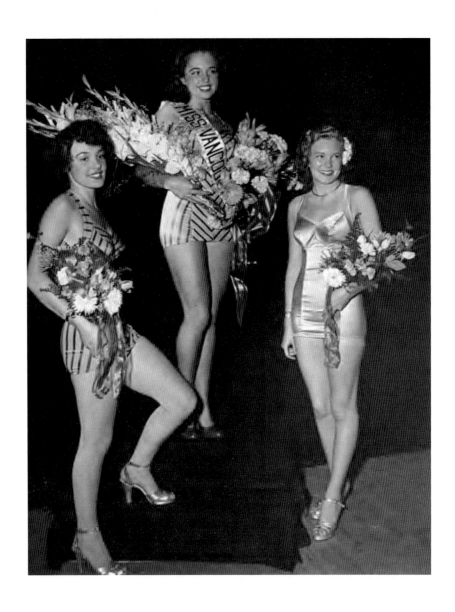

Miss Vancouver and the Runners Up, 1948. Note the "little to the imagination" covering of the body. City of Vancouver Archives, CVA 180-4355 A.A. Ray, 1948.

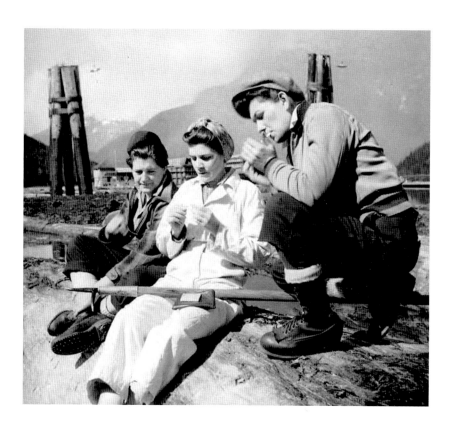

Women loggers smoking cigarettes on a break, April 1943. The fear of modernity would be typified by these loggers – women working in what had been a man's job, wearing clothing that accentuated anything but their femininity, smoking and more than that rolling their own cigarettes. Practitioners would see such women putting bodily health at risk as they took up a masculine role. Richard Wright, National Film Board of Canada. Still Photography Division, R1196-14-7-E, WRM 3442, e00761561, Library and Archives Canada.

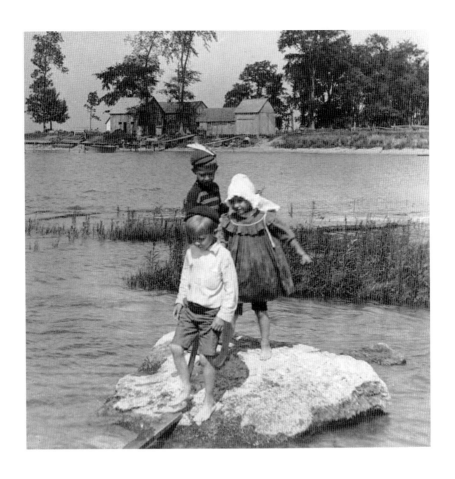

Bill, Helen, and Rowley Murphy at Fisherman's Point, Lake Erie, near Dunnville, Ontario, ca. 1898. Physicians seldom discussed the young childhood of girls or distinguished it significantly from that of boys. This photo of the Murphy children reflects the freedom many young girls experienced before puberty. Rowley Murphy fonds, Rowley Murphy prints, C 59-3-0-9-1, 19913870.jpg, Archives of Ontario.

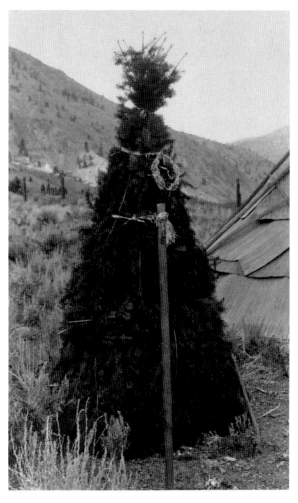

Small fir brush tipi used by a Nlaka'pamux (Thompson) pubescent girl, Spences Bridge, British Columbia. Puberty changed the expectations of girls. Across cultures, the advent of puberty was the beginning of a new phase in a girl's life. In these three photos, the significance of puberty was reflected in the traditional customs of Aboriginal young women in 1914 and 1950. In Euro-based cultures, the customs were ones of limitations and restraint, which continued until menstruation ended. In Aboriginal cultures limitations were offset by belief in the power represented by menstruating. Canadian Museum of Civilization, James A. Teit, 1914, 26976.

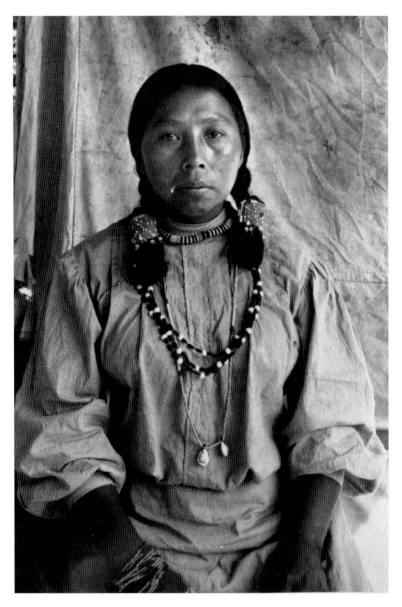

Hairstyle worn by Nlaka'pamux (Thompson) pubescent girls towards the end of the puberty training, Spences Bridge, British Columbia. Canadian Museum of Civilization, James A. Teit, 1914, 27054.

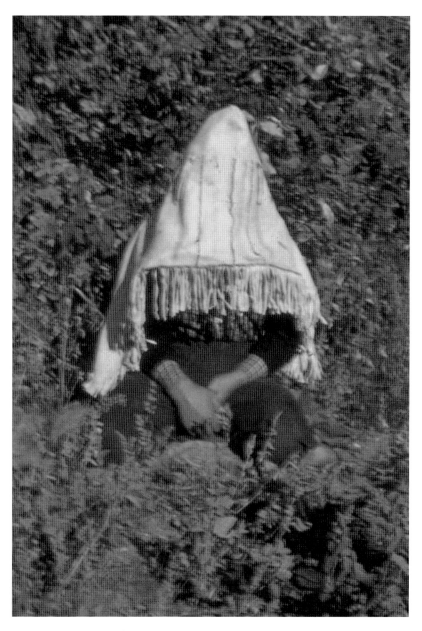

Mamie James in puberty hood, September 1950. Canadian Museum of Civilization, Catharine McClellan, S71-921. **Coloured.**

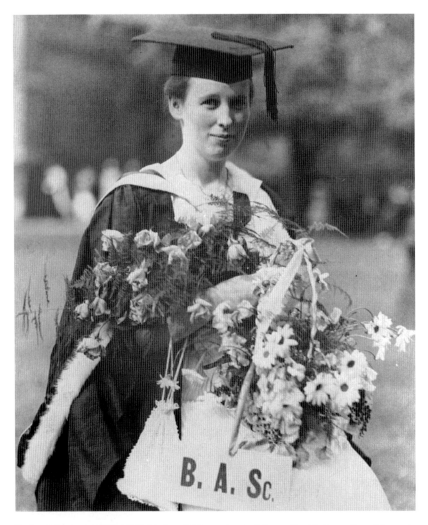

Esther Marjorie Hill, 1920. Esther Hill graduated from the University of Toronto in 1920 with a BA Sc. She became Canada's first woman architect. In the early part of the century Dr A. Lapthorn Smith advocated curtailing the education of women. For Smith, educating women such as Hill represented a physical danger to their health and to their ability to engage in domestic activities and fulfill their roles as wives and mothers. B1986-0106/005P, Digital Image No. 2002-17-4MS, James and Son Photographers, University of Toronto Archives and Records Management Services.

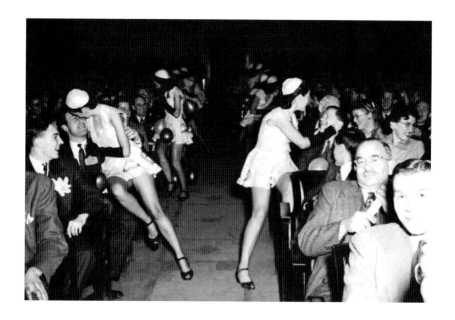

Daffydil Night, December 1948. Chorus girls are in the aisles flirting with members of the audience. If Dr A. Lapthorn Smith worried about the education of women, what would he have thought about the Daffydil Night of drama and music by students? Here were girls on display, men ogling them. Such dress and antics by young women suggested a more public sexuality. B2003-0001/046-2, Digital Image No. WFM 046-2, Walter F. Mackenzie, University of Toronto Archives and Records Management Services. **Coloured.**

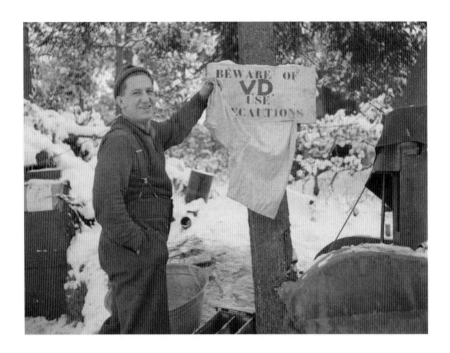

Private Louis Dufour of the Essex Scottish Regiment standing beside a venereal disease warning poster, Groesbeek, Netherlands, 24 January 1945. In the arguments of practitioners, public sexuality could lead to a rise in venereal disease with consequences for men and women and any children they might have. Doctors more than other Canadians knew the toll that VD took on bodies, especially those of women. And unlike the military, which emphasized the danger of "loose" women to their male recruits, doctors tended to assume the "guilt" of husbands. Lieutenant Michael M. Dean, Canada. Department of National Defence PA-137657, Library and Archives Canada.

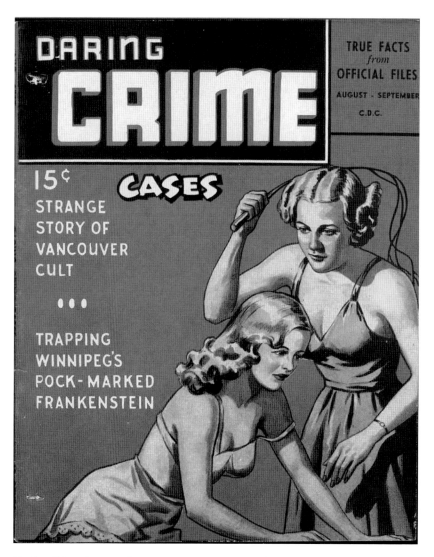

Daring Crime Cases, vol. 1, no. 6 (August–September 1943). Despite the increasing recognition of women's sexuality, the medical profession as a whole was generally very conservative about what it was willing to see as healthy and normal. The covers of true crime comics pushed the bounds of acceptability even as the stories inside had fairly traditional plots in which women challenging the sexual norms of society were punished. Cover, Norman Book Co., nlc-10130, Library and Archives Canada. **Coloured.**

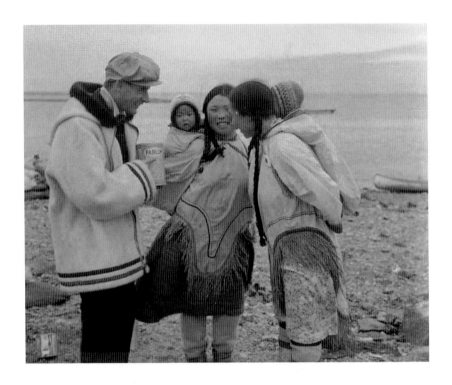

Representative of the Department of Indian Affairs S.J. Bailey explaining the benefits of pablum to two Inuit women with babies, Repulse Bay, Nunavut, 1948. Doctors were willing to provide advice to women on all sorts of topics. How and what to feed their children was one. Here Inuit women are being encouraged to feed their infants pablum, a creation of doctors at the Hospital for Sick Children, Toronto. Motherhood was no longer to be instinctual but rather scientific with doctors as the experts. At the time this photo was taken, the health of the Inuit across the North was in dire straits. S.J. Bailey, PA-167631, Library and Archives Canada.

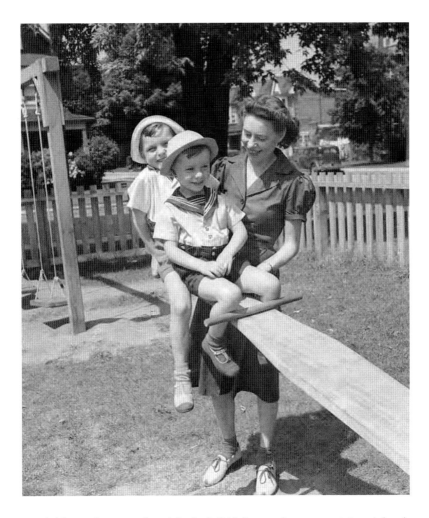

Two children whose mother, Mrs Jack Wright, works at a part-time job, play on a seesaw with a day nursery worker, September 1943. An apparently cosy wartime family until the description informs the onlooker that the mother figure is a nursery substitute for a working mother. Canadians were willing to accept wartime work by mothers but it was not something with which medical commentators were happy. Forty years into the century and physicians still believed that the domestic world was the healthiest for women. National Film Board of Canada. Still Photography Division, WRM 3831, PA-116141, Library and Archives Canada.

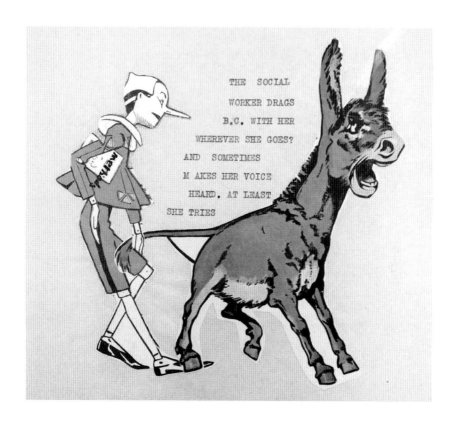

A.R. Kaufman was a major supporter of birth control in Canada. In his papers were scrapbooks consisting of cartoons (drawings) worked into the subject of birth control by members of the Toronto Art School. One series consisted of cutouts from the story of Pinocchio as B.C. (Birth Control). This image is an example of the cutouts and the message attached. A.R. Kaufman fonds, GA 173, series 4, box 1, file 22, University of Waterloo Library.

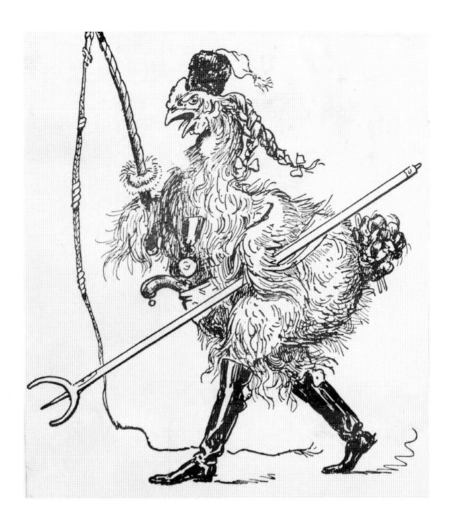

Another cartoon used to appeal to Kaufman by the Toronto Art School depicts a very ferocious version of Birth Control. The caption for the cartoon is, "In her dreams Birth Control arms itself for conquest. Nothing shall stand in its path. The Medical profession shall be subdued at once??????????" A.R. Kaufman fonds, GA 173, series 4, box 1, file 23, University of Waterloo Library.

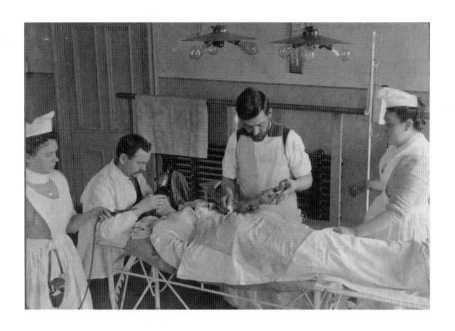

Operating Room, Montreal General Hospital, 1899. This surgery room from the turn of the century depicts quite a different vision from that apparent in the operating room of today. What it represents is the expansion of surgery as the favoured response to many ailments of women. McGill University Archives, PR009155, RG MGH, School of Nursing.

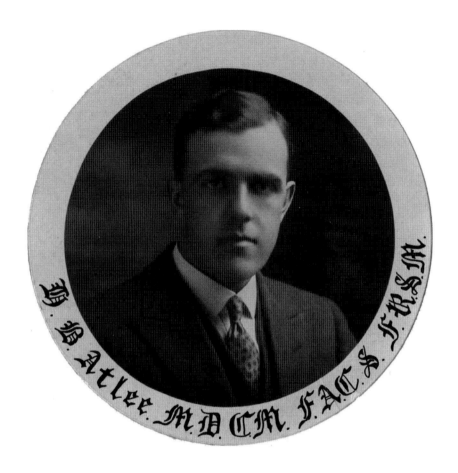

Dr H.B. Atlee. Dr Harold Benge Atlee was one of Canada's most prominent obstetricians and gynaecological surgeons, a larger-than-life figure to his students in his opinions about women and the limitations of their lives because of their bodies. Dalhousie University Photograph Collection, #73-589, Courtesy of Dalhousie Archives and Special Collections, Halifax, N.S.

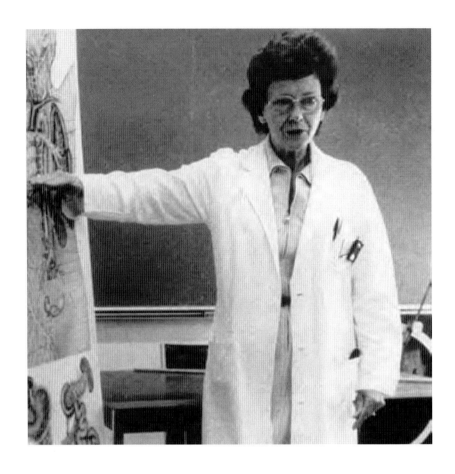

Dr Mildred Vera Peters, 196?. Dr Vera Peters graduated from the University of Toronto's Faculty of Medicine in 1934. She was a key figure in the Canadian move away from the Halsted radical mastectomy to less invasive surgery. B1996-0019/001(07), Digital Image No. 2001-77-219MS, Vera Peters fonds, University of Toronto Archives and Records Management Services.

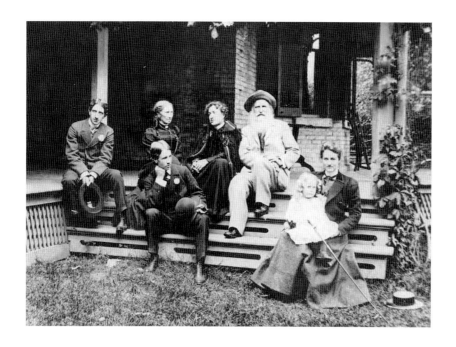

Dr Richard Bucke of the London Asylum on the steps of the Superintendent's House, ca. 1900. As superintendent of the London Asylum Dr Bucke approved of gynaecological surgery on "insane" women taking place there. While always insisting that the surgery was for physiological problems, the goal of "curing" women's insanity was clearly uppermost in his and like-minded doctors' actions. PA-135690, Library and Archives Canada.

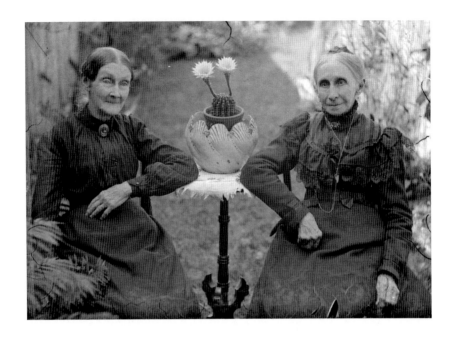

Two older women seated outside on either side of a flowering cactus (1898–1920). These elderly women at the turn of the century are a reminder that even by 1900 women were outliving men, giving the lie to the notion of the biological inferiority of the female body. Marsden Kemp fonds, C-130-5-0-0-198, 10013303jpg, Archives of Ontario.

This would suggest that the use of abortion by women was just part of their nature. Yet medical records suggest individual reasons that physicians were not always willing to acknowledge. In the case of Mrs Mavis Denton, although she already had one child that child was only one and one half years old and its birth had been a difficult one. Perhaps the memory of the birth trauma was such that Mavis Denton could not face another pregnancy, at least not yet.[71] While it is impossible to know what was in the minds of these women, their records suggest that historians need to examine what women themselves thought of childbirth and their own bodies, especially what limits they placed on what those bodies could withstand. Abortion crossed marital, class, religious, and ethnic boundaries. Many women resorted to it when desperate and if their attempts failed, infanticide could be a possibility.

The reasons for women aborting were complex and defy generalization. What was clear to physicians was that despite abortion's illegality, despite the moral rejection of it in public discourse, too many women felt they had no other choice. While rejecting the act, some practitioners could sympathize with the individual motivation behind it, particularly after the early years of the century. Neither did all physicians generalize women who aborted. They were more sympathetic to the "good" girls who had gone astray. They were hostile to what they viewed as the promiscuity of some young women. As for married women, promiscuity among them did not seem open for discussion. Instead the medical literature focused on the economic reason for abortion, reasons that the Depression heightened.

Assessment of Fertility Control Methods

The fact that many women were using birth control and too often resorting to abortion made physicians want to make sure that Canadians understood which birth control methods were best and which were dangerous and to warn women against abortion unless done by a reputable physician and for therapeutic reasons. Assessment was the area in which physicians exerted expertise. It allowed them to express that expertise to one another and provided a source of information for popular writers to present to their readers as "scientific" fact.

In his 1907 text J. Clifton Edgar rejected birth control based on the "detriment to the health of the participants." The irony is that these medical reasons were couched in the most tentative language. Couples practising birth control would have their health injured "to a certain extent."

Vague in the extreme, it left the door open to all sorts of fantasies on the part of the reader. When Edgar decided to list the possible specific consequences of birth control, however, his tentativeness disappeared and he recited a list that any reader would think was a necessary consequence rather than a possible consequence: in a woman – oophoritis, endometritis, leucorrhea, dysmenorrhoea, sterility, metrorrhagia, cancer of the uterus, neuroses, spinal irritation, neurasthenia; in a man – related health consequences. The birth control methods specifically mentioned as objectionable were "coitus interruptus, coitus reservatus, simple or artificial douching after coitus, wearing of coverings for the penis or obturators for the uterus." All were deemed antiphysiological and many untrustworthy, the latter acknowledging that some forms of birth control were effective. What Edgar meant by antiphysiological was often defined in male terms, focusing on the condition of the penis. He encouraged his readers (other male physicians) to explain to their women patients that the sex act consisted of three distinct stages. The first was when the male organ became erect; the second consisted of the orgasm; and the third when the penis became flaccid, which he insisted must occur within the vagina. Another text argued withdrawal could result in posterior urethritis and nervous symptoms in men.[72]

As already noted in the chapter on motherhood, women often resorted to extended breast feeding as a birth control tactic, one that physicians disliked.[73] In addition, Charles Reed's edited work dismissed the vaginal sponge, "womb caps," and condoms as "damaging," not physically damaging, but rather symbolic of "a psychic state inimical to the perfectly normal performance of the copulative act."[74] If physicians could not oppose birth control on physical grounds, they could on psychological. The normal performance of the sexual act was one in which no effort at birth control should be made. Such "medical" reasoning included social/cultural/moral aspects. Separating them from the medical was not possible because at times what was deemed medical was based, in part, in long-held beliefs that had become givens. In his 1912 textbook *A Text-Book of Obstetrics*, Barton Cooke Hirst recognized that some women were using a form of rhythm method to avoid pregnancy, an undependable method since he believed women could ovulate at any time and that sperm could last for more than three weeks (untrue) in the fallopian tubes. Dr P.C. Murphy of Tignish, Prince Edward Island, blamed douching for a perceived increase in ectopic pregnancy. As he made clear, "Given the relaxation of the tissues, following the natural orgasm, with a syringe bulb against a flaccid os; the well directed stream of water, and you have the proper physical conditions for driving semen and ovum to an unnatural place for impregnation."[75] Murphy's assessment had details that seemed missing in many of the descriptions of birth control methods and it was in the details that the credibility of the medical profession's knowledge often lay. Noteworthy about the listing of birth control methods was its negativity – the focus was on what didn't work. Left unsaid was what did work.

By the 1920s that had changed. J.S. Fairbairn, author of the 1924 *Gynaecology with Obstetrics: A Text-Book for Students and Practitioners* was quite typical in rejecting some forms of birth control and accepting others. He seemed willing to endorse medicated pessaries as long as they did not contain "poisonous antiseptic or other chemical" that could harm the internal tissue. Similarly, he viewed douching as harmless as long as the solution was not strong. The safest method, however, was what he called the "Dutch womb-veil," which he believed was successful in restraining the "enterprising spermatozoa." He even believed that a woman of "average" intelligence could remove and reinsert such a cap. Other items inserted into the vagina such as tampons and sponges he found problematic since he believed that too often women forgot about them until they had been left in too long and began to smell. He did grant, however, that they were safer than intrauterine devices, which could result in septic endometritis (inflammation of the inner lining of the uterus).[76] What concerns such as Fairbairn's suggested was in the post–World War I years the morality of birth control was fading into the background, although it would never totally disappear for some, and the medical safety factor becoming paramount. Many physicians still focused on what they saw as the problems of male contraceptives, in particular coitus interruptus and the use of condoms. Not all dismissed condoms, however. Harry Sturgeon Crossen and Robert James Crossen were willing to endorse the use of condoms "if the husband is cooperative and careful." Like Fairbairn they also approved of the diaphragm for women over other methods.[77] Others recognized that breast feeding did inhibit conception, although it was not totally dependable.[78] Physicians were choosing among types of contraceptives and debated among themselves about their value.

In 1942 Percy E. Ryberg published *Health, Sex and Birth Control*, which delineated in detail the various options before married couples. He assessed each form of birth control: rhythm method, sponge tampon, pessaries, jellies and cotton swabs, suppositories, condoms, coitus interruptus, abstention, and douching. Countering those who advocated abstention as the only moral form of birth control, he rebutted that abstention was really no different from other forms of birth control. If marriage was for the purpose of procreation only, then allowing the ovum to pass out of the body each month without being fertilized was no different from preventing it from being fertilized – the outcome was the same. The most-used method, he believed, was coitus interruptus. Although popular, he concluded it was unsatisfactory because of the interruption of pleasure at its height. Similarly condoms, while an excellent contraceptive, lessened both a man's and a woman's pleasure. The woman was denied both the seminal fluid and "the delicate interplay between her own sensitive vagina and the male organ." The douche Ryberg felt was the method most generally used by women, but he did not recommend it wholeheartedly. Neither did he feel restriction of sexual expression to the safe period was practical since couples simply could not regulate when they would desire one another and also because a woman's sex drive might very well be strongest when she was most liable to become pregnant. Ryberg did not approve of the widely advertised suppository but admitted that a sponge tampon was effective and could be made at home, and thus had cheapness to recommend it. He also approved of the use of spermicidal jelly especially in conjunction with a diaphragm pessary.[79] L. Carlyle Lyon, an English physician writing in the *Canadian Medical Association Journal*, rejected the "safe" period for different reasons than Ryberg; it had to be adjusted to the individual cycle of the woman and few women could keep track of their cycles:

> One is usually struck by the indifference to her menstrual functions exhibited by the average intelligent women, even among the so-called educated classes. She can seldom recall, with any degree of accuracy, the exact date of onset even of their *last* period. She has, occasionally, random jottings in a diary, but this is seldom available when she visits her medical advisor. The time thus wasted by doctors throughout the world (especially those like myself who are interested in teaching women contraceptive technique) in an attempt to arrive at some idea of the nature of individual women's cycles, must be incalculable![80]

The quote is fascinating for what it implies. First is the assumption that women should not be indifferent to when they menstruated. That they were suggests women may not have seen a monthly period as anything significant, at least not to the point of keeping track of it. Lyon clearly did. Second, that "even" educated women did not keep track of their periods suggests the assumption that class in patients mattered. Uneducated women could be expected not to keep track of the timing of their periods – more, however, was expected of educated women. Third was the wasting of a doctor's time – it was valuable, not the patient's.

Medical assessment of abortion methods were informed by who performed the abortion – the woman, the abortionist, or an ethical practitioner. In the early years of the century the focus was on the infections that criminal abortion could cause, resulting in future sterility, the need for gynaecological surgery, or death from peritonitis or septicaemia. Certainly physicians worried that in the use of instruments, which many women seemed to favour, there was always the danger that the woman would insert the instrument too forcefully and perforation of the vagina or the uterus itself result,[81] or laceration, haemorrhage, and peritonitis.[82] In subsequent decades doctors argued that women who aborted themselves or the abortionists who helped them simply were not skilled. In addition induced abortions were more dangerous than spontaneous ones.[83] In the case of douches of lysol, carbolic acid, etc., there were "caustic effects, followed by excoriation, ulceration and absorption." Drugs could also have toxic effects and result in damage to the kidneys and liver. If they did not result in death, permanent invalidism could result. Potassium permanganate tablets in the cervical canal and vagina could result in "punched-out ulcers at the point of contact."[84]

Physicians certainly had a vested interest in seeing that abortion outside the medical establishment was controlled if not eliminated. But it cannot be denied that many of their fears were real. Women were dying. David M. Eddy has analysed how physicians deal with complex problems by simplifying them: "A physician can ... draw on a number of simplifying heuristics. Anyone uncomfortable dealing with probabilities can use the heuristic, 'If there is any chance of (the disease), the (procedure) should be performed.' If one cannot estimate the number of people to be saved, one can use the heuristic, 'If but one patient is saved, the effort is worthwhile.'"[85] With abortion the heuristic device was simply the reverse. If there was any chance of death or complications from abortion, then the procedure should not be performed. If one patient died, that was one too many. In the case of abortion, doctors focused on women dying and ignored the lives these women would have lived if they had had the child. In following such logic, physicians were able to feel they were taking the "high" road, what was in the best interest of women (and society).

Medical Behaviour

Nevertheless, some practitioners did perform criminal abortions. Others railed against the abortion laws. The biographer of Harold Benge Atlee, one of Canada's foremost gynaecologists and obstetricians, noted Atlee was frustrated by the situation in which many women found themselves and felt the law needed to be changed to allow legal abortion by skilled practitioners.[86] Patient case records often reveal a lack of professional moralizing over the issue when doctors faced women who had undergone abortion. They also reveal the apparent lack of difficulty in accessing abortifacients from physicians to bring on women's periods. All these stances suggest historians need to rethink the idea of physicians' public opposition to abortion since they suggest that in private some physicians identified with women rather than the law.

As we saw in the discussion on criminal abortion, many physicians harboured the fear that if left to their own devices women would abort for frivolous reasons. When left to physicians to determine when abortions were necessary, the indicators were much different – medical abortions were acceptable to save the life of the mother or to preserve her health. The interpretation of when the mother's life or health was in jeopardy was not always clear, however, and that gave physicians a certain amount of latitude. Nonetheless, even in performing a therapeutic abortion, physicians had to take care so that their motives would not be suspect. One 1902 article warned readers that abortion should not be induced without consulting another practitioner.[87] A consultation would give protection from prosecution and maintain a physician's good name, both professional and public. Yet such a scenario was out of step with many physicians' medical practices, which were in small towns or isolated communities where colleagues were not always available. Such advice also assumed that the practitioners had the luxury of time to consult whereas sometimes that simply did not exist, at least not if the woman's life was to be saved.

The medical indicators for therapeutic abortion tended to be physical conditions that a pregnancy would make worse. In 1901, Dr Lapthorn Smith expressed concern about the number of women he saw going insane as a result of uraemia, a toxic condition originating in the kidneys that the added stress of pregnancy could cause. To prevent this, he cautioned physicians, after they had consulted with one or more of their colleagues, to abort such patients to prevent the kidneys from becoming permanently damaged.[88] Other conditions such as the pernicious vomiting of pregnancy also justified therapeutic abortion.[89] The difficulty with medical indicators was that there was no agreement on them. In the case of a previous insanity caused by pregnancy, many physicians believed that a subsequent pregnancy indicated abortion should be done. Alfred Galabin and George Blacker in their 1910 text argued the opposite – that the abortion itself could induce the insanity and thus it was not worth performing if it meant losing the life of a child. In a review of contemporary medical literature *The Canada Lancet* pointed out that abortion in the case of a woman with fibroids should not be done, suggesting that perhaps some physicians were doing it. One of the indicators for abortion that was most discussed was tuberculosis. On 18 June 1914, Mrs Harriet Scott, age 40, entered the Royal Victoria Hospital, Montreal, for "the emptying of the uterus." On 4 July she was discharged to go to Saranac Lake, a tuberculosis facility. Dr D.A. Stewart from Ninette, Manitoba, was very adamant about the need to abort in the case of advanced or active TB. Even in those women where the disease was "quiescent," at the first sign of symptoms, he advised the pregnancy be terminated. On the other hand, Dr Adam Wright argued that physicians involved with tuberculosis patients were too prone to abort; their job, he argued, was to cure the tuberculosis, "not interfere with nature."[90]

Some of the factors of concern in the early years continued in the years following World War I while others were dropped or modified and still others added. What was different was the increased willingness of physicians to discuss therapeutic abortion. In part, this willingness came from the Bourne decision in England that specifically allowed therapeutic abortion to save the life of the pregnant woman. Canadian physicians comforted themselves that the decision also covered the situation in Canada.[91] Among the medical indicators listed for a medical abortion were previous insanity of pregnancy, extreme vomiting of pregnancy, kidney disease, heart disease, pernicious anaemia, leukaemia, chorea, melancholia, carcinoma of the uterus, Addison's Disease, acute diabetes, epilepsy, mental limitations, and TB.[92] Old age was also an indicator. Gertrude Roswell's mother was 45 when she gave birth to Gertrude. Because it was her first child she had to go to several doctors before she found one who agreed to deliver her. Others thought she should abort since they deemed her too old.[93] As we saw above,

TB remained an indicator, although perhaps more nuanced than it had been. Most felt that abortion of a woman with TB until the fifth month was safe, but afterwards there was not much difference between the stresses of abortion and those of labour. In 1941, the Medical Committee of the Sanatorium Board of Winnipeg agreed with Wright's earlier view of doctors using TB as a too-frequent abortion indicator. Indeed, when abortion did occur in the case of a woman with TB, some believed that, more often than not, it was for nonmedical reasons. As one physician pointed out, "[I]t is often easier to terminate the pregnancy than to remove the social and economic difficulties." Others, too, had raised the fear that the indicators for abortion were becoming too flexible.[94] Some insisted that the profession needed to be as specific as possible about what the medical indicators for a therapeutic abortion should be in case some physicians hid behind the smokescreen of "general health unsatisfactory," which clearly some were doing.[95]

In 1938 George W. Henry described a situation that he had difficulty endorsing. A woman who already had two children she couldn't support found herself pregnant. Wanting to terminate her pregnancy, she entered a hospital that refused her request despite the fact that she had had two episodes of mental illness and that insanity seemed to run in her family. The refusal was based on her "good physical health." Apparently, she was not sufficiently depressed at the time to attract attention. In the mid 1940s, Dr Richards recalled a case with which, as an intern, she was familiar. The patient was an "older woman [who] suffered from intractable 'Hyperemesis Gravidarum' [a severe form of morning sickness]. She begged the obstetrician who was on the public service to do an abortion ... He refused ... because 'she just doesn't want this baby, that's all.' She eventually died in the second trimester of 'acute yellow atrophy of the liver.'" That Richards remembered this woman 50 years later testified to the horror she felt about the situation. Mrs William Wyatt, age 38, was two and one half months pregnant with her first child when she entered the Kitchener-Waterloo Hospital on 20 January 1945. Her record read, "Patient has been very nervous because of family responsibilities she has worried a great deal, and has slept poorly ... and it was thought a therapeutic abortion was indicated." Clearly physicians could be much less dogmatic in their treatment than historians have suggested and also what the public medical literature suggested.[96] What these scenarios indicate is that therapeutic abortion indicators were seldom absolute and that physicians were forced to make decisions for which reasons were not always clear and indisputable.

Birth control did not present the same kinds of dilemmas for practitioners. Many of the women interviewed testified to the willingness of their doctors in the 1930s and 1940s to assist them with birth control. Gertrude Roswell seemed part of a trend of women who before they married went to a physician to be fitted with a diaphragm. She had had sexual experience before marriage with a man who had used a condom, but with marriage Roswell felt a diaphragm was the way to go. She certainly did not feel that she would have any difficulty in getting a diaphragm fitted by a physician and even when she was having sexual experiences before marriage did not feel that her physician would refuse her birth control, although she anticipated that a lecture might attend it. Jane Rutherford, married in 1942, also remembered going to her physician to be fitted with a diaphragm before her marriage. Geraldine Mitchell had always taken responsibility for birth control even before she married. Indeed, her husband simply assumed that she was wearing a diaphragm. Betty Mackenzie, too, was fitted with a diaphragm and made it clear that morality was not an issue – she simply did not want children at that point. Many of these women lived in urban centres so that access to birth control and doctors who were supportive may have been more available. They were also women knowledgeable and strong enough to ask their physicians for help. Not all women were. Dorothy Atkinson, for example, was too shy to ask.[97] Some physicians even went beyond the pragmatism of providing birth control already available. They experimented to expand the forms of birth control that could be considered: hormone control, immunization by spermatoxins, and temporary sterilization by means such as heat, roentgen-rays, and diet. The physician of Betsy Lawrence, for example, tested both Lawrence and his own wife with a "new" spermicide. Both became pregnant.[98]

Conclusion

Several conclusions emerge from this examination of fertility control. First is the incredible shift that occurs in the medical discussion of birth control after WWI and the way it took place in tandem with what many patients and Canadians were demanding. Second, if access to birth control was a hit-and-miss affair for Canadians in general, access to training on it for practitioners was equally hit and miss. Third, birth control was an issue on which the profession was divided. It was one of those issues in which pressures other than the medical came to bear: its illegality, personal morality, social attitudes, and religious beliefs. The medical discussion of birth control and its connection to eugenics was an important one in that it constituted an underlying context for general reactions to birth control. It revealed the way in which medical, gender, race, class, and moral issues could become intertwined. For a profession that tried to appeal to science for its grounding, internal divisions on birth control were uncomfortable. Internal divisions were even more so on the topic of abortion.

Abortion was publicly and privately considered more reprehensible than birth control. Nevertheless, the frequency of abortion revealed to all the desperation and determination of many women not to give birth to an unwanted child. The medical literature contains descriptions of why women were willing to resort to abortion with differentiations made between single and married women and the former as either good girls and those of easy virtue. In later decades the moral condemnation lessened somewhat as the economic situation of both unmarried and married women loomed larger than in the previous decades because of the economic downturn of the 1930s. What did not change and indeed may have increased was the repugnance at the abortion methods chosen by women and the potential physical harm those methods could cause, harm that reinforced doctors' conviction that abortion must remain within the control of physicians. Doing so would lessen their vulnerability to pressure and would allow them to make *medical* decisions rather than social ones. But in private practice, the story was somewhat different with some physicians being willing to expand the meaning of medical to include social or economic health.

8 "The ... mischievous tendency of specialism": Gynaecology

Winnipeg's J.N. Hutchison summarized woman's situation. Her female system was a source of "strength and power" but "if neglected and mismanaged [her organs] retaliate on their possessor with weakness and disease."[1] Such a view revealed the centrality of the reproductive/sexual system in physicians' understanding of women's health. The system was strong but strong in a way that dominated the well-being of women for if it weakened, became ill, broke down, then woman's very life was compromised in a variety of ways.

This chapter examines the specialty of gynaecology and what some saw as the "mischievous tendency of specialism."[2] Up to this point, the chapters have followed the normal life cycle of women and the kinds of challenges it presented to women and practitioners. Here we return to the thrust of the first chapter on the broader social perception of women's bodies as weaker than men's. Within medicine, the focus of that vision underlay the specialty of gynaeoclogy. The chapter begins with a brief look at the history of gynaecology, its emergence as a specialty, its emphasis on surgery, and the demands placed on those who practiced it. Following is a description of the perceived general weaknesses of women's bodies and specific disease/illness causation that physicians and specialists alike emphasized; the problems encountered in the patient/doctor relationship when that relationship was based on the most private and intimate parts of a woman's body; and the difficulty in examining women and determining a diagnosis. The chapter ends with a general overview of treatment offered to women, both medical and surgical, and the glimpses of patient agency that often emerged when surgery was the treatment advocated. All these topics reflect the interconnection between gender and medicine and especially the specialty of gynaecology.

History of Gynaecology

The practice of gynaecology resulted in conflicts with other specialties and within gynaecology itself. During most of the first half century gynaecology was closely tied to the specialty of obstetrics. Both focused on the reproductive/sexual system of women, but whereas obstetrics stressed the system's physiological nature, gynaecology emphasized its pathological elements. Joint professorships in both specialties became more common in the early years of the century and while they made a certain amount of sense, they represented an uneasy alliance. Obstetricians worried that gynaecology's emphasis on the pathological resulted in a surgical orientation that was influencing their own field. At the same time, they believed their skills were superior in that they were more qualified to treat gynaecological disorders than gynaecologists were equipped to deliver babies. For their part, gynaecologists mentioned how often the childbirth practices of their obstetrical colleagues caused problems in women that they had to fix.[3]

Gynaecology's surgical orientation also brought those advocating it into conflict with general surgeons and those within gynaecology who supported a more medical approach to treatment. General surgeons had long believed surgery was their prerogative and, at the very least, if gynaecologists were going to perform surgery within their own speciality, then they should familiarize themselves with general surgery first.[4] In response A. Lapthorn Smith, surgeon at the Samaritan Hospital for Women in Montreal, argued that in a vaginal examination only an "experienced gynecologist" should use the sound (a slender instrument for insertion into body passages) to ensure safety. Smith was specifically concerned about general surgeons who were undertaking procedures in which they were not trained. William Gardner criticized general practitioners for the same reason. He also went further than Smith in distinguishing skill, suggesting that experienced gynaecologists didn't need a sound; their touch examination was enough.[5] Within gynaecology, critics of the surgical orientation suggested that it weakened "accurate diagnosis and medical treatment" and that surgical gynaecologists were too interested in the high fees they received for performing surgery. But even medical gynaecology had its critics, one being that its practitioners too often were so engaged by the problems their patients presented that they believed that healthy women were in the minority, another that they failed to acknowledge that their skills were not the only ones that medicine had to offer women.[6] The turf wars between gynaecology and other specialities and within gynaecology itself continued well into the century.[7]

Underlying the speciality of gynaecology was belief in the centrality of the reproductive/sexual system in women's bodies. Its organs were "among the marvels of creation," and determined women's health both physiologically and psychologically. The ovaries, for example, played a key role in procreation and early in the century physicians speculated that they also secreted "something" that was "essential" to women throughout their lives. Belief in these secretions led to therapies based on ovarian preparations and, in the words of W. Blair Bell, brought "gynaecology and obstetrics into the domain of biochemistry."[8] They also varied in size in different women and in the same woman at different times of her life.[9] Pelves came in various shapes as well. There was a sense that the Caucasian pelvic type was the norm: "The pelvis of the Australian is nearly circular in horizontal outline, and in Bush women the antero-posterior exceed the transverse diameters. The pelvis of the Laplander is small."[10] The meaning of the shapes was unclear and there was little sense that different ones posed different problems except perhaps needing to be kept in mind during childbirth, but the normative aspect of one group of women over others made the latter appear "curious" and "different" and somehow inferior. Whatever the meaning of the shapes, the physician needed to understand the variety and determine what was healthy and what was not. The "discovery" of sex hormones, too, changed the medical landscape and, according to Nelly Oudshoorn, "enabled gynaecologists to draw the human body more and more deeply into the gynaecological clinic." In 1923 researchers demonstrated the effects of estrogen and in the 1930s details emerged on the chemical closeness of estrogen and progesterone. The reproductive/sexual system appeared more complex than anyone had imagined. Pelvic types continued to intrigue. What once seemed fixed in number, were no longer so as radiological pictures of the pelvis revealed that "the female pelvis ... [was] a strangely variable thing."[11] Variation apparently occurred with race with what H.B. Atlee referred to as the android or male type of pelvis, the "rogue among the archetypes" being much more common in white women and the anthropoid or "ape-like" type being common in "negro" women. Such a statement did not reflect what Atlee knew to be the case, that is, that anthropoid pelves had an occurrence rate of 23.5 percent in white women as well. He did not hide the knowledge – it was present in a chart he presented – but in the narrative description it was overlooked, which permitted a negative categorization of black women. By 1949, the pelvic shape was no longer being connected to race, but rather to the lack of vitamin D as the woman was growing up.[12]

As the medical understanding of women's bodies expanded so did the field of gynaecological surgery, aided by the introduction of antiseptic techniques and the use of anesthesia in the late nineteenth century. Hospitals reported increasing numbers of gynaecological surgeries performed. The Vancouver General Hospital listed 703 gynaecological surgeries in 1912 and 1105 in 1918. In 1925, the Royal Victoria Hospital, Montreal, reported 681 gynaecological surgeries being performed, in 1933, 1279, and by 1940, 1970.[13] If the early period of surgery was enabled by the safety that antiseptic techniques could provide, towards the end of the period under review it was the sulfanilamide family of drugs that confirmed the abilities of surgeons to ensure the safety of their patients through controlling the spread of infection better. These years consolidated the rise of the gynaecological surgeon as a separate specialist within gynaecology and surgery.

Surgical literature is similar to an adventure tale, in which surgeons are at centre stage. Patients came to them more often than not through referral, with one physician who wouldn't do the surgery asking another to do so. It was the surgeon's expertise that was necessary. Second, the reproductive system was the focus; not only was it significant physiologically but its proper workings were of social and personal importance. Third was often the performance of a complex procedure. The image of the surgeon as a man in control was a familiar trope. Atlee's reputation as a gynaecological surgeon was, in part, based on the quickness of his surgeries. There were reasons for this since he had been trained at a time when there were few expert anesthetists and management of surgeries tended to be poor. In that kind of situation the faster the surgery, the better chance the patient had. But the speed and his surgical technique also reflected the man, a larger than life individual. His biographer described one case in which he was performing a hysterectomy when he perceived that the woman's gall bladder contained stones. He closed the hysterectomy incision and made a new one further up on the abdomen and removed the gall bladder. While finishing off that procedure his intern noted a lump in the patient's breast. Atlee examined the breast and determined the lump was malignant and proceeded to perform a radical mastectomy on the breast.[14] The self-confidence that such procedures demanded is difficult to imagine. Atlee determined what was wrong with the woman and proceeded to take out whatever parts of her body that he had judged to be problematic. How the patient felt about it on awakening is unknown.

Despite their confidence, surgeons lived in an uncertain world. They had to determine not only what the problem (or problems) were, but also what needed to be done and how, knowing that for the same problem there were many approaches, often with varying results. The decision to operate or not was just that, a decision that had to be made not only taking into account the physical problem that needed to be dealt with and what the norms of treatment were or were becoming, but also the patient herself and her situation. In addition, there was an ebb and flow in treatment modalities. What were seen as problems changed as did treatment. Keeping up to date was not easy. Those trained in one era were not always aware of the latest findings of medical scientists and even when they were, it was often unclear how their findings impinged on medical and surgical practice. What did it all mean for the practitioner faced with a patient who was suffering? What hadn't changed to any significant extent was the overwhelming perception of the weakness of the female system. It provided the context in which the scientific advances and the innovations in treatment and surgeries occurred.

Weakness of the System and Its Causes   ·

Perusal of hospital statistics in the early years of the century reveals that women tended to be underrepresented as patients and that gynaecological disorders, compared to other medical problems, were a minority of cases. Nonetheless, doctors at the time believed women's bodies were more at risk than men's because their various organs of generation were both more numerous and complex and hence their functioning demanded more energy. Montreal General Hospital's *Annual Report* for the year ending 30 April 1901 noted 210 gynaecological cases containing over 90 different categories of problems.[15] Each problem was subdivided into variations, which made the lists seem even longer and more encompassing and reinforced the image of women having problematic bodies and those bodies being poorly designed. Indeed, one 1901 textbook had to assure its readers that the diseases of women were not increasing and that "the Anglo-Saxon woman is not degenerating."[16] She may not have been degenerating, but compared to her uncivilized sister or the females among the lower animals, all of whom experienced pathological conditions, the perception was that "civilized" woman of the early twentieth century did so even more.

The notion of the ill health of women only increased over time. In 1927, L.M. Morton of Yarmouth, Nova Scotia, reminded colleagues, "[I]f not for the ills of the 'Female of the species,' the Doctor's income would be seriously handicapped." The disorders under the heading of gynaecology in the literature remained numerous; hospital reports delineated with care the various "female" organs that were prone to breakdown, and advertisements in medical journals emphasized the disorders that could accompany all the transitions of women's lives. The Montreal General Hospital's *Annual Report* for 1928 noted the pressure that gynaecological patients placed on the facilities in the outpatient department. At mid century, Walter C. Alvarez warned medical students that in their practices they would meet women with "puzzling" ailments. No cause would be found because there was no cause beyond "poor nervous heredity and 'the contractor's having put in poor materials.'"[17] That the large majority of women came to hospitals for reasons linked to the fragility of the human body, not the female body, was lost in the discourse. Gynaecology's focus was on the problems of the latter.

The perceived causes of women's gynaecological problems varied, but three stand out: lifestyle, childbirth, and iatrogenic causes. Taken together they were all-encompassing in that both body and society worked against women's health. No one would deny that lifestyle can affect health (for good or ill), but focusing on it allowed physicians to envision a world in which women would be healthier if only they followed the advice given to them by their doctors. Much of that advice encouraged women not to challenge their traditional roles or engage with modernity. We have already seen this in the perceived dangers posed to women who ignored their destiny of being wife and mother or those who engaged in advanced education. Physicians tended to believe that women maintaining their traditional role in society did not experience stress. But if the changing customs of civilization hurt women, they also saved them from the customs of "savage conditions."[18] Noted in previous chapters, beyond general issues of the strain and pressures of modern civilization, practitioners focused on specific aspects of life that were problematic such as luxurious living, overexertion, and excess sexual stimulation.[19] Over time, new lifestyle issues were emphasized such as alcoholism, the use of birth control, and abortion. Older ones continued revealing deeper concerns. In the 1940s some commentators were still suggesting that not marrying and not having children could be a problem due to psychic stress.[20]

As we have seen, marriage could bring its own dangers in the form of venereal disease. It also brought with it the likelihood of having children and childbirth was a major physiologically based cause of women's ill health.[21] As well, the care women received in childbirth could be and often was problematic. In his 1900 text on obstetrics, David James Evan made a point of referencing "the great numbers of women who throng the gynaecologic clinics"; he placed the blame for their health issues on physicians not practicing the "antiseptic method" of directing labour. Whether woman's body or her physician's lack of care was to blame, the case records of many women revealed how childbirth took its toll. In 1905, Mrs Terrance Moore, age 46, entered the Victoria General Hospital, Halifax. She had married at 18 and had already given birth to 14 children, the youngest of whom was 7 months. Mrs Joan Slater was 63 when she entered the Royal Victoria Hospital, Montreal, on 30 April 1906. For the last 30 years she had suffered from prolapse of the uterus, a result of the birth of her third child. Although operated on 18 years previously little improvement had occurred and she was now getting worse.[22] While such cases became less common, the focus on the obstetric art and childbirth as a cause of gynaecological troubles did not. E.K. Maclellan, a Halifax physician, opined in 1935 that childbearing and its problems were the origins of gynaecology.[23]

If many physicians acknowledged that the medical care provided women in childbirth had resulted in iatrogenic-caused disorders, the problem was not confined to obstetrics. Commentators mentioned "the applications of irritants, forcible dilations; injections of fluids into the uterus; pessaries; exploratory punctures" that were part of general medical treatment and care of women. There was also concern about dirty instruments and hands and the problems that sounds could pose in internal examinations.[24] Physicians recognized that medical fads came and went and that often in the early years of use, a procedure could be "attended by ... abuses."[25] Neither did such abuses abate. In 1936, Ross Mitchell reviewed an article on haematometra (accumulation of menstrual blood in the uterus) in the *American Journal of Obstetrics and Gynecology* and summarized the findings for readers of the *Canadian Medical Association Journal*: "Increasingly frequent improper uterine curettage, improper application of radium to the cervix, the use of caustic and heavy cautery tips in cervical cauterizations, ... are stressed as important factors in the increasing frequence of acquired haematometra."[26] Physicians could too easily succumb to the excitement of new "advances" and get caught up in the bandwagon effect resulting in treatment that could harm.

Whether through lifestyle choice, childbirth, or physicians, women were at risk. Indeed, any examination of medicine and women makes that clear. But what was the solution? Women could make better choices, but some of the harmful choices made were rational ones given their circumstances. Childbirth was part of a woman's life and in a world where birth control was illegal it was difficult to avoid. Any medical treatment came with its own risk. Certainly practitioners did not want to do harm. Indeed, they spent a great deal of time worrying about the patient/doctor relationship and how to best do what was in the patient's interest. Physicians recognized that their relationship with their patients was crucial to the healing process and given that the focus of gynaecology was on the most intimate part of a woman's body and the physician was more likely than not a man, it was often an uneasy one.

Doctor/Patient Relationship

The area that generated much discussion of the female patient/male doctor relationship was the internal examination: whether to do it, who should receive it, and how to make women more comfortable with it. Such examinations "invaded" the most private parts of the body, raising issues of morality, sensitivity, and skill. A central question in the early years was whether a physician should perform an internal examination on a virgin and, if so, how to do it in a way that was least upsetting for the patient and safest for the physician. While few physicians at the turn of the century considered the examination of a virgin the "moral rape" that earlier generations had, some still saw it as problematic.[27] A rectal exam was a possible alternative but the only way it was better was because the rectum was not endowed with the cultural baggage held by the vagina. Another way of avoiding a vaginal examination was the rather impractical suggestion of having the mother examine her daughter. If an examination by a physician was unavoidable, then perhaps an examination under anaesthesia would lessen a young girl's pain and moral shock.[28]

While examinations on virgins posed specific problems, the non-virginity of other women did not make the issue of respectability and morality disappear. How do you exam the "holy of holies," the "delicate ground"?[29] Physicians were aware that women did not like to discuss what they considered private problems let alone submit to a vaginal examination. But practitioners agreed that in those cases when an examination was needed, a woman must consent and, if she did not, some experts suggested refusing to treat her.[30] Generally, however, physicians had faith in their ability to convince their patients; the appeal to rationality would be successful and overcome modesty.

Once they deemed an examination necessary, physicians focused on the best way to proceed. Some suggested talking with the woman first – a verbal examination, so to speak. While a physician might consider it a waste of time, a verbal exam would make the woman more comfortable with and trusting of the physician. The setting for the physical examination should provide ease of sight for the physician; thus a bed or couch would not be good venues. They also might be too suggestive. A table or some firm surface was best, even though William Gardner acknowledged many women were uncomfortable lying on such a surface, "especially if the practitioner be young."[31] Nevertheless, physicians' needs had to have priority.

As physicians accepted the need to do an internal examination, the concern about it subsided, even with respect to examining a virgin. H.B. Atlee was rather blasé about the issue and instructed his students that while the presence or absence of the hymen should be noted, absence of it did not mean lack of virginity and the presence of it did not mean virginity.[32] Physicians needed to take care about making false judgements about a woman's virginity, but the virginity itself was not a medical concern. The public, however, still saw examination of a virgin as problematic. As already noted, when Gertrude Roswell was in high school, her periods were so heavy that her mother took her to see Dr Marion Powell who did an internal examination, an occurrence that appalled Gertrude's mother since she feared her daughter's hymen might be broken during the process.[33] Physicians were well aware of the continued hesitation on the part of many women about the vaginal examination. Yet protecting their modesty during a vaginal examination was not an easy task. The woman was usually in the lithotomy position with her thighs pulled up to the abdomen and her legs flexed away from one another. Atlee's practice was to place a sheet over the patient's knees not only to preserve her modesty, but also to prevent her seeing the instruments that might be used in the examination. Atlee was a teacher and, at times, his determination to have his students remember his teachings outweighed consideration for the patient. For example, in trying to emphasize the importance of the vaginal and rectal exams, he wrote a poem entitled "The Moving Finger," which had as the last line of every verse the statement "Please don't – oh don't – forget to Stick a finger up her ass!" What message he thought he was sending his students was unclear, but it certainly did not express any kind of sympathy or respect for women. Nevertheless, he was willing to acknowledge the problem of male physicians treating women patients and one of his women students recalled that he predicted that the future of gynaecology would lie with women doctors.[34]

Women patients were seldom in any position to object to their treatment. Dr Richards recalled that when she was in medical school she was "appalled at the cruel & insensitive treatment of women," especially public ward patients who were open to the gaze of medical students. On one occasion she remembered that a young woman brought into the examining room complained when the physician inserted a speculum into her and he "remarked, crudely – 'Don't complain about that, you've had something bigger than that in there and I bet you liked it.'! There was profound silence in the room as the medical students were shocked – and this was a role model!" Her reaction and the reaction of other women physicians on the issue of physician/patient relations was to hope that women doctors would empathize more with their female patients than men doctors did, but until that day, many women probably shared the experience of Dorothy Atkinson. When having a first internal exam during pregnancy, the doctor didn't explain the procedure and she didn't ask. "In those days," she recalled, "I thought that doctors were gods more or less and you just lay back and let them do it."[35]

The vulnerabilities presented by the male doctor/female patient relationship went beyond the internal examination. Some practitioners warned their colleagues that women patients were impressionable, so a little subterfuge did not hurt: "[D]on't cure your female patients too quickly. No woman as a rule is willing to submit to treatment unless she has been convinced that her's [sic] is a complicated case."[36] Doctors could be judgmental, especially towards uncooperative patients. Mrs Letitia Danvers, age 24 and married only two months, entered the Royal Victoria Hospital, Montreal, on 24 November 1913 suffering from pain in her lower abdomen, leucorrhoea, and burning and frequence of micturation. She was diagnosed as having double salpingo-oophoritis (inflammation of uterine tube and ovary). The treatment offered was relatively noninvasive – bed rest, an ice bag to the abdomen, douching, and use of tampons. Nevertheless, she went home against the wishes of her doctors. In trying to come to terms with this recalcitrance, the writer of the case record, instead of understanding why a young bride might want to go home, deemed her "of low mentality hysterical and gives very foolish reasons for wanting to go."[37] Physicians could not help but admire some of their patients more than others. One 1928 text described the "plucky" woman who could undergo a dilation and curettage on a doctor's office table. Less admirable were the "chronic invalids or semi-invalids [who] complain of a multitude of pains and aches" and whose actions wear down "the patience of their husbands and relatives."[38] Some physicians also ignored some patients more than others – those with leucorrhoea and lesions of the cervix, and especially those they suspected of having a sexually transmitted disease.[39]

Physicians controlled access to information. In terms of what to tell patients, some physicians considered silence acceptable. The authors of one 1930 text on the diseases of women put forward the case of a woman in which a myomata (a benign tumour of the uterus) was discovered during an examination for another ailment. The authors instructed their readers not to tell such a patient about it – it required no treatment – but rather to monitor its size. They were, however, to "explain the condition to the husband or other responsible relative, that your skill be not called in question should the patient be examined by some other physician and the presence of a tumor announced."[40] In this case, the attitude was paternalistic, saving the woman from worrying, but, at the same time, letting her husband or someone else "responsible" know as a means of protecting the physician's reputation. The woman herself was clearly not "responsible."

While much of the secondary literature on the doctor/female patient relationship has focused on the way in which the patient was treated and the kind of power that physicians had, we should not assume that physicians were always aware of having that power or at least not in all situations. And as we saw in the chapter on sexuality, physicians themselves felt vulnerable when faced with "excitable, emotional, women" and their sexual imaginings.[41] Certainly the male doctor/female patient relationship was fraught, but the challenges had to be overcome in order for a diagnosis to be made.

Diagnosis

Diagnosis in gynaecology faced a practitioner with particular issues. Certain diagnoses could place a woman's reputation at risk. At a time when pregnancy was not a straightforward diagnosis, physicians warned one another about the dangers of assuming a woman was pregnant when she wasn't.[42] Another challenge was knowing what the normal or healthy reproductive system should look like. As we have seen, there were different pelvic types and within Western medicine the "Caucasian" pelvis was deemed the norm.[43] An early article in the 1900 *Canada Medical Record* reminded its readers that the uterus was "a very movable organ" in that its shape could be affected by distension in the bladder or rectum and by coughing or vomiting, leading the physician to make an incorrect diagnosis of retroversion or some other displacement. But how serious was displacement? In the *Annual Report* of the Montreal General Hospital, for the year ending 30 April 1901, the gynaecological report of the outdoor department listed various displacements that had been seen: anteflexion, anteversion, procidentia, prolapse, retroposition, retroflexion, and retroversion. It would seem that there were so many ways uteri could be "abnormal." And if abnormal, surely problems would ensue.[44] The physician needed to understand the variety and determine what was healthy and what was not. Nonetheless, the boosters of gynaecology were confident that their specialty "had the advantage of employing very exact methods of diagnosis."[45]

New testing procedures could certainly offer the possibility of greater diagnostic precision but they also increased expectations of what was possible to diagnose and the ease of diagnosis. Pregnancy became easier to diagnose with the Zondek-Aschheim test that came into use in the 1930s. Nevertheless, mistakes still occurred.[46] In the 1940s, radiological examination as a diagnostic aid was available, allowing the physicians to "see" what could not be seen otherwise.[47] But some of the fundamental problems remained. What was normal in the sexual/reproductive system of women? What was a normal position for the uterus? What was the meaning of abnormal and did being "abnormal" matter if it did not pose a problem? There was little consensus. Some physicians remained convinced that uterine displacements were problematic. Others were less sure.[48] The variations of the pelvis also remained an issue with some physicians acknowledging five different "parent" shapes, each of which had variations more difficult to identify, let alone determining, the reasons for those variations.[49] Without that understanding, being able to discern the normal from the problematic abnormal became a guessing game.

Treatment

Assuming a diagnosis was able to be made, a specific treatment followed. But it was not always easy to determine the right treatment or to be sure that women would be able to accept its demands. Some practitioners realized that for working women the best treatment for a particular condition might not be possible because of the financial situation of the woman and her need to continue working.[50] Extended bed rest was possible for the wealthy; for the poor it was not. W.G. Colwell reported in the *Dalhousie Medical Journal* of 1939 that while hormonal treatment for uterine bleeding could be successful, it often took time in order to be successful and that it was expensive: "In the public wards of the Victoria General Hospital [Halifax] the disadvantage is apparent and so these cases are treated by some form of hysterectomy." As one 1944 text summarized: "[T]he patient's social and marital status are factors often quite as important in guiding [the surgeon's] decision as are the pelvic pathological findings."[51] Working women simply could not afford to have less invasive treatment, which could be more time consuming and require financial means both to pay for treatment and to assume an invalid role for some time during the treatment period and afterwards. On the other hand, working women were also more at risk when surgery was performed since often they could not afford to take the time from work or their household duties to build up their strength and health before the actual surgery occurred.

As well, physicians had to keep the needs of the society in mind and their own moral judgements about the role of women in that society. Treatment also varied depending on the training of the practitioner. The medical or surgical focus of the physician could influence what he thought would be in the best interest of his patient, what would work, and also what treatment he was most comfortable advising. What almost all agreed on, however, was to try and avoid interfering with the ability of women to bear children.

Medical Treatment

In the early years of the century, a variety of medical treatment options existed that were a continuation of those used in the late nineteenth century. Some the woman herself could implement such as patent medicines that maintained their allure despite medical criticisms of them as dangerous and lulling the patient into a false sense of well-ness.[52] When women did consult with their doctors, some of the advice could be minimal. Some advocated exercise such as cycling, especially for dysmenorrhoea and other problems women faced. Of course, not all women could afford a bicycle or even had access to one. Douching was a minimal treatment when left in the hands of the patient and was advised by both general practitioners and specialists for cleansing and treating leucorrhea, vaginitis, and cervicitis. Medicines that may have been the medical equivalent of patent medicines were advertised freely in many of the medical journals. These were treatments that did not take any particular skill to use once a physician had determined the efficacy of them in any particular case. An advertisement for "Wyeth's Elixir," a uterine sedative, exhorted "the intelligent practitioner" to use the product for "various kinds of pain incident to the diseases of the female sexual organs."[53] Such an advertisement not only appealed to the sense of pride a physician took in being an expert ("the intelligent practitioner") but also to the belief in the widespread nature of women's problems. It was an easy, noninvasive way of handling a myriad of complaints.

Medicinal sedatives were still being advertised in the postwar years for uterine disorders as well as neuroses, the conflation of the two together being a comment on the belief that the reproductive system and the mental health of the woman were somehow interrelated. Other treatment came from the necessity of using what was available. In 1936 L.R. Morse from Lawrencetown, Nova Scotia, reported on "A Morning Visit to a Rural Hospital" detailing one patient with double salpingitis (inflammation of the fallopian tubes) for whom surgery was not possible and so bed rest and application of "dry heat" became the options chosen. Other treatments came from experience, learning from what had worked in the past or for others.[54] At times, practitioners were sensitive to the situation of the woman patient. Harry Sturgeon Crossen and Robert James Crossen in their 1930 text sympathized with the fatigue of women as a result of caring for their families and household and how rest could be all that was needed. They also acknowledged the unlikelihood of many who worked for a living being able to manage to rest.[55]

Some treatments were more invasive than others. In the first decades of the century, bloodletting, often seen as a treatment of the more distant past, was still considered helpful for cases of various inflammations of the cervix. And cupping or leeching could help with the throbbing pain of subacute ovaritis. The use of electricity in medicine occurred almost as soon as electricity was available. Its use in gynaecology was in various types of ovarian, pelvic, or uterine congestions and for neurasthenia. The use of pessaries to support or reposition the womb had a long history. Their use, even in the early years of the century, however, was contentious and remained so.[56]

In addition to tried and "true" treatments, new ones emerged. One was radiation. Gynaecologists were intrigued very early on by its possibilities for metritis (inflammation of uterine lining), pruritus (itching) of the vulva, chronic pelvic cellulitis (inflammation), chronic salpingitis, and epithelioma (tumour) of the vulva, although not all physicians agreed on its use in each case.[57] In later years many physicians deemed radiation use as conservative treatment, in many cases offsetting the need for surgery.[58] Not all were willing to see radiation or X-ray as the saviour of women and worried about its cost; its impact on childbearing women and the children they would bear; and the likelihood of it bringing on premature menopause, which was not a problem for older women, but certainly for younger women.[59]

As we have seen with other problems such as infertility, another new treatment for gynaecological disorders was hormonal. A primitive form of it appeared in the early twentieth century – what was known as organotherapy. Physicians sensed that certain organs secreted substances that were necessary for health. The ovary in women was one of those organs and ovarian extract used.[60] When the sex hormones became better known in the 1920s, physicians began to endorse hormone therapy with enthusiasm, encouraged by manufacturers who began to advertise their various preparations. In July 1931 an ad appeared in *The Nova Scotia Medical Bulletin* for "Theelin, Female Sex Hormone in Crystalline Form." It informed physicians that "the therapeutic indications for Theelin are functional amenorrhoea and scanty menstruation, artificial menopause and sexual frigidity ... delayed puberty, lack of sexual development, and functional sterility." Over time, the list for the uses of "endocrine extracts" became longer,[61] extending the gynaecological gaze over other parts of the body. Despite the excitement over hormones, physicians were still coming to terms with their use. Some practitioners reminded colleagues that many of the early claims for ovarian extracts had proven false and so physicians had to be wary of the bandwagon effect. Links were being made as well between estrogen treatment and the development of some cancers.[62] Despite such warnings, many practitioners took up hormone therapy and saw in it the future of medical gynaecology.[63]

The sulphoamide drugs were also performing wonders, and by 1945 penicillin was available more widely. Certainly not everyone was "easy" to treat. Two physicians who studied the experience of gonorrhoea in women at the Division of Venereal Disease, Vancouver, noted that for those with pelvic inflammation the tendency was that those who had to work "during the acute state of their infection and through their menstrual period ... showed a higher incidence of pelvic complications. Blondes did not seem to have the same degree of natural resistance as did brunettes."[64] While the reasons for the former may have been self evident, those for the latter were not and remained unexplored. What was important was what occurred not why, for in some respects physicians could not change the why. The new drugs were welcomed, no matter what the variation in rate of response. Compared to surgery, drugs offered a less invasive response[65] and they represented optimism that venereal disease was treatable and that all that was needed was an early diagnosis and immediate treatment to offset the long list of horrendous consequences.

Surgical Conservatism

Within medicine, surgery is the most radical of solutions. While surgeons appeared to be the daredevils of gynaecology, underlying the specialty was a strong conservative orientation to preserve the childbearing abilities of women as much as possible. Many worried that too much surgery was being performed, leading to a redefinition of skill to include a surgeon who did less not more. While the focus of conservatism was on preserving ovarian function, two surgeries – the hysterectomy and sterilization – countered that orientation. Each had its own challenges and reflected different aspects facing the gynaecological surgeon. But the surgeon was never alone. He was accompanied by the patient, the woman who feared and hoped for what the outcome would be. Who these women were and how they were treated varied, but they were the true heroes of surgery.

Those espousing the conservative surgical stance feared too much surgery was occurring. In 1902, Hamilton's L.W. Cockburn suggested that gender was a factor: "When watching a surgeon ... cut away ovaries and tubes for adhesions, thickening, cirrhosis or cystic degeneration, the thought has often occurred to me as to how the operator would relish having the corresponding organ in his own person so unceremoniously whipped off!"[66] The real skill in medicine was the right treatment for the right disorder; this was easier said than done. For retroversion alone, S.M. Hay from Toronto Western Hospital estimated that there were at least 50 different operations – some good, others no longer used.[67] A physician's decision to operate was also determined by whether it morally/socially made sense to do so. Fashioning a vagina in a woman who did not have one but who did menstruate made sense; doing so in a woman without a uterus and thus for whom a vagina would be "merely ... an organ of copulation" did not.[68]

The concern that too many unnecessary gynaecological surgeries were being performed continued. Harold Atlee had given a great deal of thought to the surgery being done and, like Cockburn, argued that if ovaries had been located on the outside of the body as were the testicles of men, fewer of them would have been removed. He queried whether the golden age of the surgical "conquistador" was coming to an end. After all, the surgical technique could be "possessed" by any graduate in medicine and, unfortunately, that seemed to be occurring. Brian D. Best from Winnipeg also agreed about the unnecessary surgery being done and listed several reasons for this: "lack of surgical conscience; ignorance of gynaecological physiology and pathology; inadequate appraisal of the psychological and socio-economic aspects of pelvic complaints; incomplete or hasty investigation with inaccurate diagnosis."[69] By criticizing others for not doing a good job you placed yourself on the side of the angels.

The predominant concern for gynaecologists was removal of ovaries. The recommendation of the conservative surgeons/practitioners was to preserve as much of a healthy ovary as possible so that the woman would still be able to reproduce. When Miss Bertha Crandell, age 17, entered the Victoria General Hospital, Halifax, on 17 September 1900, she was suffering from endometritis, erosion of the cervix, anteflexion, and slight enlargement of the fundus. Surgery was performed and her right ovary was found to be cystic and thus removed. Her left ovary was slightly cystic and so it was punctured and stitched with cat gut to leave her capable of having children.[70] In addition to maintaining the reproductive potential, practitioners considered the ovaries important for other reasons. For Hay, their removal often left "the patient irritable, nervous, morbid, hysterical and neurasthenic." Remove them and you removed a woman's sense of self; she would become old before her time. Practitioners also debated whether the removal of ovaries lessened a woman's interest in sex.[71]

The importance of the ovaries and the significance of removing them raised the issue of the surgeon's skill and its meaning. For those espousing it, conservatism demanded skill. When discussing ovarian and fallopian tube problems as a cause of sterility one commentator argued that it took more skill to decide which ovary (or tube) and which part to remove than it did to remove both ovaries and tubes.[72] Skilled physicians knew when to operate; unskilled ones did not. Skilled physicians were those who did not take the easy route, the taking out of ovaries and tubes, which required "but little thought and a moderate amount of surgical skill."[73] Not all were agreed about the nature of surgical conservatism, nor the kind of picture that was being depicted of the adventuresome surgeon as taking the "easy" road to treatment. Indeed, those espousing surgical solutions often judged their skill by the radicalism of their surgery. Most outspoken was A. Lapthorn Smith, who did not feel the need to adopt a conservative approach. In many cases of what appeared to be one diseased and one healthy ovary he had left the "healthy" one intact only to find that subsequent surgery was necessary to remove the second organ. To counter the "conservatives" he made a point of saying that after removal of both ovaries women were often much stronger despite popular opinion to the contrary. But as with most everything in medicine, Lapthorn Smith's surgical decisions depended on the condition being treated: for ovarian prolapse he only removed the ovary that had enlarged and dropped. It also depended on the age of the patient, for at times even Smith succumbed to leaving a young woman with the ability to have a child even when he felt that ending it would have been better. The economic situation of the patient was an additional factor. Smith was willing to remove ovaries for the pain of dysmenorrhoea in young working women when no other treatment had worked, for it allowed them to hold down employment and "to get fat and well."[74]

What emerged in the interwar period and beyond was increasing emphasis on the psychological impact of ending the ovarian function. As one 1928 text explained, "Women ... regard menstruation, during the normal reproductive period, as one of the insignia of sex, and its regular function has, therefore, a psychic as well as physical value." An article by Karl Stern, assistant professor of psychiatry at McGill University, in a 1948 issue of *Chatelaine* explained that artificial menopause often led women to become "emotionally disturbed" due to the "symbolic meaning" of their loss. Nurses, too, found that the psychological aspect was important in the care of women undergoing such surgery.[75] Part of the psychological impact was the belief by some practitioners that the ovarian presence was linked to sexuality and as in the early years the issue was debated.[76] But whatever the reason for concern about the removal of ovaries, as late as 1948 critics raised the alarm that the "promiscuous removal or destruction of healthy ovaries" was occurring.[77] The language was rhetorical, but it separated the good physicians from others.

Compared to removal of ovaries, the hysterectomy was a more significant surgical procedure, in part because it not only removed the uterus from the woman but also, at times, included the removal of the cervix, ovaries, and tubes. Lapthorn Smith not surprisingly had an opinion on hysterectomies similar to his opinion on ovariotomies. He saw it as the best response to fibroids of the uterus as opposed to a myomectomy, which was simply a removal of the growth. The hysterectomy guaranteed that there would be no need for a subsequent surgery. At a time when any kind of abdominal surgery was a serious risk, Smith's concern was well taken. Limiting the number of surgeries for Smith defined what was conservative, not what was removed. He also argued that since most women with fibroids of the uterus were either unmarried or older, the ending of childbearing did not loom as large for them as for other women and for that reason he did not support leaving in the ovaries or the tubes.[78]

The concern and debate about hysterectomies strengthened after the first two decades of the century. E.W. Mitchell of Toronto listed the perceived advantages of the more limited hysterectomy for benign tumours of the uterus – less invasive, a lower mortality rate, and a better convalescence. In addition, the chances of the vaginal vault prolapsing were less. Significant in his mind, given the discoveries of the time in endocrinology, was that saving the ovaries or an ovary to ensure a more even menopause.[79] Certainly how close a woman was to menopause was a major factor in determining whether the hysterectomy would include the removal of the ovaries. A medical roundtable in 1950 made it clear that the age of concern was 40. After 40, the perception was that the ovarian "function" was lessening and so removal of the ovaries during a hysterectomy was acceptable. It would prevent future ovarian cancer and the belief was that after menopause the ovaries served no function.[80]

The skilled doctor was the one who did not wait to operate but did so before the situation of the patient became worse. But when was that point reached? Postmenopausal bleeding suggested potential cancer and so physicians deemed a hysterectomy conservative surgery, conservative in that its goal was to save a life. Barbara Watts, class of 1939 at the University of Toronto, pointed out, in a way with which Lapthorn Smith would have identified, that preserving some ovarian tissue in the surgical removal of endometriosis was possible but that it still could result in future surgery being necessary. In addition, the success rate for radical surgery (hysterectomy and removal of ovaries and tubes) was higher than for the conservative surgical response, 95 percent compared to 70 percent.[81] For Watts, a radical hysterectomy was the best surgery and the most temperate.

Sterilizations

Hysterectomies or removal of both ovaries were procedures that ended the ability of a woman to have children. But that was not their purpose. With sterilization it was. Sterilization struck at the very foundation of what many Canadians felt was woman's destiny and the purpose of marriage and sexual relations. It was one of the most serious medical procedures physicians could do, not because of the danger it posed to the health of the patient but because of the perceived social consequences of such surgery. Physicians tended to be very careful about discussing sterilization in the literature, making sure that everyone understood that permission was necessary before such an "extreme" measure was taken.

One of the most difficult decisions faced by physicians was when the birth of the child endangered the health and even the life of the mother. In the early years of the century, the child was often sacrificed – by performing embryotomies (mutilating the foetus) – if unable to be delivered vaginally due to disproportion between the woman's pelvis and the size of the child. Caesarian section was the only hope of saving both mother and child and while it did put the mother's life at risk in the early years, it had the advantage of allowing the physician to sterilize the woman at the same time so as to prevent future conception and thus avoid the spectre of more embryotomies.[82] Mrs M., age 26, was pregnant for the first time. She had been in labour for 30 hours before being admitted to the Women's Hospital, Montreal, and repeated efforts to birth the child, who was very large, even with the use of forceps, failed. Embryotomy was not a possibility since the woman's uncle, a priest, was present and he forbade it. As a result, physicians performed a C-section and the child was born alive, although subsequently died. What is interesting is that in the report, specific mention was made that "this patient was not

sterilized," intimating that the usual routine would have been to sterilize such a patient. Other childbirth problems could also raise the issue
of sterilization. One woman, age 37, admitted to the Women's Hospital,
Montreal, in 1906 had had 7 pregnancies, with each successive birth
more difficult than the last. Her present labour had been long and hard
with little advance being made and so a C-section was performed and
at the request of the woman sterilization occurred at the same time.[83]

In the very early years of the century, the expectation that a woman
needed a C-section (for what ever reason) and the belief that C-section
would be necessary in subsequent pregnancies often resulted in the
willingness to perform sterilization. As the dangers of the C-section
receded, some practitioners argued there was no reason that a woman
could not undergo several surgeries thus "making the operation of sterilization unnecessary and ... as a routine measure distinctly unjustifiable."[84] In response to such an attitude, in 1913 Kennedy C. McIlwraith
pointed out that the C-section was still more dangerous than vaginal
birth and because of this the woman had the right to be consulted about
sterilization. But he admitted the risk of the surgery was not one that
warranted abortion.[85] The sterilization debate was becoming a discussion of under what conditions sterilization was appropriate.

Many of the discussions of the early years continued. Physicians
were sensitive to the need to have the patient's consent and that of her
husband if surgery was going to result in sterility. In 1943 one woman
coming to the Kitchener-Waterloo hospital had to sign a form of consent
as did her husband stating that "I hereby authorize Dr ... to cut both my
fallopian tubes to render me sterile so that I will not be able to become
pregnant again at any time."[86] Two aspects of the consent process stand
out. First was that the wife as well as her husband had to agree and that
the description of what was going to take place and the result was clear.

Sterilization was a serious procedure in its social repercussions and
so it should only be undertaken when the woman's health was at risk.
As we saw in the chapter on abortion, some physicians were willing to
perform abortions and then sterilize women for whom pregnancy and
childbirth were life threatening. In such situations, sterilization was
deemed preventive medicine by many. The willingness of physicians
to sterilize for health reasons is also seen in the continued association
between sterilization and C-sections. Annual reports of hospitals
tended to distinguish between C-sections without sterilization and
those with sterilization. For example, at the Royal Victoria Hospital,
Montreal, there were 40 of the former done in 1930 and 10 of the latter.

The Burnside Lying-In Hospital reported that between 1925 and 1939 of 343 C-sections performed, 149 were accompanied by sterilizations.[87] But while the connection may have continued, many physicians were feeling that C-section did not pose the danger that it once had and that sterilization was not something that should be automatically considered.[88] More adamant was the public hostility towards sterilization as a birth control method, the reason being, in part, that the state had an investment in maintaining the ability of people to reproduce. Nonetheless Gérard Bouchard has suggested that by the 1940s numbers of women in the Saguenay area of Quebec were having hysterectomies for birth control reasons.[89]

Patient Issues

All of these concerns, debates, and critiques reflected the desire to help patients. Yet in the discussion to date the patients have appeared relatively silent. But they weren't. Patients decided when to seek medical help, and they could define or limit what physicians could do. They had power to consult and to refuse surgery, and they had the right to know what was happening to them. Medical records reveal many women who were reluctant to seek out medical assistance and waited significant periods of time before doing so. There could be many reasons for this. The ability of many women to endure discomfort for long periods before seeking medical help implies that women accommodated their bodies and only when the accommodation broke down, when women lost what control they had over their bodies, were they willing to relinquish even more control and face surgery. When a chronic situation transformed itself into an acute situation, they sought medical help. Pain was acute, discomfort was not. Being able to accomplish one's tasks, even with some pain, was chronic; not being able to was acute. But women made the decision and clearly when they did would vary depending on their circumstances. Mrs Gaeton Laforce, age 59, entered the Montreal General Hospital on 3 January 1950. She had suffered from falling of the womb for 19 years, but had coped with it on her own. What had changed was that for the month leading up to her seeking help it had been falling more frequently. She no longer could cope.[90] A hospital stay faced any patient with financial costs, but for a woman, whether a paying or charity patient, it also necessitated making arrangements to ensure that her home and/or family was cared for while she was gone. For many women a hospital stay meant separation from friends and families and for those who lived out of town the separation was even more wrenching. Women could be particularly reluctant to seek out gynaecological treatment. Gynaecology was very much a surgical specialty and the prospect of undergoing surgery was understandably frightening. The surgery was even more so when it is remembered that gynaecologists did not just repair but often removed. Almost all aspects of a woman's reproductive system could be and were removed – uterus, cervix, ovaries, fallopian tubes. The variety of gynaecological surgeries was a physician's cornucopia.

Patients did have the right to refuse treatment. Mrs Aurora Cameron, age 19, reflected the endurance of patients as well as their spirited refusal at times to follow advice. She was 17 years of age when she gave birth and after that began to have a pain in her lower abdomen on both sides. The attack did get better but kept returning. She had also experienced a "whitish discharge" since the birth and her period was excessive and irregular. The record of her surgery in 1921 described what surgeons found on opening her abdomen: "Uterus found pulled or pushed well over to left. Upper abdomen packed off. Left fallopian tube distended to 1 in. in diameter and pus filled was removed. Left ovary seat of cyst about size of small hens egg removed." After enduring all this, perhaps it was just too much for her and her record states, "[T]o certify that Mrs. Aurora Cameron has left this hospital against the advice of her attending surgeon."[91]

Physicians were not particularly sympathetic about noncompliance for it challenged their authority. Surgeons especially disliked patients who tried to dictate to them about the limits of the surgery performed. Sir Comyns Berkeley and Victor Bonney raised this in their 1942 text and concluded that a surgeon simply could not be compromised before surgery. Commitment to the patient to perform only limited surgery could be an unfortunate choice and one that a good surgeon would be hard pressed to follow.[92] Such patient recalcitrance was socially more difficult to take from a woman patient. As we have seen, in many hospitals, women did not sign their consent for surgery forms – their parents or husbands did so for them. Thus women were infantilized somewhat by the process, which reflected a wider societal view of women. When a woman resisted, it was unexpected and unwelcome.

Case records suggest at times patients could be very vague about what had been done to them. For example, Jane Granger, age 30, entered the Montreal General Hospital on 6 January 1902 complaining of pain to the point of keeping her in bed. Her case record read: "[S]he had some operation in M.G.H. three years ago next March – when she believes an ovary was removed and the uterus ventrofixed."[93] Her vagueness about what surgery she had undergone suggests a different way of understanding her body than the medical. She had a problem, saw a physician, and went to a hospital to have surgery to fix it. From her point of view that was all she needed to know except that the surgery did not seem to have worked. One could suggest that her attitude shows considerable faith in the medical system and what physicians could do for her. It also revealed high expectations of treatment and disappointment when it did not work. The lack of knowledge of their bodies was a problem for many women but was one that was increasingly becoming public. In the May 1949 issue of *Chatelaine*, the author of an article on hysterectomies explained to readers the nature of the surgery and informed them that it prevented future childbearing and ended menstruation, but that it did not necessarily mean the removal of ovaries or the onslaught of the menopause. What the author was trying to do was to end the kind of mythology surrounding hysterectomy that had existed for some time, that after a hysterectomy a woman was no longer a woman. That such an article appeared in the magazine reflected women's interest in a procedure that clearly was becoming better known.[94] Women talked about their surgeries and wanted to understand, and were becoming more consumer savvy.

Patients were the heroes of their own stories as they underwent incredibly serious and complex surgeries. Mrs Perle George, age 40 and married for 20 years, entered the Royal Victoria Hospital, Montreal, on 9 June 1903 suffering from backache, headache, pain in the right side, frequency of micturition, and some leucorrhoea. The backache and abdominal pain had begun seven years previously when she gave birth to her last child. Three years later she began to feel a "moveable mass in right loin." She had given birth to 10 children, which meant that she had had her 10 children by the age of 33 and in 13 years of marriage. She was diagnosed with chronic endometritis, relaxed vaginal outlet, and lacerated cervix, for which she underwent dilation, curettage, amputation of the cervix, and repair of her perineum. Mrs Annette Mobley, age 32, entered the Kitchener-Waterloo hospital on 13 January 1943. Her patient record described her recent medical history. In 1929 at age 18 she had an appendectomy; five years later she had a nervous breakdown. Two years after she had peritonitis, a result of ovarian inflammation. In that year she had her left ovary removed and the next year her uterus removed. In 1943 she was suffering from pain in her hypogastric region. She had part of her hymen removed.[95] Such women and many others testified to the incredible strength and endurance of the "fragile" sex.

Conclusion

The history of gynaecology has turned out to be a history of medicine in that gynaecology cannot be understood without understanding its perceived connection with obstetrics and other specialties. Neither can it be understood without an appreciation of the speed at which knowledge about the female cycle emerged in the interwar years and beyond. That doctors have difficulty keeping up with the changes in medicine is one of the few constants of their profession. Change is inherent in medical science and it increasingly fed medical practice. What didn't seem to change all that much was the perception of the body that was gynaecology's focus.

All the above played into the doctor/patient dynamic. Certainly physicians had a view of women patients that often reflected the gendered norms of women in the wider society. They were aware of the vulnerabilities to both physician and patient when the former was a man and the latter a woman and the focus of both was the most private aspect of a woman's body – her reproductive/sexual system. Debates over this issue and on how to best treat their patients – medically and surgically – were ongoing and exposed the turf wars to which the surgical choice led: the choice to go with a tried and true procedure versus one that was new and often promised more than it could deliver, the increasing complexity of the surgery and its limits, and the critique of surgeons as medical practitioners. Within what appears the irreducible current of surgical dominance was the rhetoric of conservatism. It was a rhetoric, however, shifting in meaning depending on who was writing. Such a concept would be one that would be familiar to postmodern analysts. It was certainly a contingent concept, varying with the age of the woman, her economic status, and the organ (or part) being removed. The concept encompassed the skill of the surgeon or practitioner and, because it had a commonsense appeal, even those who were fully supportive of surgical solutions could reinterpret conservatism to include what it was they did; it was integral to seeing themselves as skilled. The reasons for supporting the conservative approach were reflective of the value system of the time: protect a young woman's ability to procreate; the lesser need to protect an older woman's reproductive system; the assumption (perhaps accurate) that the psychological impact of much of the gynaecological surgery done was serious enough to be seen as a counter indication to some surgery; and the conflicting opinions about surgery's impact on women's sexuality and the concern about surgery bringing on a premature menopause. Underlying the discussions was the need to determine what was good practice and to be able to articulate that practice.

9 The Womanly Body: A Cancer Threat

The images of cancer are not positive. Early in the century physicians considered it a "dreaded disease" with an "insidious nature," resulting in "suffering and great mortality." Even when doctors considered the curative rate improving, Canadians remained caught in their fear of cancer, as its incidence rate continued to increase with thousands of Canadians dying from it each year.[1] This chapter examines the way in which physicians dealt with cancer in women, focusing specifically on cervical and breast cancer.[2] In doing so, several common themes with respect to the two cancers emerge. First was the way in which doctors perceived women's bodies as problematic. Cervical and breast cancer suggested that women who met their womanly obligations to marry and have children were at risk, as if there was a design flaw in their bodies. Second was the feeling of urgency in treating cancer leading to a sense that the body was guilty until proven innocent. Third was a consequence of the second, the drastic nature of treatment. Women's bodies became a battlefield on which doctors fought the enemy – death in the guise of cancer.

Cancer's Historical Context

As infectious diseases came under control and their mortality rate declined in the first half century, cancer loomed larger with mortality rates second only to diseases of the heart.[3] The widespread and deadly nature of cancer led physicians to seek general explanations of susceptibility, be they diet, class, heredity, race, or even civilization. For example, an editorial in *The Canada Lancet* of 1907 argued that cancer was more prevalent among the "well-to-do and well-fed" classes and using this perception as a way of explaining causation posited the notion that cancer would strike at those organs of the body receiving more blood than others. The class component was difficult to maintain, however, as statistics gathered increasingly suggested that cancer recognized no class boundaries, and was increasing "in all civilized countries." As for race, one turn-of-the-century American text pointed out that one out of every hundred whites (men and women) died of cancer – only one of every three hundred blacks did. At times culture seemed more powerful than race, although linked to it. E.E. Montgomery in his 1912 *Practical Gynecology* noted that cancer was increasing and that researchers had attributed this to type of diet.[4] Cancer statistics revealed women had higher rates of cancer of the peritoneum, intestines, and rectum. Men suffered from cancer of the cheek cavity and from skin cancer. Sometimes physicians recognized a particular gendered behaviour being at fault. For example, cancer of the lip was found more in men due to their habit of smoking "dirty, short clay pipes." The body itself also meant that most breast cancers occurred in women and cervical cancer existed only in women (as did prostate cancer in men). Age was also a factor in that cancer deaths in women occurred about 10 years earlier than in men, at age 55 rather than 65, but after age 65 men's deaths soon exceeded women's.[5] Whether convincing or not, physicians used such factors both to advise preventative measures and identify people at risk.

Canadians had difficulty ignoring cancer's existence – its visibility increased and the public efforts to overcome its threat increasingly organized. As early as the 1920s, L'Institut du Radium in Montréal provided treatment for those with cancer. In the 1930s Saskatchewan introduced legislation to establish the Cancer Relief Act; the Canadian Medical Association (CMA) responded to a request from its Alberta affiliate to study the problem of cancer throughout the country; the government of Nova Scotia announced its intention to establish a "Cancer Institute"; the Ontario Institute of Radiotherapy (with clinics eventually in Kingston, Toronto, and London) opened in cooperation with the provincial Department of Health to provide cancer treatment on a more centralized basis; and the British Columbia Cancer Society was founded. In the 1940s, Alberta introduced the Cancer Treatment and Prevention Act and the Provincial Royal Jubilee Hospital in Vancouver reported with pride in its *Annual Report* that it had purchased a "400 K.V. Deep X-Ray Therapy machine" for use in cancer treatment.[6]

The more organized approach to cancer treatment was a reflection of societal concern about the disease and also a belief that if enough resources were poured into treatment and research then science would find a cure.

Cancer was a frightening disease and physicians resorted to heroic measures to treat it. The perception in the early part of the century that inoperable cancers far exceeded the operable led to the adoption of a variety of treatments, most of which proved of little use: "injections of alcohol, turpentine, acetic acid ... venom of cobra, the application of calcium carbide and the administration of certain drugs, e.g., thyroid extract." Patients and practitioners alike touted new treatments, and some practitioners also turned to alternative treatments that appeared to have some glimmer of scientific respectability. The 1934 *Canadian Medical Association Journal* abstracted an article that suggested using fresh human placenta and ovary "plus certain special sera" and blood transfusion resulted in an increase in general cancer cure rates of 25 percent when such methods were used in conjunction with surgery and radiation.[7] The respectability in this case was the addition of something new to approaches that already dominated cancer treatment. Surgery as a therapeutic had long existed and its underlying rationale as cancer treatment was in removing the cancer through cutting out diseased and suspected diseased tissue or organs. When supported by the theory of the localized origin and growth of cancer – that it began with one abnormal cell which duplicated and spread centrifugally to surrounding tissues – the logic of surgery became almost irresistible.[8] It explained cancer in a way that allowed physicians to act and patients to understand. The results of surgery could be seen and it appealed to the interventionist philosophy of western medicine.

Radiation therapy – X-rays or use of radium – was a twentieth-century therapeutic. North Americans used radium sparingly in the early years because of lack of supplies and cost but by the 1930s it had come into its own, with the CMA Committee on Cancer reporting in 1933 that clinics for diagnosis and radium facilities were available in eight provinces. By 1947 there were 55 X-ray and 33 radium treatment centres throughout the country.[9] While some medical pundits worried that radiation was being depended on too much, others opposed its use for political/vested reasons. For example, in Winnipeg some physicians were treating their cancer patients surgically rather than sending them to the Manitoba Cancer Relief and Research Institute (MCRRI) for radiation treatment because they disliked MCRRI's control over radium in the region and because nonphysicians ran the institute. Opposition also came from those who disliked the quick rise of radiation and what appeared to be a threat to surgery's dominance. Opposition to the Institut du Radium and its assertive self-publicity came from surgeons in Montreal who felt threatened by any suggestion that radiotherapy might remove patients from them for benign disorders or obviate the need for surgery in cancer patients.[10]

With two "acceptable" treatments available, physicians urged the "facts" about cancer be publicized to encourage Canadians to consult their doctors when danger signals appeared. Too many delayed because of fear; the cost of treatment; indifference; family responsibilities; denial; or, in the case of women, modesty.[11] While understanding the reasons Canadians delayed seeking medical help, doctors considered them negligible compared to the death that awaited them if they did not. As a result, underlying the medical concern about "delay" was a tone of frustration on the part of many physicians. From their perspective, such individuals were not acting according to medical rationality. Even when patients sought medical advice, surgeons complained that too many general practitioners did not take the symptoms presented to them seriously enough.[12] But it was easy for surgeons to blame general practitioners. Surgeons tended to see patients once the disease had advanced and so perhaps were not as understanding of the diagnostic problems faced by general practitioners as they might have been. They also did not acknowledge the emotional trauma for general practitioners having to tell someone they probably knew and whose family they knew that s/he had a potentially deadly disease.

Cervical Cancer

In 1902 A. Lapthorn Smith, professor of clinical gynaecology at Bishops University, noted that in his early practice not a week passed by without a woman coming to him

with the cervix a mass of cancer, and the broad ligaments full of the same disease, so that it was impossible to draw the uterus down, even as much as a quarter of an inch ... At that time nothing was attempted for the relief of these patients except to keep them as free from pain as possible by means of opium or morphine suppositories. The smell was so horrible that their friends and relatives might well be forgiven for praying for their death. And when death at last came, either from sepsis or hemorrhage, every one, including the patient and doctor, was very glad.

Such a death was a "happy release." While the point to Smith's article was to suggest that things had changed by 1902, the reality was that the image of the "old" days that he conjured up was still in evidence.[13]

Frequency and Causation

Cervical cancer was one of the most common cancers in women. In the 1940s, W.G. Cosbie of Toronto estimated that it was the second most common site of cancer in women. And its mortality was high – second only to cancer of the breast for female deaths from malignancy.[14] Women who conformed to the norms of society – who married and had children, especially those with many children – were most at risk.[15] If the body was made to have children, as so many physicians suggested, there seemed to be a design flaw. The focus on childbirth was appealing because it fit a broader understanding that physical trauma caused cancer, in this case to the cervix. Indeed any trauma to the cervix could be dangerous and so no woman was exempt even if she had not given birth.[16] The trauma theory in the early years provided both patient and physician with a reason for the cancer appearing where it did. While not disagreeing with the trauma theory, some practitioners in the early years focused on other factors. Some noted, for example, the emotional pressures many women experienced that might lead to cancer: worry about money, illnesses of husband and children, grief over the death of family members, for widows "the depressing monotony" of their lives, and becoming older. Physicians were willing to grasp at any seeming correlation – even being well nourished.[17] But, it could be asked, what has all this to do with cancer of the cervix uteri? Why were the pressures focused on the cervix rather on some other part of the body? Few answers were forthcoming. Neither were the contradictions among doctors' views debated or reconciled.

Many of the beliefs of the early years of the century continued with new ones being added. Trauma to the cervix remained a popular explanation. Some practitioners emphasized not only the problems that arose from childbed experiences but also at times blamed poor obstetric care for the cervical lacerations that too often went unattended and became sites for cancer. In 1935, Eleanor Percival, a Montreal physician, took up the class origins of cervical cancer, arguing poor women lacked medical care and that private patients received superior care in child-birth so would not have as much childbirth trauma that could lead to cancer. She also noted that Jewish women seemed to have lower rates of cervical cancer than did other women. The reason given was culture since among Jewish women "any discharge is considered 'unclean' and is therefore cared for." For women who did not have children, some physicians blamed "chronic infection and developmental abnormalities." One Niagara Falls physician in 1934 argued that women practising birth control could develop endocervicitis, which he claimed could lead to cervical cancer. Others attributed the cancer to heredity. Age seemed less significant than it had been. While some linked cervical cancer and menopause, others noted that a significant percentage of cervical cancer occurred in women between the ages of 36 and 40, the years before menopause.[18]

Making correlations were ways physicians had of understanding causation. They noted the women who were more susceptible to cervical cancer and speculated on the risk factors that led to cancer's development in such women. But despite the interest in who would get cervical cancer and in causation, there was no significant debate about either. Risk factors were put forward as fixed and added to over time. Nonetheless physicians hoped that by accumulating what they perceived was information about cervical cancer they would eventually determine its cause. Their speculations paved the way and also reflected their desperation to understand in the hopes that understanding would allow them to treat their patients more successfully. For men of science, not understanding was not an option.

Diagnosis and Prevention

While who developed cervical cancer and why were interesting questions for practitioners, they gave much more attention to diagnosis and prevention. As with many cancers, doctors were concerned that women and their colleagues understand what the early signs of cervical cancer were. Agreement existed throughout the first half century that any unusual genital bleeding, especially after menopause, was a sign about which to be concerned with respect to the cervix.[19] Such bleeding was suspicious with an early estimate in 1900 being that in 95 percent of cases it indicated a malignancy of some kind, perhaps an exaggeration to prove the point. Just over 30 years later the estimate was that post-menopausal bleeding was a sign of malignancy in about 50 percent of women.[20] The trouble was that many women did not consider irregular bleeding unusual and often attributed it to the onset of menopause or some other cause, menstrual or otherwise. As a result, too many women did not consult their physicians early enough in their disease for treatment to be successful. Exacerbating the delay was lack of pain to warn women that something was amiss and women's reluctance to seek out regular pelvic examinations. Harold Atlee's response reflected the frustration of his colleagues. He argued any irregular bleeding should be presumed to signify cancer until proven otherwise. If a physician could not satisfy himself that a woman did not have cancer then he should send her to a cancer clinic and if she refused to go he should inform her relatives. Atlee's fear was that cancer developed so quickly that delay was irresponsible. Women's bodies posed a threat and physicians were in a race against time, and often the patient herself, to save her life.[21] Even if the woman did consult her general practitioner, however, he might not have responded. As late as 1947 estimates by one official with the Manitoba Relief and Research Institute was that general practitioners in the province saw cancer of the cervix rarely.[22] That being the case, they could easily misinterpret the symptoms of the cancer for something else.

Diagnosis and treatment of "minor" ailments was part of the prevention of major ones. W. Blair Bell, professor of gynaecology and obstetrics, University of Liverpool, looking back on his work in the early years of the century noted that he advocated "every badly infected cervix should be repaired or removed, for it is doubtful whether cancer occurs in an uninjured uninfected, virgin cervix."[23] Such a stance linked itself to the belief in trauma causation. By the 1920s, prevention was more than fixing what was obviously wrong – it was monitoring women, especially those who had had children, through yearly or half-yearly physical examinations to see if there were any observable changes in the cervix. The purpose was not to wait for the cancer to start, but to prevent it from starting by eliminating precancerous conditions – cervical lacerations, cervical erosions, leucorrhoea – that could only be discerned through an internal examination and treated. Such check-ups reminded women that their bodies were potential sources of danger. Nonetheless examinations were the first line of defence and the medical literature urged both physicians and women to understand this.[24] Such urging reflected how "normal" the internal examination had become from the point of view of physicians and how problematic they considered the female body.

Pelvic examinations elicited strong reactions from female sufferers and even some practitioners. A 1922 educational manual for physicians noted, "Too often the disinclination of the patient and the indifference of the physician combine to postpone this examination until too late for cure of the disease."[25] In 1932 only 40 percent of Saskatchewan women consulted their physicians with respect to cervical cancer in an early stage; in 1939 the figure was still only 54 percent. In a history of the Toronto General Hospital, Dr W.G. Cosbie pointed out that with regard to the treatment of cervical cancer no methods of early diagnosis had been established and that in the late 1940s more than 60 percent of the patients coming to the Cancer Institute had advanced lesions, which lowered the survival rate to 35 percent.[26] Without an examination, early diagnosis could not occur so it was the woman's responsibility to see her doctor and her doctor's responsibility to do an internal examination. Certainly G.C. Maloney felt that compared to uterine cancer, cancer of the cervix was easy to detect since the cervix, unlike the uterus, was not hidden from gaze but easily accessible through a medical examination.[27]

Even if the woman underwent an internal examination, not all physicians agreed on the significance of the so-called precancerous conditions and how precancerous they really were. Neither was there a way to distinguish noncancerous from precancerous and so the lack of consensus meant diagnostic prevention varied. Only a biopsy could provide a conclusive diagnosis, and even it could only "catch" the cancer at an advanced stage.[28] While biopsies were invasive procedures, in her study of cancer in Ontario Barbara Clow has determined that physicians were using them more on cervical lesions than on any other form of "neoplasia."[29]

The real advance in diagnosis was the Pap smear. In 1928 Dr Papanicoulaou, a Greek-American physician, presented a paper on diagnosing cancer with a vaginal smear and observing single malignant cells that had been cast off from the tumour into the vaginal secretion. His findings were not immediately taken up in large part for the reason expressed by Maloney – the physical access of the cervix.[30] With the wider acceptance of the vaginal smear test in the 1940s, however, diagnosis for cervical cancer became more straightforward. Canadian J. Ernest Ayre was a strong advocate and in his description of how a cervical smear worked became almost poetic: "The cervical smear is taken from the surface of the growth and so it is very much like a surface biopsy, and has been compared to raking a lawn – the leaves gathered up may be shrunken but they still possess the identity of structure of the mother plant. So it is with cancer – the cells shed from the surface are identical to those in the growth."[31] What the Pap smear offered was an earlier diagnosis based on screening. The smear was fast and easy to do and once the reliability issue (false negatives and positives) were overcome it was preferable to biopsy. Canadian women were fortunate. Canada was at the forefront of early detection and began setting up screening clinics in the late 1940s with British Columbia being in the vanguard. Yet as already noted, screening reminded women of the danger their bodies posed to them. Screening clinics also charged a modest fee for the exam, which meant that poorer women did not go even though these were the women less likely to have or to consult their own physicians and have an examination.[32] Even with the significant advances in diagnosis, some still believed the message of early detection and the need for examinations was a difficult one for physicians to accept.[33] Certainly the challenge of getting apparently healthy women to come in for what was still an unwanted and rather personal examination was one factor as was the time this would take from a physician's already busy schedule. Prevention for many physicians and patients was what the latter could do for themselves, not what physicians could do for them. Physicians' work was treating patients who were ill.

Treatment

In the early years of the century, the only hope for treatment and cure was surgical – that is, removing the part of the body the cancer was attacking. The real question was how much of the reproductive system to remove. For cervical cancer, while some surgeons removed the cervix, many preferred the removal of the uterus as well feeling that it was an easier procedure and guaranteed a better chance of eliminating all the cancer.[34] The mortality rate from the surgery itself was considered minor (at five percent), but the recurring nature of the cancer was discouraging. Perhaps it was this high rate of recurrence that resulted in some doctors allowing the disease to run its course without resorting to surgery. In that case, they provided the woman with palliative care in the form of opium or morphine suppositories. Curettage and cauterization also could make the last years of the woman's life more bearable.[35] Even with surgery, cervical cancer survival rates were not high. In 1917, for cases deemed operable (maybe only one quarter to one third), only one quarter to one third of those might be "cured."[36] Surgery was a treatment of desperation and was largely confined to the early years, eventually being superceded by radiation.

In the early years of the century, when cervical cancer was inoperable or recurring, some practitioners resorted to X-ray or radium therapy.[37] It was in the postwar period, however, when radiation came into its own. By the end of the 1920s, so convinced were physicians about the promise of radium that in the 1929 *Annual Report* of the Royal Victoria Hospital, Montreal, the report of the Department of Obstetrics and Gynaecology could confidently state, "The improved radium results in carcinoma of the cervix lend support to the view that radium is the logical treatment of this condition." By the early 1930s, the Toronto General Hospital had specially designed radium applicators for use in treating women with cervical cancer. In Manitoba, the MCRRI in Winnipeg reported the most common condition for which its radium was used was cervical cancer.[38] Radiologists were understandably excited and A. Stanley Kirkland, a radiologist from St John, exuded confidence when he declared that "radium has proved itself the master of carcinoma in the cervix." Cosbie announced that in North America radium had consigned surgery "to the realm of history."[39] If an exaggeration, some certainly believed that the results of radium treatment approached what the best surgeons could do. Seldom did physicians get a case detected early enough for surgery and, in any event, surgery had a high recurrence rate. Radium allowed later stages and recurrent cases to be treated.[40] In 1936 Gordon Richards, one of Canada's leading radiologists, estimated a survival rate (of five years) of close to 30 percent. Some practitioners, however, questioned the hyperbole surrounding radiation treatment and the survival statistics. Joseph Colt Bloodgood, a Canadian practising in Baltimore, reported in 1935 that a 33–40 percent cure rate was misleading for it only included those women whom doctors felt could be cured. Given that most women coming to be treated for cervical cancer were not good candidates, the cure rate was exaggerated.[41] Nevertheless, the literature claimed cervical cancer radiocurable.[42]

Despite the performance of radiation, supporters of surgery remained. In the 1930s, high surgical cure figures were claimed and debated.[43] In 1948 *Modern Medicine of Canada* published the opinion of Dr Meigs, clinical professor at Harvard, who acknowledged the decline of surgery for cervical cancer for good reasons. In noting that medicine did not stay still, he felt it was important, nevertheless, to reconsider surgery's decline, arguing that with advances in surgery – blood transfusions and antibiotics – "the surgical attack should again be tried to determine if some cases of cervical cancer would not be better treated

by this means." In an attempt to walk the line between surgery supporters and radiation advocates, M. Lederman, deputy director of the
radiotherapy department, Royal Cancer Hospital in London, England,
suggested that surgeons and radiologists cooperate to determine which
treatment was best for the individual patient instead of letting the decision be made by the expertise of whomever she happened to go to see.[44]
Unfortunately, little detailed discussion of this appeared in the medical
literature.

The repercussions of treatment choice could be severe. In their 1930
text *Diseases of Women*, Harry Sturgeon Crossen and Robert James
Crossen described the surgical treatment for cancer of the cervix uteri:
"By 'radical operation' is not meant any particular form of operation,
but any operation that removes all tissues likely to be involved in that
particular case. As to what tissues may be removed, by those skilled
in pelvic work, that is well known." Then they listed what could be
removed. The cervix was the minimum but in some cases "the lower
part of one or both ureters may be removed, or a part of the whole
of the bladder, or a part of the whole of the rectum. Also, the pelvic
connective tissue generally with its contained lymphatic vessels and
glands, may be cleared out to the soft structures of the pelvic wall, and
the enlarged lymphatic glands about the iliac vessels may be extir-
pated." For the Crossens, the attitude seemed to be, "Let's see what we
can remove and still have the woman survive." Little discussion in the
medical literature occurred about what the repercussions of removing
these various "parts" would be, nor the consequences to the patient's
future life, although some did raise the issue of whether "marital relations" could survive such surgery.[45] As for the consequences of radium,
as J.D. McQueen of the Winnipeg General Hospital noted in 1934, they,
too, were not harmless:

> local necrosis, fistulae, fatal infections, alarming anaemias, may and do
> result from injudicius dosage and application. Only by familiarity with,
> and attention to, the many details in the technique of application can these
> complications be avoided. Inadequate dosage, on the other hand, accom-
> plishes little and brings the use of radium into disrepute.[46]

Even applying it was uncomfortable with a probe being inserted into the
vagina and the woman being asked to lie still for hours while she was
"bombarded" with X-rays. If using radium, then either her vagina was
packed with radium or radium needles were inserted into her cervix.[47]

Nevertheless, it would appear that radiation had a lower mortality rate than surgery; the patient recovered from the effects of it better; and in some cases it allowed the woman to still bear children, something that surgery prevented.[48]

The treatment of cervical cancer did change with time. Radiation, which was new in the early years of the century, had become the treatment favoured. What had also changed was the significant improvement of diagnosis through the Pap smear. It is because of these two shifts that the optimism about curing cervical cancer and other cancers became more believable.

Breast Cancer

A similar optimism in breast cancer treatment was more difficult to maintain. In a 1934 *Canadian Medical Association Journal* article, British surgeon Geoffrey Keynes noted the dominance of William Halsted's radical mastectomy in the treatment of breast cancer:

> There are few departments of surgery in which practice has become so thoroughly standardized as in the treatment of carcinoma of the breast. The work of Halsted and his successors has grounded so securely the principle of operation, and the results have been relatively so good, that for many years there have been no two opinions as to how to deal with a carcinoma of the breast.[49]

The dominance of Halsted's surgery continued well after mid century. The result was women with breast cancer faced the prospect of significant body mutilation.

Frequency and Causation

At the turn of the century, after uterine/cervical cancer, cancer of the breast was the most common cancer in women. Even more significant, breast cancer death rates in Canada were high: 4.5 per 100,000 in 1914 and 13.2 per 100,000 in the early 1920s. By mid century, the death rate had climbed to 56 deaths per 100,000. Gordon E. Richards, director of the Ontario Institute of Radiotherapy, Toronto General Hospital, pointed out that in 1947, 1500 deaths per year were attributed to breast cancer. Nonetheless, like cervical cancer, breast cancer was not a common complaint in general practices. In 1947, estimates by one official of the Manitoba Cancer Relief and Research Institute suggested "that the average practitioner saw a cancer of the breast once in nine years."[50]

Historians have debated whether physicians perceived breast cancer risk linked to women's "essential nature" rather than outside factors such as trauma or the "dangers of civilization."[51] In the literature Canadian physicians were reading and writing on breast cancer both views existed. Because breast cancer occurred predominantly in women, physicians often looked to women's bodies as a causal explanation and determined it was their improper use or nonuse of those bodies that accounted for the development of breast cancer. In turn, their actions were very much linked to concerns about "civilization" and its creation – the modern woman about whom physicians, along with many Canadians, seemed concerned. Trauma also was a factor, although the trauma did not have to originate outside the body. It could happen as a result of the body itself.

In a 1912 study of cancer in Ontario, John Joseph Cassidy, editor of the *Canadian Journal of Medicine and Surgery*, reported the belief by some that cancer was especially liable to attack parts of the body "which had survived their usefulness," among which were the breasts of women after menopause. In the 1928 *University of Toronto Medical Journal*, E.A. Keenleyside noted that breast cancer was a disease of women much more so than men (80:1) "owing to the larger size of the gland in the female, its periodical functional activity, and to the greater incidence of disease of other kinds in the female breast." He estimated that 80 percent of women with breast cancer were or had been married and 70 percent had had children. The most common age was between 40 and 45.[52]

Keenleyside's descriptions were typical of how physicians used correlations to give an impression of understanding disease etiology. In Keenleyside's listing, it would seem that the relative larger size of the gland in women than in men was a factor of significance. Does this mean a woman with a larger "gland" than other women would be more prone to breast cancer as well? That issue was not addressed. Keenleyside's point that 80 percent of the women suffering from breast cancer had been married and of these 70 percent had had children would lead the reader to assume that marriage and childbearing were somehow related to breast cancer. Yet most women married and had children, and most of those women did not suffer from breast cancer. Keenleyside's statistics are not incorrect, only evidence of co-relationships not cause and effect relationships. Indeed, six years after Keenleyside's publication, the relationship between marriage and cancer posited with such statistical assurance came under scrutiny and was deemed "a statistical fallacy."[53] It was not marriage per se that was the crucial factor but fertility and its extent.

The childbirth link reinforced belief in trauma causation, although its linkage to breast cancer was unclear other than through breast feeding. In 1939, M.A.R. Young of Lamont Hospital, Lamont, Alberta, noted that breast cancer was rare in Ukrainian women and explained that Ukrainian women tended to nurse their children longer than was usual among most Canadian women. But Young also raised other possible factors. Slavs were "probably the purest racial entity in Europe today" and since they seldom married "out," perhaps breast cancer might have a racial and a hereditary dimension. Neither did Ukrainian women seem as susceptible to "civilizing" trends as other women. They did not wear corsets, brassieres, or other breast supports. They worked outdoors in the garden and fields; in essence they were more "natural" women.[54] The portrait was of a stereotypical peasant woman, hardly what most Canadian women wanted to be or what most in society would see as the epitome of Canadian womanhood.

The issues raised by Young reflected wider societal concerns. As already noted in the chapter on motherhood, breast feeding was declining and experts, recognizing its value in ensuring the health of infants, were trying to encourage women to breast feed and to do so longer. The cancer argument was simply another reason that supported physicians' endorsement of breastfeeding – it was good not only for the infant but also for the woman herself. Young's description of the Ukrainian-Canadian woman as more "natural" than her Canadian sisters had embedded within it concerns about the "civilizing" aspects of modernity that seemed to be destroying the traditional role of women, a prospect that many Canadians found disturbing. Unlike many cancers, breast cancer did not seem to be blamed on specific lifestyle factors. But in the emphasis on the need for women to breast feed and breast feed longer, a more traditional view of women's role in society was being endorsed to some degree and a modern one, if not rejected, at least challenged. The challenge, however, had limits. While practitioners were arguing that breast feeding was good for both infant and mother, as the chapter on motherhood and breast feeding indicated, they also were uncomfortable about what they saw as extended breast feeding.

In the 1930s and 1940s, some physicians began to make a link between the female hormone estrogen and breast cancer. The linkage, while disturbing, was at least confirmation of some tenuous cause and effect and helped offset the sense of uncertainty in the medical literature. While the CMA remained neutral on the issue, others responded with warnings against giving estrogen to women with high rates of family breast or genital cancer.[55] Some physicians so strongly believed the suspicions about the estrogen/breast cancer connection that they advocated removing ovaries as a palliative approach to breast cancer.[56] Noteworthy is that the fertility, breast feeding, and estrogen theories of causation contradicted the apparent relationship between breast cancer and older women. Breast cancer did not appear frequently during the years when fertility, breast feeding, and the presence of estrogen were of moment. That being the case, it suggested that breast cancer was a delayed disease or one with a long incubation.

Diagnosis and Prevention

While accurate diagnosis was important for all cancers, physicians were not agreed on the best diagnostic method for breast cancer. They debated the advantages and disadvantages of clinical examination versus biopsy, revealing a profession that was dynamic in its argumentation. The debate also highlighted practitioners who were more comfortable with the tried and true rather than the "new," especially when the latter meant relinquishing some control of the diagnostic process to others.[57]

Clinical diagnosis was the oldest and most familiar diagnostic tool. Based on sight and touch it had been the bedrock of medical diagnosis for centuries and depended on the physician knowing both the signs of the disease and his patient. I have already noted how few cases of breast cancer general practitioners actually saw. Nevertheless, in the early years of the century, because women often presented themselves so far along in the disease that the signs of breast cancer were clear, diagnosis would have been easier than later became the case. Diagnosis early in the disease was more difficult. As a result, when women did seek advice early in the disease, the practitioner could too easily keep his patient under observation too long or dismiss her concerns.[58] Similar to cervical cancer, complicating the situation was the need to be aware of precancerous conditions that might exist and the debate over what was precancerous. For example, chronic mastitis had long been a reason for some to remove breasts. Yet in 1934 Max Cutler in his paper before the Annual Meeting of the CMA in Calgary argued that mastitis was too general and vague a term on which to make such a decision. Fourteen years later Margaret MacLachlan, a new graduate of the University of Western Ontario, gave her opinion that chronic cystic mastitis rarely changed into a malignant condition.[59] In addition to precancerous conditions, physicians had to consider the age of the woman, with women over the age of 40 who presented themselves with breast symptoms being particularly suspect.[60] Such factors needed to be considered before making a diagnosis but what weight to give to each of them was unclear as the perceived importance of each changed over time. Consequently, diagnosis at the clinical level was becoming increasingly complicated and difficult.

If clinical diagnosis was the traditional diagnostic method, biopsy was newer and engendered debate within the profession. It consisted of two types. A quick frozen biopsy (developed in the late nineteenth century) occurred in a surgical setting in which the surgeon, after removing a section of the tumour, waited in the operating room for the pathology diagnosis before proceeding. The result was one-step surgery, a situation in which the patient would enter the operating room not knowing whether she would awaken with both breasts or not. A second form of biopsy was more detailed; it could involve the local doctor, and resulted in two-step surgery. A tissue sample was taken and sent to a laboratory for analysis, and the results reported some time later. If surgery was indicated, it would be scheduled. Such a process gave the patient time to accept the idea of having cancer, if that is indeed what the biopsy showed. She would undergo surgery knowing what would happen. It would also allow for more careful biopsies without the pressure of a surgical timetable.[61]

Criticism of biopsy emerged in the interwar period, a reflection of and reaction to more being done. It also was a reaction against the use of "accessory aids to diagnosis" instead of effective clinical diagnosis.[62] In 1924, Alexander Primrose, dean of medicine, University of Toronto, argued that not only was a "quick section" potentially dangerous in spreading the cancer, it was also unreliable since it did not let the physician know whether there was cancer beyond the section being tested. For Bloodgood, concern that a biopsy could spread the cancer was easily met. Combine it with "irradiation," which would both stop the cancer from spreading due to interference with it and allow time for the diagnosis to be made. The latter would help overcome the problem of having benign tumours misdiagnosed as malignant and vice versa. Bloodgood's procedure would allow for a two-step surgery and thus give time for the woman to become accustomed to a firm diagnosis of breast cancer. If she did not have cancer, however, it would mean she had been exposed to "irradation." She would also have undergone significant surgery since Bloodgood's idea of biopsy could be extreme. He described what should be done in a case of a woman who presented symptoms of tumour of the nipple. The decision was to do "an immediate biopsy, and this biopsy should consist of the excision of the nipple, the areola around the nipple and all the nipple and breast tissue beneath, continuing until a complete zone of the breast tissues is removed."[63] If some physicians, like Primrose, were wary of the consequences of biopsy, others also pointed out that the science of medicine as represented by biopsy was fallible – false positives and negatives could and did occur. N.E. McKinnon of the Department of Epidemiology and Biometrics, University of Toronto, blamed the wider medical culture of cancer phobia for influencing pathological diagnosis in the direction of false positive test results;[64] that is, those reading the biopsies were influenced by the "rather safe than sorry" attitude that was so common in the treatment of cancer.

The advent of biopsy did not do away with clinical diagnosis. After all, a physician's examination had to turn up some clinical evidence before he would advise a biopsy. In some circumstances a biopsy seemed redundant, the diagnosis was so obvious. Of course the circumstances varied from physician to physician and patient to patient. Some practitioners remained attached to the benefit of clinical diagnosis even when faced with an opposing tissue diagnosis. It was a commitment to the experience of medical practice rather than its theory. Even Primrose didn't discount biopsy; for cases where a malignancy seemed unlikely and when a pathologist was on hand, it was insurance against a faulty clinical diagnosis, but he didn't privilege it. But as J.G. MacDougall of Halifax pointed out, clinical diagnosis, even in an incision form, was only as good as the physician who did it.[65]

As with cervical cancer, physicians feared women with breast cancer were not seeking help early in their disease. But delay was understandable. The breast is not just "any" part of the body. As philosopher Iris Young has explained, the chest is "a center of a person's being in the world and the way she presents herself in the world so breasts cannot fail to be an aspect of her bodily habitus." The breast has long held deep meaning in western culture – as a source of life in providing milk to an infant and as a source of sexual and emotional bonding with a partner. Society has endowed it with the essence of womanliness, of sexual identity.[66] Simply going to a physician for a breast examination was problematic and physicians recognized that many women still remained hesitant to expose themselves to a "stranger."[67] In 1934, Montreal physician E.M. Eberts described how to examine the breasts of a patient. The sexual overtones, of which Eberts seemed unaware, are striking as is the objectification of the woman's body:

> The patient, stripped to the waist, should be examined in the sitting position in a good light. Inspection should be first from in front ... One should then stand behind the patient and observe the relative fulness of the breasts from above; and, passing the hand over the shoulder, manipulate and draw out the nipples, noting any difference in pliability or degree of prominence when erect ... Then [roll] the base of the nipple between the thumb and forefinger.[68]

Women, especially older women, might well feel hesitant about undergoing the examination Eberts described. And if modesty wasn't enough, breast cancer treatment faced women with the possibility of breast removal. For every woman who underwent such surgery, many more would have heard about it and their hesitancy in seeing a physician and perhaps having their worst fears confirmed is understandable. They needed time to absorb the possibility of cancer and to deal with the immediate response of fear.[69] While physicians' focus was clearly on convincing women about the seriousness of cancer and the need to consult their physicians as quickly as possible, some acknowledged that not all physicians took their responsibilities as seriously as they should. As with cervical cancer, this realization reflected a divide between surgeons and general practitioners.[70]

Treatment

The seriousness of breast cancer pushed physicians to prove themselves through action, and medicine had seemingly found its best practice – the Halsted radical mastectomy. Not all women were suitable "subjects" for the surgery, however, since it was a curative procedure, the success of which was dependent on diagnosing the cancer early, not often possible. Nonetheless, the focus on the radical mastectomy in the medical literature tended to mask that fact. The literature stressed the significance of the surgery and enthusiasm for it appeared to increase over time, in part as a reflection of the increased literature on it being published. The discussion emphasized the urgency to operate sooner rather than later and eclipsed a concern about the surgery's aftermath, as did the attitude that surgery was the safest action even when a diagnosis of breast cancer was unclear.

Much of what we know about the history of breast cancer and its treatment has been generated by the concern regarding cancer rates in recent years, the activism it engendered against the radical mastectomy, and the attempt to explain its dominance in breast cancer therapy.[71] Yet we still do not know what percentage of women with breast cancer underwent the radical mastectomy. It had pride of place in the medical literature and represented a drastic response to a deadly disease. But the fact that we do not know how many women experienced it suggests that care must be taken in assuming its dominance at the therapeutic level. Radiation therapy as an adjunct to surgery was very much accepted in Canada and some Canadian physicians mounted challenges to the radical mastectomy. If the historiographical literature on the United States is to be believed, both distinguished the Canadian situation from the American.[72]

The Halsted radical mastectomy consisted of removal of the entire breast around the malignancy, the lymph nodes under the arm, and the pectoral muscles under the breast. Named after William Halsted (1852–1922), first professor of surgery at Johns Hopkins University, the Halsted radical was a version of the mastectomy that physicians had performed for centuries. Other surgeons had done surgery as extreme as Halsted, but the point and difference of his procedure was its routineness. Surgeons were not to make decisions about what to remove – they were to operate as Halsted prescribed. In the words of A. Stanley Kirkland, the radical mastectomy was "a monument to the persistence, skill, ingenuity, thought and dexterity of generations of surgeons."[73]

The urgency surrounding surgery is nowhere seen more than in the work of James Bell, professor of clinical surgery, McGill University, and surgeon to the Royal Victoria Hospital, Montreal, perhaps the Canadian physician most extreme in his written views. In the 1900 *Montreal Medical Journal* Bell described his approach to a woman presenting herself before him with a breast lump:

A simple incision will detect a cyst or a chronic abscess, but if the simple incision does not make the diagnosis clear, I do not hesitate to advise the removal of the whole breast, with the understanding, that if a microscopic examination shows evidence of cancer, a more extensive dissection will follow within a few days. And if in serious doubt, I do not hesitate to recommend as wide removal as if I were certain of the diagnosis, even though the microscope may subsequently show that disease is not malignant.[74]

Bell believed that the consequences of cancer were so serious that even before a definitive diagnosis, the breast should be removed. If the postoperative diagnosis proved him wrong then so be it – better to be safe than sorry. In being safe, uncertainty became controllable. But there were consequences. Little mention is made in the published literature on breast cancer of the consequences of the surgery – restricted movement on one side of the body, a sunken chest, and often "milk arm," a chronic and painful condition.[75] And the woman would have lost a breast. Bell certainly didn't see breast removal as an issue and neither did many others. The 1901 *Annual Report* of the Royal Victoria Hospital, Montreal, revealed that breast amputations had occurred for the following conditions: multiple cysts of the breast, cystic adenoma of breast, multiple abscesses of the breast, fibroma of the breast, and depressed nipple, as well as for cancer of the breast.[76]

Removal of the breast was not even the worst of it. Bell noted that in some cases "portions of the bony wall of the chest have been removed," although he admitted that "there is a limit to this procedure, and it can never be either very safe or very satisfactory." But he was willing to push the limits, as when he argued that at times the arm should be amputated as well, even while recognizing that his colleagues might not agree. Bell asked that surgeons not close their minds to it if this was the only way to save the patient's life. Nowhere did he suggest that there might be too dear a cost to be paid for life and comforted himself and others by stating that, although the recurrence of breast cancer was high after breast removal, advances had been made.[77] Few physicians accepted Bell's extreme views on surgery, but Halsted's radical did remain the conventional "curative" approach throughout the interwar period and beyond. Complications resulting from the surgery were at times recognized in the later period, but in general those side effects took second place to the immediate need for the surgery.[78]

The rush to operate, however, could lead to unnecessary surgery. Harold Burrows in his 1923 *Mistakes and Accidents of Surgery* recalled errors made in removing breasts and then discovering that the condition was noncancerous. His response: "[S]uch a mistake is not likely to cost the patient her life, although the error is unfortunate for the patient and disquieting to the physician." On finding a breast lump, one Ontario woman in 1934 did what physicians urged, she went to see her doctor. He advised surgery and she agreed, and he removed the breast with the lump and the healthy breast as well fearing "it would only be in the same condition in a year or two." Only after the surgery did the pathology report reveal she did not have cancer.[79] The cure for breast cancer was radical surgery and the more radical the better. The stakes were high in the game of cancer and better a woman lose her breast unnecessarily than physicians be too cautious. For the woman the situation was, as Burrows put it, "unfortunate." Such women were the casualties of the war against the disease.

While the radical mastectomy remained the dominant approach to breast cancer, at least as reflected in the medical literature, X-ray and radium became therapeutic aids to surgery. They also permitted a challenge to the radical and engendered considerable debate, which reflected both the openness of the profession and the defensiveness of individual practitioners about their own area of expertise.[80] Canadian physicians were not slow to realize the opportunities provided by radiation in the early years. But the interwar years and after consolidated its use. *Annual Reports* of the Victoria General Hospital, Halifax, indicate that few radium treatments were given for breast cancer; X-rays revealed a different story. In 1933–4 there were 1304 X-ray treatments; by 1939–40, 8136; and by 1948–9, 14,288. Of these 232, 2442, and 3194 respectively were for breast cancer. Elsewhere radium was more popular. The Toronto General Hospital had a specific radium unit for the treatment of neck and breast cancer.[81] While the use of radiation treatment had increased, care needed to be taken, for such treatment had severe side-effects, among them headaches, vomiting, nausea, and reddening of the skin. Dr Vera Peters at the Ontario Institute of Radiotherapy, Toronto, was particularly sensitive to the precautions radiologists needed to take to lessen radiation sickness, to care better for the skin, to keep track of blood counts, and to be aware of the psychological needs of any individual undergoing radiation therapy for any kind of cancer. Nevertheless, the experience of some women led them to believe that the treatment was worse than the disease. Clow describes an Ontario woman, M.A.M., whose postoperative experience with radiation for reoccurring breast cancer was so horrendous that she finally rejected further radiation: "I was already burned to the bone ... and terribly weakened by the effects [of radiation]."[82]

Despite some of the problems with radiation treatment, its supporters were excited by its results. In 1926 Gordon Richards argued that postoperative radiation decreased breast cancer recurrences by

25 percent.[83] By the mid 1930s, W. Alan Curry wrote that three options were available: surgery only, radiation only, or a combination of both. Surgery in cases where the cancer had spread too far afield was not recommended. For cancer believed "curable," Curry preferred a combination approach with radiation occurring both before and after surgery. Others may have differed over when the radiation should be given but agreed that the combination of radiation and surgery had improved survival rates.[84] Increasingly, the challenge went out that surgery should not stand alone. Not all surgeons were convinced. Neither were they always pleased about sharing the limelight. Over time, surgeons had emerged in the profession as heroic figures of medicine. Certainly the Halsted procedure was heroic surgery. Radiation, even as an aid to surgery, challenged the image (and at times the reality) of the surgeon being in charge. In 1939, Halifax physician J.G. MacDougall asserted that in the hands of a good surgeon, radiation either before or after surgery was not necessary.[85] Surgery could stand alone. But increasingly it did not.

In 1934, Geoffrey Keynes's seminal article appeared in the *Canadian Medical Association Journal*. In it Keynes queried the necessity of Halsted's radical mastectomy and suggested that in early growths of cancer the radical operation could be obviated with the use of radiation. Other British physicians, too, had come to the same conclusion and by the late 1940s urged an end to the radical.[86] A few Canadian physicians joined the British opposition. While significantly influenced by the surgical thrust of the American medical profession, the cultural ties with Britain and at times their own postgraduate experiences overseas meant that the alignment of Canadian physicians could not be predicted or generalized. In the same year that the *Canadian Medical Association Journal* published the work of Keynes, J.A. Gunn, associate professor of clinical surgery at the University of Manitoba, wrote, "I regard the use of radium alone, as a substitute for operation, as occupying a hopeful position, and I now offer patients the choice between operation (with radium) and treatment by radium alone."[87] If proven over time, radiation would limit the mutilation of breasts.

In 1944, Vera Peters published an article in which she expressed strong support for radiation similar to her Winnipeg colleague, except her findings were supported by careful clinical analysis based on case histories at the Ontario Institute of Radiotherapy, Toronto. For breast cancers deemed inoperable and incurable she argued deep radiation could make a certain percentage of them "operable." What wasn't public at the time was that after the mid 1930s, Peters began to use an alternate treatment to the radical – a lumpectomy followed by local radiation – on many women who had refused a mastectomy or were considered too advanced in their cancer for surgery. She followed patient histories, comparing them with those who had had mastectomies (of any kind) and discovered no difference in outcome. Indeed, in some cases women who had undergone less invasive surgery lived longer.[88] While her findings and the publication of them were in the future, her work in the 1930s and 1940s reflects the willingness of some Canadian physicians not to follow medical orthodoxy as represented by the radical.

Conclusion

The barrage of literature on cancer meant that more Canadians were diagnosed earlier, which meant that they lived with the knowledge of having cancer longer. If they delayed consulting a physician early in their disease, the literature of the later period, which was difficult to ignore, made it clear they were to blame if their treatment was unsuccessful. Doctors warned their patients and one another that in the case of cancer, they could not afford to temporize. Cancer killed. With cervical cancer, the target appeared to be women who had had children – their bodies had done what they were designed to do and they were paying the price. Despite the dangers of cervical cancer, physicians maintained an optimism that it could be beaten *if* caught in time. Thus many physicians advocated a regular monitoring regimen that could only have emphasized to themselves and their patients the danger posed by women's bodies to women's health and survival. As for treatment, half-measures were not acceptable. If cancer was diagnosed or suspected, action was needed right away. The body was to be treated as guilty. Delay was dangerous. The urgency to respond to cancer resulted in heroic treatment. In the early years, surgery was the treatment of choice, and specifically radical surgery, often a hysterectomy. In the later decades radiation had become the main therapy. Both treatments, either separately or together, had harsh consequences for the patient.

For women with breast cancer the situation had also changed somewhat over the half century. The curative treatment of choice remained constant – the radical mastectomy. There may have been some challenges to it but they did not usurp its dominance. Radiation worked as an adjunct to surgery and was only just being seen as a possible substitute. Thus women who feared they had breast cancer were aware of what was in store for them. Indeed, their experience had become more alienating. Whereas early in the century a woman might have seen only her general practitioner, by mid century in her search for a cure she was visiting a number of different physicians and professionals – chief among them the surgeon and radiologist – most of them strangers to her. And what was the result of all those changes? The incidence of breast cancer was apparently increasing and the one "curative" treatment had not improved its survival rates significantly.[89]

10 The Mind's Health

Harold Atlee wrote movingly in the interwar period about the way in which women's lives could result in various neuroses. He acknowledged the

> tremendous inhibitions they lived under with regard to sex up to the time of marriage, and the difficulty they labor under to achieve full satisfactions in the career field of this man's world. From the time they are little girls there are so many things they may not do that their brothers may. Once they menstruate and begin to take an interest in the opposite sex, the pressure put upon them to preserve their virginity is tremendous. When they go to work, as most modern girls do, they find that with few exceptions the plum jobs are for men, and that for doing the same work they receive considerably less than the male wage. As a result when they marry so many find it difficult to sufficiently release themselves from their long built up sex fears to enjoy life in bed; or to find the same satisfactions in looking after a house and babies that they saw men achieve in the field in which they once worked. So their unconscious mind tricks them into seeing whatever escape they can find.[1]

His words are reflective of the issues explored in this book and in this chapter. Atlee and others saw women as limited by both their bodies and society. Not surprisingly practitioners saw those bodies as fragile and prone to breaking down as a result. But it was not only their bodies that did so; their minds did as well.

Mental illness is of interest in a study of women and their role as patients. First, psychiatry and its ideas became increasingly influential in modern society and more than other types of medicine, psychiatry was defined by norms in society that constantly shifted. Second, psychiatry defined what a healthy self was and in doing so expanded physicians' sphere of expertise. Third, interest in it went beyond the purview of specialists. The medical belief that the body and all of its aspects, including the mental, were interrelated meant that most physicians engaged in discussing mental health and the wide spectrum of disorders they thought exhibited deviation from it. Fourth, the definition of mental health was often gendered, as were its causes. We have already seen in the literature on puberty and menstruation how physicians saw women as more emotional than men. When that went too far it could be labelled as a mental or psychological ailment or disorder. As with many physical ailments to which women were perceived to be prone, myriad "causes" connected to women' bodies and their lives could result in mental symptoms. Not surprisingly, some treatments were gendered as well.

Background and Categories of Ilness

As far as the gendered nature of mental disease went, determining the sexual division of those suffering from nervous/mental disorders is impossible. Statistics on the "minor" manifestations are unreliable. When incarceration occurred, men outnumbered women, except in asylums in which numbers of beds were allotted evenly. When parity was not enforced, men's more violent symptoms compared to women's ensured that they would be incarcerated in an attempt to protect society and to hide violent lunatics from public notice. As for why people developed mental illness several medical models existed in the past to explain the process. Edward Shorter has suggested that before 1870 a reflex model dominated wherein one aspect of experience in part of the body resulted in consequences in another in a reflexive way. By the latter part of the century, experts had put forward two new medical paradigms. The first was that nervous symptoms were the result of organic disease of the central nervous system. Such a view, Shorter contends, dominated until WWI. The rival theory was that nervous symptoms were psychological in origin and could physically affect the body, a belief that dominated the second half of the twentieth century.[2] All three theories, however, overlapped in the first half of the century and physicians often took what they wanted from each. And given the gendered view physicians had of bodies, minds, and lives, all of the theories would have imposed a gendered perspective of mental illness.

Of more concern to most physicians than any theory of mental illness were its symptoms. Indeed, for much of the period under study, symptoms determined categories of mental illness and their severity. Of least concern were individuals suffering from "nerves," people who exhibited emotional upset but not to the point of needing any long-term treatment. In the first half of the century, women and their nervous dispositions were a given both in the medical world and wider Canadian society.[3] Of special concern were young working-class women. Given the pressures young women were already facing as a result of changes in their bodies, practitioners saw added pressures such as employment as especially problematic. Doctors' testimony at the 1907 Royal Commission investigating the labour conflict at Bell Telephone in Toronto repeatedly noted the pressure young women operators experienced with the result that their nervous systems were under considerable strain. It was no wonder that at times they broke down.

More serious than "nerves'" were emotional disorders that could interfere with leading a "normal" life. Two such conditions were neurasthenia and hysteria, both forms of neurosis. As a "functional" disease neurasthenia was a catchall diagnosis with a broad range of symptoms and causes.[4] Barbara Grosvenor, age 31, entered the Victoria General Hospital, Halifax, in February 1921 suffering from pain in her right ear that seemed to move to the right side and then to the back of her head. Diagnosed as neurasthenic, her case record also reported "suspect[ed] intracranial growth." Moira Webster suffered from dysmenorrhoea; she was not given an internal examination at the hospital but was still diagnosed as neurasthenic. The case notes on Mrs Eleanor Ritchie, age 51 and widowed, who entered the hospital in 1931 with the designation of neurasthenia, stated, "She is distinctly the neurasthenic type ... The patient has been in this hospital several times. The diagnosis in each case has been neurasthenia. This time she returns complaining of various pains, none very clear cut and wandering from place to place."[5] In the late nineteenth century neurasthenia was depicted as a middle-class ailment, brought on by the pressures of modern life and particularly experienced by businessmen. Over time, however, the general medical literature was less unanimous on who was more susceptible – men or women. While Carvell MacIntosh in a 1939 article in the *Dalhousie Medical Journal* complained both men and women neurasthenics wasted physicians' time, he blamed women in particular for seeking attention through their neurasthenic symptoms.[6]

Similar to neurasthenia but more intense in symptoms was hysteria. Originally connected with the Greek belief in the ability of the womb to wander within the body, it was a diagnosis that was female in designation. Its symptoms of loss of control over the emotions – crying, shouting, pointless laughter – appeared to be female more than male and indeed few cases of male hysteria were diagnosed in the early years of the century.[7] Class was believed to determine who experienced hysteria with the "lower classes" exhibiting more equal distribution of hysteria between the sexes. Women of the middle and higher classes exhibited more cases, due in part "to the absence of healthy occupation, partly social custom, which so markedly limit the activities of women, and partly to the ignorance of sexual subjects, and in older women to repression and perversion of the sexual instinct, and particularly to any cause, surgical or otherwise, which may direct their attention to the reproduction organs."[8] In the interwar period and beyond, while some insisted that hysteria was not just a female disease, it still appeared in hospital statistics more in women than in men with the most well-known clinician of his day, William Osler, remarking that women were its "chief subjects" even while admitting that men were not rare sufferers from it.[9] Diagnosing hysteria was never easy and like neurasthenia it could be a catchall label and the diagnosis could occur with seemingly little evidence.[10]

Mania was a significant designation that could result in incarceration. At the turn of the century, alienists considered women more prone than men to experiencing acute mania. According to Toronto's Daniel Clark this was a result of women generally being more nervous and emotional than men. Mania, then, was simply the extreme expression of a "natural" tendency in women. As one 1919 text claimed, they were "more noisy, more excitable" and more troublesome than men during their maniacal episodes.[11] In the interwar period, mania was still used in the medical language of mental illness. In 1931 E.C. Menzies, assistant medical superintendent of the Verdun Protestant Hospital, Quebec, described with sympathy a patient of his, an unmarried woman of 35, who had limited education and who had spent her life taking care of her father. Bright and sociable, she had recently "began to act strangely, became excited, disturbed, noisy, and had to be removed to the hospital where she threw things about and was very violent and destructive. In this phase the patient was diagnosed as suffering from mania."[12]

The flip side of excitability was depression or melancholia. In the present day, depression is diagnosed more in women than in men, at least in terms of who seeks help for it and who is medicated for it. Although depression was experienced by both women and men in the past, one of the divisions was linked to a specific life stage: involutional melancholia, a depression associated with menopause. While modern studies have not shown any rise in depression during and as a result of menopause, the belief in it was significant, especially in the early decades of the century; even after WWI, involutional melancholia was still a category used by some.[13] Other diagnoses than the ones listed emerged in the mental health field, such as those influenced by Freudian categorization, but not with as much discussion of them in the general medical literature. For some practitioners, diagnosis was a guide and little else. Daniel Clark believed categorizing was a fool's errand. The medical superintendent of the Nova Scotia Hospital, Halifax, W.H. Hattie, agreed and argued that in general practice, the terms mania and melancholia would do.[14] Even in later decades the urge to classify symptoms continued to appeal to the medical interest in making sense out of chaos. By classifying, there was a sense of coming to understand the problem. But there remained a sloppiness of categories and understanding well beyond the early decades of the century. Some lay and medical commentators, for example, tended to conflate mental illness with mental retardation, particularly when the arguments were about keeping such individuals separate from the rest of society.[15] One physician at the end of the period under study pointed out that insanity was a term that included categories as "different from one another as a sore toenail is from pneumonia."[16] Whether the various categories and subdivisions within them aided physicians in understanding the problems of their patients is unclear. Equally unclear were the actual meanings of some terms used because they shifted with time and with the person using them. Clearer is that what physicians focused on and how it was often gendered.

Causes

The gendered aspect is nowhere seen more than in causation. But determining causation was fraught with problems. Most categories of disorder did not have a firm causal base and were more descriptive of symptoms. Consequently, the tendency was to emphasize correlations to suggest causation; however, a correlation that seemed to exist for one patient did not always seem to work for another. The point here is not to analyse how correct or incorrect the medical profession was in its view of causation, but rather to illuminate how their views reflected their own gendered perception. Not surprisingly, the main cause that physicians focused on was the physical. Physicians were trained to discern the physical origins of problems and they perceived the body and the mind as capable of influencing one another. Any disease or crisis could, in theory, result in mental distress because of the pain it caused, the worry and stress it created, or the reflex action it had on the nervous system. Over time, additions were added to disease causation, making it seem as though there was increased understanding of the causation. What follows is an examination of causes that had strong gendered aspects.

Heredity

Alienists saw poor heredity as a significant predisposing cause of mental disturbance. Indeed, some considered a racial connection between hysteria and Latin, Slavonic, and Jewish backgrounds rather than the "more phlegmatic Anglo-Saxon race."[17] Toronto's Frank N. Walker went further and warned that "mental ailments" were not only hereditary but also congenital due to the marriage of individuals of different races.[18] While heredity or race did not have a necessary gendered component, in the way hereditary mental illness was perceived it did. In the early years of the century, the gendered nature of heredity emerged in the relationship believed to exist between the health of the mother and the health of the foetus. Anything that undermined the physical or mental health of the mother could lead to mental or physical weakness in the child.[19] The consequences for women could be significant since it was not unknown for women who were deemed insane to be sterilized to offset the possibility of any future progeny. Sterilization was not performed on men to the same extent. Physicians also discussed whether in the case of pregnancy, a family history of insanity or a previous case of insanity on the part of the woman were grounds for aborting the foetus.[20] Heredity remained a focus for alienists in the interwar years even though it posed a challenge to their work. After all, if mental instability was hereditary, it negated the curative thrust of psychiatry. The belief in heredity meant marriage of those with an hereditary predisposition to mental disease should not occur. As the eugenics movement strengthened in the interwar years, the solution for some, as in the early years of the century, was sterilization of the mentally unfit, specifically the insane and feebleminded. Sterilization would "catch" women whom marital health certificates did not. Certainly studies of the 1928 Alberta sterilization law indicate that it was invoked more against women than against men.[21] While many physicians supported the eugenic solution, a few spoke out against it, pointing to the cultural and class bias of deciding who was fit and who was not.[22]

Life-cycle Transitions: Puberty and Menstruation

Passing on "tainted" heredity through the next generation was clearly a focus of concern about hereditary mental illness. But reproduction itself was also one of the life-cycle transitions that placed more stress on women's bodies than on men's. Such transitions were also more numerous for women. As we saw in a previous chapter, the notion of puberty as a stressful period dominated the medical literature on this topic throughout the first half century. In 1902, J.A. MacKenzie, assistant medical superintendent at the Nova Scotia Hospital, Halifax, was clear about puberty's threat to the mental health of both sexes but especially to girls due to the speed at which the transformation occurred in them compared to boys. If that was not problem enough, so troublesome was the sexual development in girls that Mackenzie quoted one expert who insisted that "girls who fail to exhibit some hysterical symptom at puberty are few indeed."[23]

In the interwar period and beyond, alienists were trying to be more precise about the types of mental illness that existed. Diagnoses often referred to the time when the illness arose, such as the insanity of puberty, but other than indicating the timing of the disorder, many argued that the nomenclature did not illuminate its nature. J.S. Fairbairn was a gynaecologist who believed that mental illness was the sphere of the alienist and not the gynaecologist, but he did believe that two periods of life and their mental disturbances were of concern for physicians of women: puberty and menopause. He was in good company. As we have seen, William Osler believed that hysteria occurred more in women than in men, "usually" exhibiting itself first at puberty.[24]

If puberty was a major transition, menstruation ensured that women remained at risk in a way men did not. Some saw hysterical fits coming around the time of menstruation and linked to it. One early twentieth-century textbook posited the relationship between "psychopathic manifestations" and menstrual irregularity. While believing that the former came before the latter, it was the female reproductive system that broke down and not another system in the body, reinforcing the sense of its fragility and susceptibility to influences.[25] Certainly husbands and fathers of women who experienced a mental breakdown were known to blame menstruation for it, as did asylum committal agents.[26] A.T.B. Hobbs, a physician who had operated surgically on women at the asylum in London, Ontario, noted in 1901 that "a series of nerve storms ranging in gravity from localized abnormal sensations to profound mental derangement" could occur during an ovarian malfunction.[27] The view that menstruation was problematic continued in the years immediately following World War I. Nonetheless, the emphasis on menstrual problems leading to insanity or mental instability did not seem to have as strong a following in the interwar period as in the early years of the century. A major 1935 text judged the idea that amenorrhoea could lead to "psychic symptoms" and even to insanity as "groundless."[28]

Life Cycle Transitions: Childbirth

While puberty and menstruation were life transitions and experiences that many considered stresses in women's lives, they paled in comparison to the experiences surrounding pregnancy and childbirth. Physicians viewed pregnancy as a potentially exciting cause of mental attacks, especially if the woman was already predisposed through heredity or by the sex of the child carried, or if she was unmarried, older, or anxious.[29] Some blamed pregnancy with its increased demands on the body for interfering with the blood's access to the brain and thus its ability to nourish the brain. It was, in part, a reflection of the belief that an individual had only a fixed amount of energy or vital force and if energy was directed to one part of the body, as in pregnancy, it was taken from another part (perhaps the brain).[30] The disturbances of pregnancy were on a spectrum; all women were in some way upset during pregnancy, but some crossed a boundary that separated the psychologically normal from the pathological. And if the pregnancy was coupled with economic concerns then the psychic energy of worry could add to a woman's breakdown.

Interest in the problems that pregnancy presented vis-à-vis mental disturbance continued in the postwar years and after. Any stress or extra physical effort/change could weaken the nervous system. For some, infection was the culprit leading to "toxic exhaustion."[31] But as was the case for insanity of puberty, physicians in the interwar years and beyond increasingly challenged a specific link between insanity and pregnancy.[32] What didn't change was the thin line between normalcy and pathological mental symptoms exhibited during pregnancy, as had been the case in the early years of the century. Physicians throughout the first half century believed the actual process of childbirth and its stresses could also be an exciting cause of mental disturbance.[33] Neither did the risk lessen after the birth. Nursing a child, some believed, was an act that could excite psychic disturbance and upset the energy balance of the body. In later years, others argued it was not nursing per se that was the issue but the accumulation of many childbirths followed by nursing that eventually caught up to the woman, weakening her health. Nursing was simply the final straw.[34]

Whether caused by pregnancy, childbirth, or lactation, the nomenclature of puerperal insanity was a strong one. In the early years of the century, it was a particularly significant classification of disturbance. It occurred after the actual birth of the child and so, in theory, did not include those cases in which pregnancy itself loomed large, but this was not always clear. After all, something that started with the pregnancy but went unnoticed could be intensified by the actual childbirth and postpartum period. Since practitioners deemed puerperal insanity curable, many women suffering from it were kept at home and so accurate statistics on its incidence were difficult to determine. Nonetheless, estimates were made. Daniel Clark believed that one woman in 450 who was confined with child became insane. He also made the point that puerperal insanity was not a "distinct" form of insanity since its symptoms were similar to those of other insanities. What made it different was cause only. Such a view stressed the importance of symptomology for Clark rather than causation. But the importance of this kind of insanity for others was that there did seem to be a clear cause and effect relationship. Hattie admitted that perhaps the nomenclature was not accurate but he agreed with one expert who stated categorically that "to know that a case is one that has begun after recent child-birth, is to know far more about it for treatment and for prognosis, then to know it as mania or melancholia."[35] But what caused the relationship? A favoured theory was some form of sepsis. MacKenzie speculated that it was "due to the sudden change in the pressure of the circulatory system" which affects the brain cells. Others added the importance of both social and other physical factors.[36]

The interest in puerperal insanity continued after the first two decades of the century. As before, some questioned a specific designation of "puerperal mania"; nonetheless the classification still continued.[37] As for the exact cause, some focus on sepsis remained,[38] but more significant was the persistent awareness of other factors. For example, life situation was recognized in the understanding that the economic downturn of the 1930s influenced the "incidence of childbirth psychoses."[39] It would appear that what was "natural" – having children – was fraught with danger. But then the received wisdom was that not being able to have children could also lead to mental instability as could having small families.[40]

Life Cycle Transitions: Menopause

Women who had children were at risk, women who had few children were at risk, women who had no children were at risk. And the perception of risk did not abate. As already noted, risk followed women into menopause. As will be seen in the next chapter, physicians saw menopause as a major transition in women's lives, bringing with it shifts that rivaled those of puberty. Not surprisingly, then, practitioners saw a woman's mental stability threatened by such a major disruption in life and it was one more experience that distinguished women from men. Mary-Ellen Kelm's study of the British Columbia Provincial Hospital for the Insane in the early years of the twentieth century noted that husbands often connected their wives' insanity with the onset of menopause as did male committal agents more so than female ones.[41] Many physicians agreed on the danger that menopause posed. As one physician noted, "[T]he special dangers of the climacteric period ... must be remembered." Women committing criminal acts during that period might really be suffering from climacteric mania.[42]

A. Lapthorn Smith had given serious thought to the relationship between insanity and menopause. He rejected "starvation of the brain cells due to senile degeneration" as an explanation for it provided little hope of cure. He preferred looking at the lives that many women had led as the origin of instability: the "overwork, child bearing and lactation with insufficient food and sleep." Nonetheless, he didn't deny the timing of the mental breakdown. In terms of the designation, Maurice Craig in his 1917 text *Psychological Medicine* emphasized that there was no specific mental disorder one could refer to as "climacteric insanity." Maybe not, but Craig recognized that there were certain "somatic disturbances" that often accompanied menopause and that were symptomatic of insanity: "insomnia, failure of attention, alteration of temper, irritability, changed affection towards husband, suspicions, jealousies, ... a tendency to make false accusations ... difficulty ... performing their ususal household duties."[43] The list says as much about his view of menopausal women as it does about insanity.

In the years after World War I the interest in menopause and involutional melancholia remained.[44] While there was a trend to assure women and practitioners that the incidence of insanity, breakdown, etc., did not increase with menopause,[45] notions of the relationship nonetheless persisted. In 1948 *Chatelaine* introduced the topic of menopause to its readers through an article by Robert Cleghorn, assistant professor of psychiatry at McGill University and "in charge of the experimental therapeutics laboratories at the Allan Memorial Institute of Psychiatry."[46] What message did the editors think they were sending women by having Cleghorn write the article if not that menopause and mental disturbances were related?

The threat of mental breakdown followed women throughout their lives. It did so for men as well. But the difference was that for women, many causes were focused on their bodies and those elements that differentiated them from men. Underlying the physical markers mentioned above were the frailties of the female reproductive system believed to be a source of breakdown both literally in the physical aspects of that system, but also in a more removed way in causing mental disturbances. Even while they supported classifying mental problems by their nature, that is, how they were exhibited, practitioners were reluctant to give up a nomenclature that emphasized both *when* and *why* particular insanities developed – for example, insanity of puberty, puerperal insanity, and involutional melancholia. These were descriptors that emphasized physical causation. Doctors were experts on the body and the physical and, despite the various theories of mental disease causation, they often focused on the physical as explanation even for mental diseases. Their patients, too, were more willing to admit of a disease with an organic origin or symptom than a psychological one.[47] But separating the two was never easy.

Behavioural Causes

While physical causation was a significant category of causation, specific behaviour was as well. Excess use of alcohol was generally gendered male.[48] Sexual behaviour leading to insanity was also gendered but in different ways. Sexual excess could lead to breakdown. In 1903 Ernest Hall remarked on the fact that in asylums there were more single men than married and more married women than single. In part he saw this as a consequence of the existence of venereal disease in younger men and the "ravages of gonorrhoea upon the married women." The former was a result of sexual excess in men, undermining their energy level, and the latter the result of the innocent wife being infected by her husband.[49] Venereal disease, however contracted, remained a concern in the postwar period.[50] The trope of the innocent wife remained strong. And as we have seen, these were years when some pundits were worrying about what they saw as the promiscuous behaviour of both sexes. For some women suffering mental symptoms, physicians specifically inquired about the possibility of them having contracted VD. Physicians in the Victoria General Hospital, Halifax, put down VD for one young woman diagnosed with hysteria even though she was not tested for VD. It was not deemed a cause, but simply added to the case record in the phrase "denies V.D." Whether this was because she was young (age 22) and a maid is unclear. But VD (or lack of it) was mentioned in the case histories of several women diagnosed with hysteria.[51] The message was clear, women (and men) should not experiment sexually. It was literally dangerous to their physical and mental health. But then so was sexual repression.[52] In seeing deviant behaviour – in drinking and sexual matters – as causative factors in mental breakdown, doctors could be accused of making normative judgements, bolstering the status quo, and interpreting their own value system as one insuring medical health. In some cases, their judgments would have been accurate. Alcoholism and VD could result in real problems with mental aspects. In the general medical literature both also had class and racial connections.

If the medical literature tended to see women as less involved than men in drinking and engaging in sexual excess, underlying much of the perception of women and mental illness was the image of what a healthy woman was and how she should act and how deviation from that ideal could result in mental problems. J.E. Hanna in the 1908 *Queen's Medical Quarterly*, for example, worried neurasthenia was increasing. Too often women were blaming their problems on their reproductive systems and becoming "womb crank[s]" when in truth the real cause of neurasthenia was their own behaviour. They spent too much time "running associations and clubs for the saving of wicked man." Women would be better off running their own homes and teaching their daughters how to do the same. Such a view revealed Hanna's own dislike of the middle-class women's reform movements of the time. W. Blair Bell focused on body shape. The ideal woman was plump; it was her "nature" to be so. Neurotic women tended to be thin and such women lived either a pampered life or were overworked. Here Bell covered women of all classes. Then there were the difficult cases of "neuroses," women "suffering from the unsatisfied functions of [their] sex." These were women who had reached 35–40 years of age still unmarried or sterile. And picking up Hanna's dislike of activist women, Bell exclaimed, "Such women are often found in the vanguard of the ranks of female agitators."[53] Thus Bell was able to make a linear link backwards from neuroses in women to their frustration in not being married or not being able to conceive leaving them with little else to do but to be "female agitators." Bell's and Hanna's sense of what a woman should be was clear: middle-class married with children, with her attention focused on her home, not on rights for women or on trying to reform men. This underlying ideal was often nostalgic, looking to a past where some believed women "coped" with life better than "now" seemed to be the case. Modern life was not good for women.

In the interwar years and beyond, physicians seemed more sympathetic to women. Modernity had brought telephones to rural areas, which lessened the "nervousness and insanity among the womenfolk who were confined to the house weeks on end without having even a chance to gossip with a woman friend."[54] But modernity could not offset the fatigue of women's lives or the anxiety of unfulfilled ambition. As Harold Atlee's quote at the beginning of the chapter revealed, women's lives were limited and constrained both sexually and professionally, much more so than lives men were allowed to live.[55]

In looking at causation of mental distress and illness, what emerges is how broadly practitioners reached to find answers. The most obvious focus was the body and as experts on it that should not be surprising. Heredity was the originator of mental weakness or strength for both sexes, but the heredity that came through the female side was deemed especially influential due to the close relationship between the mother and the foetus in utero and afterwards through breast feeding. But beyond heredity it was the sexed-gendered body, the female body, that seemed most problematic, again not surprising given the perceived complexity and frailty of the female reproductive system. Physicians deemed any problem in it, or even its normal functioning, as a possible cause of mental breakdown. The entire life cycle of women was punctuated by stressful episodes of sometimes long standing. And the gendered view of life ensured that behavioural aspects, lived experiences, and pressures faced by both men and women were often deemed the source of mental breakdown.

Treatment

Nonsurgical

Categories of mental disorders and their perceived causation had repercussions on treatment. Essentially treatment fell into two major groups in the early twentieth century – nonsurgical and surgical. For the general category of "nerves," treatment in the early years of the twentieth century was straightforward – adoption of a simple life, exercise, and fresh air. Patent medicines offered their help.[56] The treatment for neurasthenia addressed the fatigue and weakness of the body and could be much more invasive than for general nerves. Electrostatic treatment for the "ovarian, uterine, or the pelvic congestions" of neurasthenia and any hysterical symptoms was advocated, as were X-rays.[57] The Weir-Mitchell rest cure was an approach adopted in the mid to late nineteenth century that continued to be popular and emphasized taking the patient from her surroundings and giving her nothing to focus on but rest and nourishment. More than anything, giving up personal volition to the demands of the physician was emphasized. Ignored by most was the reality that most women could not afford to leave their work or home to take the treatment, could not easily change their environment, and might not be able to afford the food that would fatten them and bring them closer to the ideal. Nor was everyone in favour of the rest cure. In the July 1905 *Canada Lancet* William Broadbent Pritchard, a New York physician, railed against it and the way in which it took away an individual's control. The rest cure "infantalized" the patient, treated her/him as less than an intelligent adult. Fine for "real" women, it was not for "real" men.[58]

Treatment for hysteria varied as did its perceived causes and symptoms. Hysterics posed problems for physicians. Women of "indolent habits" whom some practitioners saw as more prone to hysteria received little sympathy, as did those whose hysteria was expressed in a self-centred and selfish way. More sympathy was given to young working women in whom pressures of employment triggered their hysteria.[59] At times treatment was akin to punishment if the physician believed that the patient was "malingering" or exhibiting "willful exaggeration." In those cases physicians might deem procedures "disagreeable or even painful" such as "cold baths, the faradic brush, the ... cautery," as the best solution.[60] Physicians at the Royal Victoria Hospital, Montreal, as with neurasthenia, used electricity therapy and X-rays. Others recommended the Weir-Mitchell treatment.[61]

As in the earlier decades, treatment after WWI ran the gamut from rest to hormone treatment. When causation was linked to a stressful life, a "rest cure" seemed appropriate.[62] Advertisements for nerve tonics abounded. The advertisement for Dr Mile's Nervine assured women that the tonic would relax the nerves thus lessening the lines and wrinkles in the face caused by their nervous condition. Medical recommendations weren't that different. Certainly the advertisements for Eskaphen B Elixir in medical journals explained to physicians, "One nervous woman can give rise to more diverse undiagnosed and undiagnosable complaints than a whole pathological ward." The elixir would calm her nerves.[63] The benefit of such treatment was that the patient herself had significant control over it. But even when the patient lost control, it didn't mean doctors were able to assume it.

Mrs Deborah Feist entered the Victoria General Hospital, Halifax, on 23 November 1920, diagnosed with neurasthenia. The case record indicated that she suffered from dysmenorrhoea and nausea during her menstrual period but no other physical problem. She did, however, experience moods and depression. The hospital gave her a bromide mixture as treatment, but her case record suggested a sense of frustration on the part of medical personnel. Feist would not rest and her friends did not help the situation much when they visited. Basically no one had control over her.[64] One text deemed the treatment of neurasthenia so problematic that the authors worried that physicians were too dismissive of such women, believing that the diagnosis itself was the end of treatment and that somehow the patient was to blame for her own problems.[65]

If there wasn't any apparent organic cause or consequence, the physician needed to spend time with the neurasthenic woman to find out what psychic causes and symptoms might exist. A.G. Morphy reminded colleagues that often such women were absorbed with their symptoms: they relieved them of family and household responsibilities, and gave them a status of "having puzzled all the doctors." Instead of reassuring such a woman and giving her a tonic, which too often occurred, the physician needed to have a "frank discussion" with her "to bring out her maladjustments to her life situation or to her married or unmarried or social status."[66] The psychological clearly dominated Morphy's perception of women but his advice necessitated time, which physicians and often patients did not have, and also money, which limited who could see a physician for a form of talk therapy.

Treatment for hysteria covered a broad spectrum and repeated what doctors had to offer those with neurasthenia. Patent medicines were available for self-medication. Some practitioners encouraged patients to exert their will to get better, although others believed such women needed counseling.[67] Hypnosis was even tried. Miss Mary Johnston, age 19, entered the Montreal General Hospital on 7 August 1935. According to her case record she hyperventilated when people were watching, but not otherwise. Under hypnosis, suggestions to not hyperventilate were made and she seemed better and continued to improve. Miss Verity Momaner, age 19, entered the Kitchener-Waterloo Hospital in 1941, exhibited worry over work, tiredness, and crying over minor things, and experienced some amnesia; she was diagnosed as suffering from hysteria. Taking a commonsense approach, her physicians "allowed her to rest, put [her] on a light diet and prescribed some milk of magnesia."[68] For serious cases, however, "custodial care" could result.[69]

Physicians grasped at a wide variety of treatment modalities. Given the endocrine nature of menopause, physicians were excited by the prospect of hormone therapy's ability to offset menopause's worst symptoms, which could wear down the patient and lead to breakdown. Montreal's George Reed, however, argued that endocrine therapy had been disappointing, whereas "convulsive shock therapy" had been so successful that "psychiatrists who have protested for years against this empirical and crude therapy, have at last adopted it." A review of new cases in Ontario up to 1944 suggested that women were the majority of recipients.[70]

Surgical Treatment

Patent medicine, rest cures, electrostatic treatment, cold baths, etc., were not as gendered as the most invasive of treatments – surgery. It should not be surprising given the relationship that physicians saw between the physiological breakdown of the female sexual/reproductive system and a psychical breakdown that they believed treating the former would also treat the latter. Criticism arose when some seemed to emphasize mental cure to the point that they looked for a physical cause that was not there or not significantly so. And while some historians have referred to this as a nineteenth-century phenomenon,[71] it still had adherents in the early decades of the twentieth century and after.

Given the belief that pregnancy placed extra stress on women and their bodies, the solution advocated by some was to end the pregnancy. Daniel Clark disagreed. He questioned the ethical aspect of abortion and queried whether the ending of pregnancy brought any "improvement." Others maintained abortion was just as likely to induce insanity as prevent it. It was a difficult call to make. We have seen how A. Lapthorn Smith favoured abortion for pregnant women suffering from uremic poisoning due to the possible danger of subsequent insanity. He reported on one of his patients in Montreal to whom this had occurred. When she returned home she again became pregnant and once more developed kidney failure. Smith reported the situation to the Medical Society of the time seeking opinion on whether in such a case abortion was called for to offset another bout of insanity. No one supported him in this and so he acquiesced with the result that the patient died in her sixth month. For him the lesson was clear, abortion in such cases was a medical necessity, although he did recognize that Roman Catholic physicians would be unable to do this.[72]

The issue of pregnancy-caused disturbance continued to raise the issue of abortion. Aleck Bourne's 1925 text on midwifery warned that abortion could very well "precipitate" an attack of insanity, but pointed out that "in view of the hereditary tendencies of insanity, and in the interests of the State," abortion might well be the best response.[73] In the case of insanity following birth William J. Stevens in a 1945 issue of *Canadian Nurse* explained what he believed should occur. The mother and child should be separated and the mother given sedatives. The mother was never to be left alone. Recovery often occurred within six months but recurrence was not unusual.[74] The mention of recurrence, however, laid open the possibility of a future abortion.

Some physicians advocated gynaecological surgery for neurasthenia and hysterical pain linked to uterine/pelvic disorders.[75] Early in the century W. Blair Bell saw sexual insanity in women in the form of "manhunger. " He described one consultation he had had for a 16-year-old girl (which fits the assumption that puberty was a trying and dangerous time) "who would actually write notes, take them out of her pocket and drop them for men who might be following. Her diary was a terrible document. She is now in a retreat. We have made the suggestion, for what it may be worth, that removal of the uterus and one ovary might be tried before condemning such cases permanently to an asylum." That he was willing to remove some of her sexual organs even when there was no evidence that anything was wrong with them illustrates both the desperation stemming from a fear of openly expressed female sexuality and the desire to keep a 16-year-old girl out of the asylum even if it meant surgical experimentation. Unlike some, as reflected in the international literature, he was not willing to remove both ovaries.[76]

The idea of gynaecological surgery to offset mental symptoms was not a new one in Canada. At the London, Ontario, asylum in the late nineteenth century, surgery occurred on women patients who Dr Richard Maurice Bucke, the superintendent, and Dr Hobbs, the surgeon in charge, believed had some gynaecological problem. In 1900 Bucke summarized what had been happening in London. Out of 256 women examined (almost all under anesthesia), 219 had some form of "structural disease in the uterus, ovaries or their adnexa." Two hundred of the women underwent surgery ranging from minor currettage to hysterectomies. The criticism is not that Bucke and Hobbs operated – insane women should receive the same care as the sane – but that in reporting their results the focus and excitement was on the mental improvement, if not cure, of the women and that the improvement and cure did not happen with other surgeries; that is, Bucke and Hobbs emphasized the existence of an integral link between the sexual/reproductive system of women and their brains.[77] For Bucke, there was a hierarchy of body parts and in women those of the reproductive system were easily the most significant and closely associated with the mind.

Bucke and Hobbs were not the only ones to be excited by surgical possibilities. On the west coast Dr Ernest Hall, surgeon to the Burrard Sanitorium in Vancouver, was another outspoken advocate of gynaecological surgery on the insane. In several articles he explained his position. Believing in the relationship between pelvic disease and insanity, he asked if it were not better to respond to the former rather than to incarcerate such women. Unfortunately, he was willing to push what he did beyond the practitioner's credo of do no harm. He described his approach as follows:

It has been my practice to open the abdomen only when external examination reveals disease, but a more extended experience leads me to consider intro-abdominal examination an essential part if there be indications pointing in that direction with an absence of determinable disease elsewhere.

With modern methods such an examination should have no mortality and but a few weeks confinement, and surely a disease that would remove a patient from friends and society perhaps for life justifies such careful investigation.[78]

He was advocating exploratory surgery and glossing over its consequences. His belief that insanity was the result of a physical lesion led him searching the pelvic/uterine area for it.

He reported one patient, Mrs C., age 57, confined in an asylum for two years, married with several children, whom he examined under anesthesia. All he found was a "lacerated perineum and laxity of the vaginal walls," hardly surprising in a woman who had given birth several times. He did not see any point in operating. Convinced by her "friends," however, to leave no possibility untried, he decided to do exploratory surgery and "found large varicocele of both broad ligaments with calcareous deposits and cystic degeneration of the pelvic peritoneum. Appendages were removed with as much of broad ligament as possible."[79] Thus he depicts himself as the conservative physician, influenced by the patient's friends to do a procedure he would not otherwise have chosen only to find anomalies that he had not expected. Of course the lesson he took from this case was to continue to perform exploratory surgery, a visual examination not being enough to determine whether there was a physical problem or not. By putting himself in the "conservative" camp, he perhaps hoped to lessen those who were uncomfortable with the kind of surgery he was doing and on whom. He portrayed himself then as a physician who took surgery seriously, who did not perform it needlessly, and when he did perform it, did so in a responsible way.

Some of Hall's surgery was radical. For a young woman, age 27, who suffered from "sexual" insanity and in whom he discovered "erosion of the cervical mucous membrane, with the uterus slightly enlarged," he "curretted a few fungosities, amputated the cervix, opened the abdomen and resected three-fourths of the right ovary which was cystic." He "noticed the labia majora were hypertrophied and granular in appearance, but not having a history of self abuse I did not interfere." When self-abuse was confirmed later he removed "the labia majora and minora and the mucous membrane of the vestibule to the meatus, including the clitoris." He comforted himself that others were doing similar work and that he was achieving success in relieving mental symptoms, although he admitted mental recovery was more likely

for women who had not been insane for long. He also admitted that
the results were less promising than when he first began. Nevertheless,
the main thrust of his claims had not changed, although in a 1911 article
Hall did seem to be modifying his sense of the cause and effect relationship between insanity and gynaecological disorders.[80]

A. Lapthorn Smith was also a physician who supported gynaecological surgery for mental disorders. He had, for example, determined
that ventrofixation in women with retroverted uteri who were suffering from suicidal mania could result in the disappearance of the
mania. He concluded, "[I]n my opinion every insane woman, married
or single, should be submitted to an examination under anaesthesia,
for even single women very frequently suffer from severe retroversion
and prolapse." Perhaps being aware of the dangers of needless surgery,
Smith made a special effort to remind his colleagues that removal of
healthy organs would not result in mental cure. Indeed, he knew that
some physicians had made the attempt with no improvement whatso-
ever.[81] Physicians other than Bucke, Hobbs, Hall, and Smith continued
to support the surgery. When Mrs Ruth Graftberg, age 24, entered the
Royal Victoria Hospital, Montreal, in August 1908 she was suffering
from leucorrhoea, headache, stomach trouble, and menorrhagia. The
case record noted "this patient is extremely nervous at times hysterical
possibly the repair of the cervical tear may improve this condition."[82]

Not all physicians were enthralled by gynaecological surgery on the
insane. Daniel Clark was very concerned. He estimated that only three
percent of the female insane had any serious uterine or ovarian disease. Whether he was reacting to statistics coming out of the London,
Ontario, asylum suggesting otherwise is not known, but some in the
field were vocal in specifically disapproving what Bucke and Hobbs
were doing. John H. Stand studied the surgery that had been performed
at the London, Ontario, asylum and concluded that the results failed
to establish the connections that Bucke and Hobbs had maintained.
Indeed Stand discovered that "the percentage of recoveries is lowest in
operations upon the uterus and ovaries, those organs 'most vital, most
highly organized and most intimately associated with the spiritual and
mental life.'" He also determined that in many of the recoveries that
"the personal attention" given to such patients was the curative factor.[83]

Interest in gynaecological surgery for mental problems declined in
Canada after the second decade of the century perhaps because the
criticism being mounted made sense or because there was no cham-
pion like Bucke, Hobbs, Hall, or Smith to support it publicly. In 1921

Robert G. Armour from the University of Toronto dismissed the idea but admitted that for some practitioners it was "not yet dead."[84] And he was correct. In 1933 J.R. McGeoch of the Ontario Hospital, Whitby, Ontario, reported the gynaecological procedures that occurred after examination at his hospital. He referred to two cases in which he thought "gynaecological findings and the long course of the mental symptoms might have justified a complete hysterectomy." While his report on the surgery and the procedures was much more subdued than what had occurred in the early years of the century, he did suggest that future surgery should be pursued "when the gynaecological pathology is marked, or when minor treatment such as cauterization is followed by some improvement."[85] The strongest views, however, were those against surgery as a recovery tool. There was an unease about it. In his *The Art of Treatment* William R. Houston was clear about what he had seen in the past – women's ovaries taken out in the hopes of curing their hysteria, a practice he deemed "criminal malpractice." Especially worrisome was the impact of the surgery on women already traumatized by their mental condition.[86]

In the 1940s, however, a new form of surgery was being touted – lobotomies. Lobotomies surgically altered the personality of the individual and were more often performed on women than on men. The first surgeries in Ontario occurred in 1944, performed by Dr K.G. McKenzie, a neurosurgeon from the Toronto Psychiatric Hospital. The patients were 19 women. No more surgeries were performed for four years and then from 1948 to 1952 150 more occurred, 109 of them on women, 38 on men, and 3 on patients whose sex is unknown. A similar but lesser gender imbalance occurred in the United States as well.[87] Two physicians from McGill discussing lobotomies in the *Canadian Journal of Psychology* warned their readers that the surgery did "incapacitate" patients for some employment, particularly those in which significant intelligence was needed.[88] Given the way in which women were deemed intellectually inferior to men and the limitations placed on their workplace choices, they may have seemed suitable subjects. Impairment of their intellectual faculties would not have been judged as significant as it would be for men.

What emerges from an examination of medical treatment of mental illness in women is the gendered nature of much of it. Men, too, could suffer from nerves, neurasthenia, hysteria, and more serious forms of mental breakdown. Nonetheless, the treatment of women who did was often coloured by their sex and gender and the medical focus on their reproductive system. Where it especially emerged was in the most radical treatments – gynaecological surgery in the early years and its continuation in the later years along with two new entries – electroshock treatment and lobotomies. Such procedures reflected the wider conceptualization of medicine and its practitioners' views of women's bodies (including their minds) and the weaknesses represented by them. Not that medicine and physicians did not change. Many practitioners in the later period certainly dismissed gynaecological surgery as a cure for mental illness, unlike many of their colleagues in the early years.

Conclusion

While the causes of mental illness were many, this chapter has focused on those that were especially gendered. Those surrounding the female life cycle were predominant, a confirmation of what physicians had long believed: women simply underwent more intense physical shifts throughout their lives – puberty, menstruation, pregnancy, childbirth, lactation, and menopause – than men did. Men had behaviour catalysts – alcoholism and sexual excess – but even the consequences of the latter could be played out on women's bodies. The lives women led were, at times, seen as leading to frustration and breakdown. From the practitioner's view, they were small lives, limited in choice, confined in space, restricted to responding to the needs of others. It does not matter that such a description was one-sided; belief in it was the context out of which illness causation was determined. Once diagnosis and causation were determined, physicians did what they were trained to do – they acted to bring about stability and hopefully cure. As we have seen, the treatment of mental illness ran the gamut from rest cures to gynaecological surgery to lobotomies. Some treatment was not particularly gendered, others were gendered in underlying philosophy, and still others were gendered in who tended to receive a particular treatment. The gendered nature of perceived causation and actual treatment underlies the belief in duality, in the binary of the male and female bodies. Women and men were different. Those differences lasted most of their lives. Indeed, the next chapter looks at what some in the past might have seen as the end of the binary, the end of womanhood.

11 Menopause: The End of Womanhood

In her 1916 advice manual Alice Stockham described what women could look forward to at menopause: "*Skin diseases*, ... constipation or diarrhoea, swelled limbs or joints, swelled breasts, headaches, ... dizziness, dimness of vision with floating specks before the eyes, loss of voice and aching at the base of the tongue, insomnia, strange cravings, difficult breathing, neuralgia, hysteria, etc."[1] The negativity of the list is overwhelming. Stockham's book suggests that women in the past were concerned about menopause and perceived the "symptoms" largely as physical in nature, which not surprisingly attracted the gaze of the medical profession.

Over the last 20 years, literature from the fields of anthropology, sociology, history, and the women's health movement has dominated the nonmedical work being done on menopause. Although the authors often differ in their approaches, through their arguments and their understanding of the past a consensus has emerged that at some point medical practitioners, as a result of their increased understanding of the role of the sex hormone estrogen, began to pathologize and medicalize menopause and to argue that it was an estrogen-deficiency disease.[2] What recent cross-cultural studies have revealed is that menopause is also a culturally contingent experience.[3]

This chapter begins with a study of the medical terms used to designate menopause. The meanings of such terms were often vague and, at times, contradictory, allowing physicians to conflate physiological changes with life changes. The various terms also emphasized the difficulties physicians had describing in a precise manner a process that they saw as transformative. But the lack of explicitness did not seem to be of concern. Of more moment for physicians were the factors they believed caused an early or late menopause, as if such an understanding would allow them to predict when it might occur in individual women. While these influences represented "hard" data and reflected their urge to classify, as an exercise in understanding the discussions were rather abstract. Less so were practitioners' mostly negative views of the experience of menopause and their use of it as a catchall diagnosis for myriad concerns, both physical and mental, that women brought to them, as well as their treatment of those symptoms. What emerges out of this study are several conclusions about physicians and their views of menopause. First, both the Canadian and international literature on menopause increased significantly with the 1920s. Second, the need of physicians for surety in their work was reflected both in the way they sought a definition of menopause even when they did not achieve it and how they discussed the factors influencing age of menopause as if they were presenting "facts," ignoring that, at times, disagreements existed within the profession. Third, despite what some scholars have suggested for this period, the issue of aging permeates the medical discussion of menopause.[4] Fourth, physicians in the past were sensitive to more than the physiological aspects of menopause. They had a strong sense of the impact of social/cultural influences, although how they interacted with the physiological was not always clear, just as they are not today. Last, physicians' attitudes did become more positive over time (at least to mid century) as reflected in the advice and reassurance they gave to women. Such a shift is important to recognize because as activist/scholars have pointed out, the publication of Robert A. Wilson's *Feminine Forever*[5] in 1966 signalled a downturn in reactions to menopause among many physicians and women themselves and pathologized menopause in a way that few physicians in the first half of the century ever did. And while the emphasis of recent scholarly literature has been on the feminist challenge to Estrogen Replacement Therapy (ERT) and later Hormone Replacement Therapy (HRT), many physicians themselves in the interwar period and after opposed ERT and raised significant concerns about its safety.[6]

What Is Menopause?

The first problem physicians faced was the meaning of menopause. Patricia Kaufert has argued that doctors' desire to categorize or define has led them to focus on the last menses as a universal indicator of menopause, one that cannot be recognized at the time but only retrospectively. In her study of the gendered nature of medicine, Susan Bell is not as convinced about a consensus on a menopausal indicator.[7] There certainly was little consensus in the first half of the century. Physicians used a variety of terms to designate the menopause experience. At times, each term had its own specific meaning; at others, terms were interchangeable leading to definitional vagueness. Even when a physician was clear about meaning, his colleagues did not always agree.

In his turn-of-the-century textbook Henry Byford described "menopause" as "that period of time, intervening between the beginning irregularity of menstruation and the complete cessation of the flow, with the subsequent restoration of health." Thus menopause was a process taking place over time. Others insisted that menopause referred specifically to the end of menstruation, making it a specific point in time only known after the fact.[8] Neither was menopause the only term physicians used to designate the process women underwent, although all terms one way or another encompassed the end of menstruation. Many referred to a "critical period." Less popular in Canadian writings was the word "climacteric," which suggested a shift in more than body and like the use of "critical period" denoted a crisis. An even broader phrase, the "change of life," had wider currency in the literature Canadian physicians were reading.[9] While physicians used a variety of terms and, if pressed, could differentiate among them (even if as in the case of "menopause" they disagreed about the nature of those differences), they also used them interchangeably. In the American literature she examined, Judith Houck similarly noted the variety of word usages, although she did not see problems in using terms interchangeably even when they had different meanings, nor how they reflected a profession that aspired to the sureness of science yet had difficulty attaining it.[10] But each term conjures up a different image that could lead physicians, in the words of Byford's text, "to attribute all the ills and complaints of such a patient to the menopause."[11]

While the acceptance of the role of sex hormones in the interwar years increased the understanding of menopause, the variety of terms employed did not alter to any great extent. Physicians continued to express their views with an authority that seemed oblivious to differently nuanced or even contrasting descriptions. "Menopause" was still the favoured designation. Repeating the phrasing of Byford's earlier text quoted above, one contributor to the 1924 *Diseases of Middle Life* claimed it "includes the time between the beginning of menstrual irregularity to [a woman's] complete restoration to health." Physicians also used the broader term "change of life" and William Pelton Tew from London, Ontario, recommended that women see their physicians on a regular basis until they managed to make their way through that change. As a result, the idea that menopause was a "critical" or "dangerous" age or stage continued. Physicians also continued to signify the crisis aspect of menopause through their use of the term "climacteric."[12] And, as in the early decades of the century, they did not always distinguish between the various terms. For most, the end of menstruation was key, yet terms such as "change of life" or the "climacteric" also encompassed many more aspects of a woman's life than the end of menstruation. All signalled an end to youth, which in a society that was increasingly privileging youth, made the negativity of such terms clear.

During WWII and the postwar years, there was some attempt to be more precise about meaning. "Menopause" still maintained pride of place and Percy E. Ryberg, author of the best-selling *Health, Sex and Birth Control*, made clear that the term applied specifically to the cessation of menstruation. Of course there were other reasons for the cessation of menstruation – pregnancy or some other cause of amenorrhoea – so his definition to be precise needed qualification. Less popular than before was "critical" period. Physicians were trying to encourage women not to see menopause as a crisis because by then they had something to offer women in the form of ERT. Physicians still referred, however, to the "change of life" and the "climacteric." James H. Darragh in the *McGill Medical Journal* of 1946 explained that the climacteric and menopause were used interchangeably but, in contrast to Ryberg, Darragh argued menopause really referred to a much longer period, over "several years." His understanding also differed from that of F. Gibson, resident in obstetrics and gynecology at the Royal Victoria Montreal Maternity Hospital, who claimed in the November 1950 *Canadian Nurse* that the climacteric encompassed "the transition from the reproductive period to senility."[13] While Ryberg, Gibson, and Darragh tried to be specific about their terminology, it is clear their understanding of it could differ.

The numerous terms, the vagueness of their meanings, and the contradictory understanding of some of those meanings raise the issue of communication in the first half century. If medical literature used different terms or the meanings of the same terms varied, how could medical students who read them understand what was being written? How clear was the communication between physicians? And if such communication was problematic, what can be said for the communication between physician and patient when often common understanding of terms was most likely quite different from the medical definitions? Conflation of terms, however, reflected a complex process that defied precise definition and allowed for different experiences among women.

When It Comes in Women

At what age did this complex process begin? Estimates varied from between ages 45 and 55, leading physicians to speculate on what actions determined the precise age for an individual woman. There was a sense that if the factors were controlled, then all women's bodies would behave the same, indeed that it would be better if all women's bodies did so. Physicians may have been interested in having a normative biological model of menopause, but the reality of patients and their lives introduced social and cultural factors. What interested physicians in their listing of influences (both biological and social/cultural) on the age of menopause was the correlation between them and menopause, although they did not seem able to explain or even be interested in explaining how the connection worked. But the information represented "fact," which became part of the surety of medical knowledge. Such knowledge would be the foundation of understanding, even if that understanding was in the future.

In trying to understand why some women reached menopause earlier than others, physicians in the early years of the century emphasized age of puberty as the major influence. They considered puberty and menopause the two critical periods of a woman's life and not surprisingly saw the influences on each as similar if not, in some cases, identical. They deemed each the reverse of the other, puberty building up the reproductive ability and menopause destroying that ability. Yet how the connection worked was unclear in the literature being read. Some practitioners suggested that an early puberty would lead to a late menopause, whereas others argued that an early puberty correlated with an early menopause or at least not with a late one.[14] Why physicians wanted there to be a link is unclear, but it did provide some understanding of what was happening, a predictive factor rather than a randomness with which many seemed uncomfortable.

The linkage made between age of puberty and age of menopause became stronger in later years, probably because of increased information available on the nature and workings of the sex hormones. In 1927, H.B. Anderson of Toronto argued that the symptoms of menopause were more intense at the usual time of menstruation making the connection between the two direct.[15] There was still little consensus, however, about timing. Some suggested an early puberty meant an early menopause. Even more maintained the opposite, that early puberty would lead to a later menopause.[16] One of the few texts to explain why it was significant to know how the correlations worked was the 1935 *Diseases of Women*. Understanding the timing and influence of factors on menopause could help physicians determine when the stoppage of menstruation signalled a diseased state or a natural occurrence. In 1950, F. Gibson was more specific about causation: "If the ovarian function starts early, indicating a virile gonad, its function will have a tendency to last longer." Perhaps for this reason, the literature emphasized that women with no or few children (indicating an unhealthy gonad) reached menopause earlier than those with many (the assumption being that women had no control over the number of children they could conceive).[17]

Climate was another "fixed" factor influencing the timing of menopause. If, as many physicians believed, a warm climate brought on early puberty, it brought on early menopause as well. Race, too, was influential with J. Clarence Webster, author of the 1907 *A Text-Book of Diseases of Women*, noting that menopause came earlier in Jewish than in non-Jewish women. In this example, Webster racialized a religious/ethnic group and used that racialization as proof that race was a factor influencing age of menopause. Closely aligned with "race" was heredity. While exceptions were acknowledged, there was a sense that a daughter would take after her mother.[18] No one seemed to point out that she might take after her paternal grandmother or even her father in development. The hereditary line was clear and sexed, from father to son, from mother to daughter. In the interwar period and after, discussion of the effects of climate, race, and heredity were often repeats of previous international ones with Canadian commentators joining in. For example, Gibson referred to climate and health as influencing age of menopause. He also proposed that "racial extraction appears to have some bearing upon the age of onset. Northern and Anglo-Saxon types tend to be later, while southern and oriental types tend to be earlier in onset than average."[19]

Social context or environment could influence the impact of "fixed" factors. A 1910 article in *The Canada Lancet* quoted one international authority that climate and race were not as significant in the United States as elsewhere. If, as above in Webster's textbook, race was being identified with ethnic groups, then the lack of fixedness in the racial factor in the United States was understandable. Compared to many countries, the United States, like Canada, had a significant degree of intermarriage between various ethnic and national groups. Social factors also appeared relevant in that luxurious living delayed menopause, as did city life and good nutrition, which allowed the menstrual function to continue. Almost anything in a woman's life could influence her age of menopause. Some physicians believed that marital relations delayed menopause, as did prolonged childbearing, which some considered a sign of active (healthy) ovarian functioning. Hinted at as well was that pregnancy interrupted the "normal" number of menstrual cycles thus extending the age over which they occurred.[20] The recognition of social factors suggested that medical perceptions of menopause were complex. Menopause was not "simply" a biological event; the lived experiences of women and their environment impinged on its timing.

Physicians continued to connect social conditions to the timing of menopause, revealing an awareness of factors other than the biomedical. They seemed to approve of women whose menopause was delayed since the factors influencing it could be interpreted as more positive than negative – wealth (the assumption being that the affluent were healthier), good nourishment, continuation of marital relations, and childbearing. The non-Canadian literature especially linked early menopause to women who were working class, overweight, had their children too close together, or had experienced an unhealthy confinement.[21] But the association between positive/negative factors and late/ early menopause was not consistent. For example, some argued uterine disease worked to delay menopause whereas others insisted the link depended on the nature of the health problem.[22] Neither did all physicians mention each factor or influence; rather each mentioned those he deemed most significant, adding his favourites to a gradually accumulating list.

How social and fixed factors interacted was unclear. In his 1929 textbook, William P. Graves agreed that an early puberty was linked to a later menopause. He also was convinced that upper-class women came to puberty later than working-class women, which, using his own logic, meant that their menopause should come somewhat earlier, but it didn't. He argued that menopause in upper-class women came an average of five years later than in working women. He explained this through better nourishment and "freedom from hard work." Percy E. Ryberg and others were not so confident about such causal links.[23] Nothing definite could be determined because few if any studies had been done. Nonetheless, medical beliefs were often passed down from one generation to another, repeated until something emerged to contradict them. By writing with authority, physicians were able to overlook the uncertainty of whether or how those linkages actually worked.

If the factors influencing age of menopause did not change significantly, according to Susan Bell, what did change was the emphasis on blaming individual women's prior behaviour for experiencing severe symptoms of menopause. She has argued that such blame declined with the discovery of hormones because that discovery allowed the attribution of severe menopausal symptoms to a biological process.[24] But blaming the behaviour of women continued even after the discovery of sex hormones. Physicians repeated the national, class, and race prejudices of an earlier period and added to them. In *Gynecology and Obstetrics*, a text edited by Carl Henry Davis in 1935, readers were given the same description noted above Webster's 1907 text. Some physicians went further and associated severe symptoms with personality weaknesses well into the 1940s. Evan Shute, from London, Ontario, argued that those having severe emotional setbacks during menopause were women with "life-long habits of pessimism or self-pity in egocentric personalities." The positive side was that women who were emotionally healthy had little difficulty with menopause.[25] Understanding the role of estrogen did not lessen the willingness of some physicians to look beyond the biological to explain the differences in women's experience of menopause. Indeed, in some respects they avoided the temptation to essentialize menopause (and women) and recognized a multiplicity of experiences.

General View of Menopause

Two general overviews of those experiences existed. The first was muted positivism. Doctors recognized that menopause was not a negative experience or did not have to be for most women. But – and there was a but – the focus on the positive always seemed to be phrased in a way that took away from the assurance. The second overview was a more consistent negative perspective. In seeing the body as "failing," no longer able to do what it had long been capable of doing, practitioners suggested, in the words of Emily Martin, that the "authority structure in the body" had failed. What women had taken for granted had disappeared. The medical view was full of metaphorical negativity that had embedded within it medical "facts" presented in a way that included values about the worth of women and their bodies.[26] Within aboriginal society, menopause brought access to power and influence.[27] The negativity of the literature Canadian physicians were reading and writing suggested quite the opposite.

In the early years of the century, some medical literature recognized that menopause did not necessarily pose problems for women. But the message was often conditional. Daniel R. Brower and Henry M. Bannister in their 1902 *A Practical Manual of Insanity for Medical Student and General Practitioner* were typical in noting that "in perfectly normal individuals this change ought to occur without disturbance." The question was, how many "perfectly normal" women were there? Obviously not many, since immediately following their reassuring statement the authors pointed out that such women were "rare." And whether at risk or not, women at menopause should be under a physician's care.[28] It was the physician's challenge and responsibility to determine a normal from an abnormal menopause, not the woman's. J. Clarence Webster continued his focus on race in seeing the problems of menopause as linked to race when he quoted the belief that "in races or nations that are phlegmatic, cold and apathetic, in women accustomed to life in the open air and to hard work, in savage and barbarous nations, the disturbances of menopause are slight. Whereas among emotional, passionate people, like the Latin nations ... the distressing phenomena of the climacteric are usually found."[29]

Despite the acknowledgement that menopause did not have to be problematic, at least not for all women, physicians in the early years generally stressed the problems that *could* arise. Arthur E. Giles, Surgeon at Chelsea Hospital for Women, in an article published in the 1914 *Canada Lancet* went further and connected menopause with some kind of unhealthy state.[30] Too often, physicians linked anything untoward in midlife to the menopause rather than searching for other possible causes. Joan Roberts entered the Victoria General Hospital, Halifax, on 5 October 1911. She was 41 years of age. She had stopped menstruating in April of that year and complained of headaches, pain around the heart, and swollen feet after working hard. She also suffered from fainting spells followed by shivers. On examination, physicians found her right ovary slightly enlarged and her left ovary not palpable but with a thick band on the left side. She refused the surgery her doctors suggested. Despite the recognition of some kind of ovarian problem, the final diagnosis was "debility at menopause."[31]

Canadian physicians tried to be and were somewhat more positive in the interwar period and beyond. Writing in 1931, W.H. Hattie impressed upon his colleagues that too often physicians still believed the extreme negative beliefs of earlier years. Doctors had a responsibility not only to remove those views from the medical literature (which he felt they were doing), but also to promote a more "wholesome" outlook among women themselves. He pointed to the obvious fact that menopause was a "universal phenomenon." A year later, the Commissioner of Mental Health for Alberta, C.A. Baragar, argued that menopause was "merely ... another physiological change when [women] will escape the monthly inconvenience of menstruation and pass into the calm and peaceful period of late middle life."[32] The idea of a "calm and peaceful period," however, may not have appealed to all women with its suggestion of retirement.

A muted but still positive view of menopause was expressed in a 1946 international nursing text written by two Canadians, Archibald Donald Campbell, gynaecologist and obstetrician-in-chief, Montreal General Hospital, and Mabel A. Shannon, supervisor of the gynaeco-logical ward, Montreal General Hospital. They assured their readers that 15–20 percent of women did not experience "abnormal menopausal symptoms" whereas the other 80–85 percent who did experienced them only on a sporadic basis. What is interesting about this quote is the term "abnormal" for symptoms that the majority of women experienced and how the supposedly optimistic statistics carried a negative message. As Mary Poovey has commented, statistics are not unmediated. They make whatever is being measured important even when it may not be and certainly not in the broader experience of women's lives.[33] In stating that 15–20 percent of women did not experience "abnormal menopausal symptoms," Campbell and Shannon emphasized the abnormality of menopause and its problematic nature for women. Understanding both how the negative image emerged and the problematic nature of statistics on menopause, Drs Cleghorn and Stern, assistant professors of psychiatry at McGill University, highlighted a simple but important reality for the readers of *Chatelaine* in 1948 – statistics on the problems of menopause were gathered from women who sought the help of physicians. They did not represent those women experiencing no or little difficulty and who did not consult their doctors.[34]

Despite the attempts at being more optimistic, physicians often perceived menopause as the end of a woman's active phase of life. In 1919, W.H. Roberts compared puberty and menopause and found "the one contains the promise and our only assurance of the continuance of the human race. The other ... that the die of life has been cast." For others it was the beginning of old age, a time when women should cut back on their activities. There was a sadness to middle age, a sense of withdrawal from activity, but commentators did not see it as particularly dangerous, which some American scholars have suggested they did.[35]

Symptoms of Menopause

When physicians discussed the "symptoms" of menopause in a specific way, the reasons for their negative view become clearer. Not surprisingly, physical manifestations of menopause were of major interest to them, both changes in and experiences of the body. In the early years of the century, physicians often focused on the internal changes of the reproductive system that occurred with menopause, using a language denoting loss and diminishment. Byford's turn-of-the-century text gave what was a typical description: "[T]he vulva becomes flattened and shrivelled ... the dimensions of the vagina become contracted ... the uterine walls atrophy, the cavity diminishes ... the ovaries shrivel and shrink ... [and] their envelope becomes wrinkled." This image was transferred to the lay public through advice manuals. Women readers of *Sexual Knowledge* learned that their ovaries and uterus could "disappear altogether."[36] Given that most women would not have known what their internal sexual/reproductive organs looked like, the picture conjured up by such descriptions were left to the imagination. Physicians continued to describe the physical changes in the genital system using a language of loss throughout the interwar years and beyond. Some focused on the image of retrogression, deterioration, or disappearance, others on thinning, shrinkage, and shrivelling.[37] However, a lessening of the implications of some indicators in the postwar years did take place. In 1946 James H. Darragh, for example, argued that atrophy of the genitalia did not occur for "many years," which left the woman much as she had been.[38]

Physicians did not limit their comments to the internal physical changes of women's bodies. They also remarked on external changes in appearance. According to some physicians, when women lost their ability to procreate they became masculine. In his 1907 *The Practice of Obstetrics ... for the Use of Students and Practitioners,* J. Clifton Edgar commented on "a more angular form ... or even the development of an imperfect beard or moustache." The voice became "harsher," more like a man's.[39] Others noted the breasts became "sunken" and "flabby," the skin "sallow" and "plethoric." Weight gain occurred with the descriptors being uniformly negative: "obesity," "stoutness," "deposits of fat."[40] Neither did much change throughout the years. While one contributor to a 1924 text dismissed the connection between menopause and weight gain, his assurance was hardly comforting:

> Women who are destined to become fat usually begin to increase in weight long before the menopause, and often reach their maximum before menstruation ceases. Often the increase after the menopause is only apparent, for at that age the external tissues begin to lose their firm contour and the fat settles into irregular and baggy folds, giving the impression of increase in size though there may be no increase in weight.[41]

More accusatory was Ryberg, who told his women readers that their weight gain was their own fault, a result of lessened activity and "overeating." After the war, Cleghorn told *Chatelaine* readers that some of them might gain weight but assured them that it was not the case for most. Yet popular articles warned women that "fat begins at forty."[42] Not all physicians were as positive as Cleghorn. H.G. Oborne, writing in the 1950 *Alberta Medical Bulletin,* after lavishing detail on the atrophy of the genitalia, noted, "One also often encounters a type of obesity characterized by deposits of fat over the trochaters, mons veneris and breasts which is usually seen in castrates after the age of 30."[43] Such a statement blamed the body and put body weight beyond woman's control. Despite the continued focus on the negative physical problems that could be associated with menopause, in the interwar period and after there was a decline in the emphasis on unattractiveness contrary to what some American studies revealed and associated with a backlash against women receiving voting rights.[44] Admittedly, in his 1942 *Health, Sex and Birth Control,* Ryberg told his lay readers that at menopause a woman "assumes some masculine characteristics."[45] But compared to earlier decades, such references were rare.

   Linked to physical changes were those that could be considered experiential. Most often mentioned were hot flashes. According to David Tod Gilliam in his 1907 *A Text-book of Practical Gynecology* they were "annoying and at times almost insufferable."[46] Hot flashes remained a major focus. The work of sex endocrinologists allowed physicians to understand the role of lowered estrogen level and its link to hot flashes, but that understanding did not make flashes, in the words of H. B. Atlee, less "unpleasant" or "troublesome." But it did help physicians to connect various symptoms. As J. Ross Vant in the 1948 *Alberta Medical Bulletin* made clear, the decline in estrogen resulted in "flushes, irritability, headaches, sweats etc."[47] Estrogen seemed to be a universal explanation, yet recent studies point out that in some cultures women don't experience hot flashes despite a lessening of estrogen.[48]

Not surprisingly, given that many of the descriptions of menopause contained the suggestion that a woman's "femaleness" and attractiveness were disappearing, physicians assumed women's sexual life would also change. While some scholars have seen an increasing emphasis on the loss of sexuality in the twentieth century, in the first half of the century such a consensus did not exist.[49] In the early years of the century, medical opinions were varied and covered a wide spectrum. Some physicians described decreased interest in sexual activity as a given, others stated that the decline was temporary, and still others found that sexual activity did not decline and for some it increased.[50] Neither did a consensus on sexuality and menopause emerge in later years. Some still argued a decline in the sexual life of woman occurred, a perception they believed women had as well.[51] A few physicians argued the sex drive in women actually increased and looked somewhat askance at the idea. More common, however, were less apocalyptic views, mentioning in passing that the sex drive increased, at least temporarily.[52] Karl Stern in his 1948 *Chatelaine* article "The Truth about Menopause" similarly tried to reassure women: "We have found that in healthy, well-adjusted women there is no change one way or another; if there is a complete disappearance or a marked increase of sex desire during this time of life, it is, in our experience, usually an indication of some hidden conflict." While meant to comfort, his words might not have been much consolation to some. For women who felt uncomfortable with some of the "symptoms" of menopause and may not have been interested in sexual activity, the message was that they were not "well-adjusted." Those who might have engaged in intercourse with more abandon than they had done when pregnancy was a possibility could interpret Stern's message as suggesting hidden conflict in their lives. Nevertheless, his and others' recognition of the continuation of sexual desire after sexuality belie the argument of some scholars that women's advice literature tended to be silent on the issue of sexuality and menopause.[53]

Physicians perceived the changes to women's bodies and how they experienced them as transformative. Unfortunately, they also linked them to ill health. Disorders of appetite – indigestion, dyspepsia, intestinal problems – were an example. Accompanying digestive disorders were constipation and gas build-up. Difficulty sleeping was a problem, as was a general decline in energy, a feeling of exhaustion, and lethargy. Vague pains were mentioned as part of the menopausal syndrome. They could appear in the arms, legs, back, abdomen, breasts, or heart. Headaches were believed common as was dizziness.[54] While menopause was not a diseased state in and of itself, physicians could be very specific about the afflictions that accompanied it: leucorrhea, torpid liver, diseased kidneys, skin diseases, bronchial difficulties, gout, and impaired vision.[55] Not all women would experience each symptom or its associated ailments but that was a reality physicians seldom emphasized. And it wasn't just physicians who focused on the "endless" problems of menopause. The introductory chapter quote by Alice Stockham proved that. No matter what assurances might be made, women reading the list of menopausal symptoms Stockham provided would be overwhelmed by the negativity surrounding menopause.

And the litany continued and expanded.[56] Some went further and saw menopause as a "malady"; references to menopausal "symptoms" aligned it with an unhealthy state as did equating it with "ovarian amenorrhoea."[57] Contrary to what one American historian of menopause has suggested, the profession as a whole clearly saw menopause as problematic even if individual physicians might not.[58] But unlike what some other scholars have maintained, they did not consider it as a disease, the references to malady, symptoms, and ovarian amenorrhoea notwithstanding.[59] *Symptoms* were evidence presented by women and *signs* of menopause were medical determinants and few in number. Darragh, who referred to menopause as a malady, in his next phrase referred to it as a "trying period," which certainly suggests something other than an ailment or disease. J.A. Low, who used the phrase "ovarian amenorrhoea," was following a tendency to refer to any interruption in menstruation, whether normal or not, as amenorrhoea. In the medical literature there was a sloppiness to the language used despite attempts to choose descriptors having the aura of science and precision. Nevertheless some women internalized the medical view. Mrs Anna Stevens, age 45 with two children, the youngest being 14, was convinced she had some of the symptoms mentioned in the medical literature. Entering the Montreal General Hospital on 17 July 1945, her case record stated that "in the last 2-3 yrs she has had loss of energy, easy fatiguability, nervousness etc & believes she may be approaching the menopause." The fact that she entered hospital suggested her willingness to see her symptoms as representative of disease. Hospital physicians were not as willing to confirm menopause and instead diagnosed her as having cystocoele (fallen bladder), rectocoele (bulge from the rectum wall into the vagina), and second-degree prolapse.[60] If Stevens's physicians and others did not see menopause as a disease, disease could *accompany* menopause. Oborne believed that both hypertension and arteriosclerosis were "exaggerated" by menopause. Those writing on menopause emphasized menopause as a marker for when certain cancers occurred and the connection made created an illusion of cause and effect. Winnipeg physician Ross Mitchell was one of the few who tried to explain why disease of the uterine system could appear at menopause. According to him, during the childbearing years, many women acquired "pathological lesions of the uterus," the toxicity of which was stimulated by the atrophy of the menopause.[61] There was a chain of causation, not a simple cause and effect and certainly not a conflation of menopause with disease.

While the literature Canadian doctors were reading and writing emphasized the physical changes of menopause, the psychological/emotional/mental aspects were not overlooked. There was concern about the perceived change in the disposition of women during menopause – many seemed more difficult to live with. While such change could be minor, it signalled an alteration that physicians found worrisome. In part this may have been because menopause emphasized in a physical and emotional way that mind did not control body. Menopause disrupted what might appear to be a regular cyclicity and faced doctors with the lack of predictability and the challenges it presented for understanding women's bodies.[62] Women's bodies and emotions appeared to be experiencing instability, which in the rational world of science could be deemed frightening and symptomatic of ill health.

In the early decades of the century, A.T.B. Hobbs, surgeon at the asylum for the insane near London, Ontario, explained that the mental life of women corresponded with the stages of biological existence and shifted with each stage; menopause was the marker that defined the last stage of life.[63] At menopause, the changes evidenced were alterations in disposition or personality that at times could be quite extreme, as we saw in the previous chapter on mental disorders. Others were not as significant – irritability being one.[64] While Canadian physicians were not specifically writing about this at the time, the image had certainly become widespread in society. Jessie L. Beattie recalled that when her mother went through menopause the "normal tenor" of her parents' relationship altered and only after her mother's menopause was finished did their "happy, untroubled companionship" return. In explaining the "new" personality that emerged, one medical text used in Canadian medical faculties suggested it was a return to an earlier one. Picking up on this, the popular medical literature distributed and read in Canada emphasized the development or redevelopment of self-centredness at menopause.[65]

In the interwar years and after, physicians continued to mention mental instability, neurasthesnia, and psychological difficulties during menopause. They also commented on personality changes in that some women found themselves impatient, irritable, excitable, temperamental, and jealous.[66] Depression and melancholy remained a perceived common consequence of menopause and one taken up in the Canadian literature. As Baragar noted, it was a consequence not only of physiological changes but also a change in mental outlook linked to aging. While Jessie McGeachy argued in a similar way in the 1950 *Manitoba Medical Review*, she insisted societal factors were also part of the explanation. At menopause women experienced what later commentators referred to as the "empty nest" syndrome.[67] As noted in the previous chapter, some physicians tried to assure women and their colleagues that mental instability was not necessarily connected to menopause, an effort not always acknowledged in the scholarship on menopause. Nonetheless the connection between depression and menopause lasted well beyond mid century.[68]

The mental shifts that were perceived to come with menopause were those that Canadians could see for themselves and that women could experience for themselves. Physicians who believed in the centrality of body were not surprised that the significant physiological change of menopause could result in a wide spectrum of emotional and mental alterations. Over time physicians tried to lessen the atmosphere of a menopausal crisis but were perhaps less able to do so with the more serious mental consequences than they could with the physical, a reflection of their own unease about mental and psychological distress and that of Canadians generally.

Treatment

Given the broad spectrum of symptoms and problems presented by women experiencing menopause, treatment tended to be scattered and designed to offset discomfort. In the interwar years, however, ERT emerged and perhaps because of its later popularity many scholars have exaggerated the degree of hormonal treatment in earlier years.[69] Certainly in Canada it is difficult to know how widespread the treatment was. All we can do at this point is to acknowledge the medical discourse on the subject, part of which included criticisms of its effects.

In the early years of the century, physicians had limited means to assist women. Given the belief that women were often depressed during menopause, Byford's text advocated the need for "mental therapeutics," recommending women eliminate as much care and responsibility as possible from their lives and get involved in "amusements" and "social diversions."[70] While this put the implementation into the hands of women, overlooked was the reality that most working-class and most likely middle-class women would not be able to follow such advice. Others recommended various nostrums, such as senna and salts, or bromides to offset hot flashes. Thomas Watts Eden in his 1911 text warned that alcohol and sedatives were too often used and dangerous to women of "neurotic temperament" who might develop the drug habit. Frederick A. Cleland of the Grace Hospital, Toronto, had found that a form of ergot was helpful in decreasing the "hot flushes, headaches, palpitation of the heart and nervous and mental depression."[71] And even before the "discovery" of hormones, physicians had some sense of internal secretions in the body that might help treat menopause, what physicians referred to as organotherapy. A. Lapthorn Smith had used ovarian tablets to reduce hot flashes, although he did not find them successful.[72]

The emphasis on treating women increased in the interwar, war, and postwar years. Interviews with two physicians trained in the 1920s and 1930s made it clear, however, that there was little formal discussion of treatment of menopause until the 1940s after the ability to manufacture synthetic estrogen occurred.[73] Practitioners were still aware of the need to provide common sense recommendations to their patients – fresh air, change of scene, plain diet, and alcohol restriction. Worry should be avoided, although it was unclear how this was to be accomplished.[74] Physicians who assured themselves and their patients that the problems of menopause were greatly overdrawn still believed they had a role to play in offsetting worry. Emil Novak in his 1944 text suggested to his colleagues the importance "of reassuring the patient and explaining to her in simple language what the menopause means." Only through the explanation in "simple" language could women understand.[75]

Nerve tonics, bromides, and sedatives continued to be recommended. Lydia Pinkham's Vegetable Compound was something that women could prescribe for themselves. As one advertisement in *Chatelaine* made clear, "Pinkham's Compound helps Nature tone up delicate female systems, build more physical resistance and thus helps calm jangly nerves, lessen distress from female functional disorders and give you more PEP to enjoy life."[76] In 1933 Beckwith Whitehouse from the University of Birmingham had readopted bloodletting (used in the nineteenth century) to offset headaches, hot flashes, and vertigo. Evan Shute of London, Ontario, did not believe bloodletting would be of much use and he dismissed the use of bromides as well, seeing in them a cumulative toxic result. He suggested barbiturates instead.[77]

Some scholars have suggested a decline in organotherapy in the interwar years as a result of the isolation of two secretions of the ovary, estrogen and progesterone.[78] But before the isolation physicians continued to use it. In 1927, H.B. Anderson from Toronto explained that extracts of ovary had not been found to be valuable in animal experimentation but that "clinicians more frequently recognize their value" and that he had found them helpful "for the psychoneuroses of the menopause" and had done so for many years. In this case, Anderson was separating the art of medicine from the science of medicine and suggesting that the science was not all there was to know. The science told him that his treatment was useless; either unwilling or unable to accept that, he simply created a parallel form of knowledge.[79]

In therapy, estrogen replacement generated the most excitement. First a natural estrogen was used. H.B. Atlee complained to a meeting of the executive of the Medical Society of Nova Scotia about the numerous trade names for estrogenic preparations and noted that by the late 1930s, there were more than 100 estrogenic products on the market. A synthetic estrogen, diethystibestrol (DES), was developed in 1938 and in the United States approved for use by the American Food and Drug Administration in 1941. DES was less expensive than natural estrogen and also more potent.[80] In Canada, Emmenin, developed by J.B. Collip of insulin fame, was widely advertised and some physicians believed it helpful to women early in their menopause.[81] Advertisements in medical journals encouraged physicians to prescribe one of the many estrogen products, no matter what the severity of the menopausal symptoms or their nature – physical or psychological. Physicians such as J.C. Goodwin found estrogen replacement "remarkably successful." Despite some concern, Atlee recommended to students that replacement therapy was useful for women who were having difficulty. In 1937 Marion Hilliard, who worked at Women's College Hospital, Toronto, published an article on the use of theelin, a natural estrogen product. Her perception was that "the effect in 75 per cent of the cases was miraculous." In 1949, Dorothy Sangster told the readers of *Chatelaine* the "modern" physician with the help of "modern science" could help women overcome the difficulties of menopause through "doses of hormones."[82]

Not all physicians were enamoured. Beckwith Whitehouse in the same article in which he advocated bloodletting argued that "oestrin" could actually enhance hot flashes. William R. Houston in his 1936 *The Art of Treatment* used past experience to try and curb the inflated claims for success that were being made. Evan Shute warned of "the indiscriminate use of oestrogens." In Manitoba, Elinor F.E. Black argued that not enough was known about endocrine balance and what happened when women were given estrogen. She also noted that too many physicians learned about endocrinology from the pharmaceutical companies, hardly unbiased sources.[83] Others worried about the carcinogenic effect that estrogens had and suggested that more benign treatment such as vitamin E was more appropriate especially for those patients with cancer.[84] The link between estrogen and cancer had long been suspected and animal studies in the 1930s seemed to confirm it. By the late 1940s international literature pointed to a rise in endometrial cancer among women who took estrogen. In 1946, Darragh warned that the use of estrogens tended to prolong the menopause "indefinitely," which he argued was "insensible." He described the problems that could result from the use of artificial estrogens especially DES: "gastro-intestinal upsets, nausea, and vomiting, and headache." He also raised the connection between estrogen and cancer. He wasn't convinced the link was strong but it did exist. Louis J. Harris from Toronto also raised the fear of cancer and noted, as many had before him, that experts agreed that no woman with a family history of breast or genital cancer should be prescribed estrogen.[85]

The concerns expressed by Canadian physicians reflected the uncertain state of medical science, the difficulty physicians had keeping up with new developments, and physicians' occasional dependence on pharmaceutical companies for knowledge. Yet the support of estrogen therapy should not be surprising. Given the almost uniform negative perception of menopause, physicians believed they had a responsibility to offer something to women and the women who came to them believed they needed help. While the traditional bromides, sedatives, tonics were still available and still used, estrogen "fit" into the sense of scientific endeavour and its modern application. It appealed to the "endocrine world" that was so influential during the interwar years and after.

Male Menopause

An interesting sidebar to the medical discussion of menopause in women was what some referred to as a similar phenomenon in men. Men did not undergo ovarian changes but, nevertheless, there was some recognition that men experienced a change of life that some commentators did refer to as menopause. The reactions to the concept in the early years ranged from denial, to acknowledging the existence of a change but making little of it, to recognizing changes in men as they aged but denying this was a male menopause. Those physicians willing to discuss a male menopause seldom went into any detail. According to the literature, it occurred later in men than in women and more gradually, and was characterized by a slowing down of life, an association with mental instability, and lack of energy.[86] One of the physical changes mentioned was decline in virility, seen calmly by some practitioners as a natural part of aging and solely a physical phenomenon. More emotional was Sylvanus Stall, who in one of his many sex manuals quoted William Acton that the male menopause was the time when man noticed his virility declining "almost with a feeling of indignation."[87]

Some historians have suggested a decline of medical interest in male menopause in the interwar and wartime period. But the perceived decline was more a factor of increasing attention being paid to female menopause rather than any real shift in attention with respect to male menopause. Those willing to discuss the "disturbances" in men varied in their estimation of age of onset (anywhere from 45 to 60 years) and duration (10 months up to 4 years).[88] The latter allowed for a significant period of time in which to attribute all sorts of male difficulties to a specific cause just as in the case of women. Because there was debate over its existence, the symptoms of the male menopause were often linked to a midlife crisis phenomenon rather than something that was inherent in the body itself beyond the experience of aging. Baragar warned that after the age of 40, a man had "to revamp his ambitions and hopes and dreams." In some men, the midlife changes could develop into more serious psychological and mental problems.[89]

While the potential psychological effects of the male menopause were discussed, the major focus, as with women, was on the physical signs. Some of them were the results of aging. T.D. Cumberland noted "arterial hardening, grey hair, wrinkling of skin, loss of physical energy." To these Ryberg added "loss of the force in the water coming from the bladder," and a change in weight, hot flashes, sweating, heart palpitations, disturbed sleep, and pains in the legs. Many of these were associated with menopause in women. Ryberg also detailed the physical changes that occurred in the male reproductive organs – the "loosening of the tissues," sagging, and the losing of tone which resulted in a lessening of sexual interest and ability. Yet the opposite could also occur. Desires increased leading to "acts of indecency, attempts on young girls, homosexuality." The increased interest in sexuality was in the words of Ryberg akin to "the last hefty kicks of a dying horse."[90]

Similar themes continued into the postwar years – denial and minimal acknowledgment. Physicians who recognized a male change of life were usually quite calm about it. Stern in a 1948 article in *Chatelaine* entitled "The Truth About the Menopause" made it clear that men experienced "emotional upsets" as much as women but that they were not recognized as being connected to the "male climacterium" because men simply did not have the physical marker of this stage of life that women did (end of menstruation). Edwin Hirsch, author of a book on marital sexuality, was very open with his readers about the change of life in men. In many ways it resembled that of women – the feeling of nervousness, irritability, depression, and inability to concentrate.[91] It was a time when life was changing and stressful.

While the emotional changes were significant, the physical characteristics were equally so and as in the earlier period conflated with aging – receding hair, grey hair, weight gain, less stamina, frequency in urination, higher rates of prostate problems and cancer, and regressive joint changes. Some of the physical symptoms were very similar to those of female menopause – "dizziness, hot flushes, palpitations, headaches, aches, insomnia and depression." And the decline in male virility remained a concern. But it was not just the ability to engage in sexual intercourse that was recognized as declining but the virility of the sperm produced.[92]

While one historian of the American situation has suggested "rejuvenation therapy" occurred for men in the 1920s, little evidence of it exists in the Canadian context.[93] What had changed by the end of the 1940s compared to the earlier years was understanding the role hormones played in some of the changes men were experiencing. For prostate gland problems, testosterone treatment was claimed to be beneficial, as was the use of estrogens. Sidney Katz, writing in *Maclean's*, warned men against getting caught up in testosterone treatment, however, quoting Dr W.W. Bauer, director of the American Medical Association's health education section: "If you administer testosterone indiscriminately you give a man a false sense of youthfulness. This would be as risky as putting a high-powered 1949 engine in a tired and worn 1929 chassis and opening the throttle wide." R.A. Cleghorn, assistant professor of psychiatry, McGill University, warned his colleagues that the psychiatric aspects of the "so-called climacteric" in men was in a confused state. Hormones were related to it in some way but he advised his colleagues "to make a thorough investigation of life situations in disturbed middle-aged men before prescribing testosterone."[94]

While male menopause was recognized in the first half of the century, it certainly did not attract the attention directed at female menopause. For those writing about it, there was always a sense of introducing a topic that had received little attention and that most people did not acknowledge existed. Men did not have the physical marker of menopause that made their entrance to it clear. All women did. Given how physicians viewed female menopause, medical hesitancy regarding male menopause was not surprising.

Conclusion

Many factors influenced the medical construction of menopause. First the multiplicity of terms used to classify it tended to broaden what "menopause," "climacteric," "change of life," etc., entailed. Second, the attempt to understand the factors that resulted in an early or late menopause reinforced the perceived centrality of the reproductive (as opposed to the sexual) system for women and the view that saw menopause as an end to womanhood. Third, in perceiving menopause in this manner, physicians after the 1920s were able to conflate the physical consequences of estrogen decline with the perceived emotional consequences of the end of reproductive life. While the former could be more easily documented, the latter was assumed based on the centrality of woman's role as childbearer in society. Some women did feel menopause was a turning point in their lives. L.M. Montgomery wrote about a gate closing.[95] But if that was true, it was equally true that menopause brought with it advantages (no longer having to worry about becoming pregnant, no longer having to menstruate). But as reflected in the medical literature, the negative view dominated. Nevertheless, compared to the early decades of the century, physicians at mid century were more positive about menopause than they had been.

The treatment of menopause ran the gamut from common sense to invasive. There is no doubt ERT created excitement within the profession and held out hope to physicians of being able to respond to the needs of their women patients. Not all physicians, however, were convinced. Some worried about too quick an adoption of therapy before studies of its effects were made. And when studies did link it to cancer in animals, that raised cautionary warnings. But until a cause and effect relationship in humans was substantiated, many practitioners maintained their optimism about estrogen replacement therapy. After all, how could what women's bodies had once produced be a threat?

Conclusion

In looking at the medical perception and treatment of women in Canada from 1900 to 1950, I have been particularly interested in tracing the way in which physicians perceived women's bodies and how that perception affected the treatment offered. The two are closely related and there is no reason to suppose that is not still the case, albeit with slightly different perceptions and treatment. By looking at medicine in this way, my intention is not to measure it by any ideal concept that I may have about how medicine should work, but rather to point out how medicine in the past functioned and, most likely, still functions. What fascinates is the culture of medicine and the significance physicians have had in our society as the contact point between the individual and health care.

Medicine no longer holds the aura of prestige that it once did. Patients are now more questioning and demanding; other medical and health care practitioners are vying to share physicians' place; and the money that medicine is absorbing in government budgets has raised queries about the kind of medicine practiced and what we as a society can afford. The women's health movement has been part of that rethinking. It has exposed how a narrow view of women distorts women's health experience and, consequently, has led to closer scrutiny of medicine. But we must always remember that if medicine is under scrutiny, society is as well because the two cannot be separated. One is the reflection of the other. In some respects I use my work on medicine as a conduit to the wider society. Society shapes medicine and in turn medicine often supports society's attitudes about health, body, men, women, gender, class, ethnicity, etc., and ties them up in a scientific aura of objectivity.

Certainty and Uncertainty

A major theme underlying this study is the tension within medicine and among practitioners between uncertainty and certainty.[1] In medicine clinical practice represents uncertainty and medical science certainty. It is the belief in the science of medicine that allows practitioners to cope with the messiness of facing patients and their varied problems on a day to day basis. Science holds out hope that the future will be better, that it will have the "cures" or successes for those times when practitioners fail in their daily practice. In believing in the science of medicine, physicians are optimists and true believers. Science provides practitioners with a "perfect story" of what medicine is – a linear development of progress and an understanding of how the body works, what the body is (usually adult and fertile). The reality of medicine that this book has shown is more diverse.[2]

The visible representation of science in medicine, both for the patient and the physician, was the accumulation of information on the patient's body. Much of that information was in the form of measurements of health. Practitioners tried to gain certainty by a dependence on measurements so that a norm of body health could be reached and health and ill health differentiated. Thus a measurement, be it the size of menstrual flow or the time at which puberty or menopause began, was a way to assess the patient. Measurements, however, only mean something if they are compared to some accepted standard and when measurements outside the norm signifies illness or something problematic. Measurement takes the art out of medicine (or the uncertainty) for it removes the responsibility from the individual practitioner and places it in the medical collective, which has agreed on what the measurements mean.[3] Measurement focuses on the body not the person and the physician's task was and is to measure the body by some measurable standard of health. The problem from the patient's perspective was that her/his norm might not be the norm for health; indeed that norm could very often be that of ill health. In their desire to understand the symptoms and signs of ill health, physicians accumulated a long listing of such indicators. If physicians had encountered headaches in women going through menopause, then headaches became a sign of menopause. The list of symptoms increased with time, in part because during these years the studies supporting their significance were often not undertaken.

Medicine is interested in finding a diagnosis and then treating the ailment diagnosed so that the patient's problem is lessened. Hospital statistics reflect the concept that cure is the goal of medicine, the statistics of outcome phrased in terms of how many or what percentage of patients were cured or improved. Medicine is a curing profession. The word "heal" is almost never used. When a diagnosis is not obvious, physicians begin the search for one even if at the end of their search they sometimes fall back on ones that allow for vagueness. Examples are the use of the hysteria, neurasthenia, and even menopause diagnoses. Each absorbed a wide variety of symptoms unable to be pinned to a specific physiological cause; as diagnoses, however, they provide a heuristic device of clarification and understanding.

Measuring the functions of the body is part of the diagnostic method. As noted in the chapter on cancer, biopsies were the test of record and we have seen how, while some practitioners may have questioned their accuracy, they took on a life of their own. Whether physicians used the information from the biopsies, however, was another issue. In some circumstances experience overrode science. What has fascinated me over the years of studying the way in which medicine works is how some physicians were able to ignore some information that would seem to benefit their patients. One example was the carcinogenic nature of estrogen replacement therapy. Some worried about it, but many others dismissed the early findings as unconvincing. And maybe they were. But even as more negative data emerged, some physicians still did not accept the potential danger. In their eyes ERT offered help to their patients' more extreme experiences with menopause and unless the connection between estrogen and cancer was compelling, they were not going to change their practice. The attitude seemed to be that it was not up to those advocating ERT to prove its safety, but for its opponents to prove its harm.

The language of medicine was another way of maintaining surety both within the professional fraternity and with patients.[4] Physicians gained their power through language and their "*apocalyptic* images and warnings."[5] The development of a technical language suggested preciseness, but as we have seen, particularly in the chapters on puberty and menopause, the terms describing each were often confused and unclear. On the surface the meanings of certain words were straightforward but different physicians could have different understandings of the same terms. Nonetheless, medical "speak" increasingly dominated how even patients described their bodies and thus shaped how they saw them.

The source of practitioners' power – the doctor/patient relationship – could also be a source of their insecurity. Patients often presented their bodies to doctors in such a way that they did not conform with the descriptions of medical texts. As David M. Eddy has noted:

> If one looks at patients who are obviously ill, it is fairly easy to identify the physical and chemical disorders that characterize that illness. On the other hand, a large part of medicine is practiced on people who do not have obvious illnesses, but rather have signs, symptoms, or findings that may or may not represent an illness that should be treated ... The dividing line between "normal" and "abnormal" is not nearly as sharp as a cursory reading of a textbook would suggest.[6]

All this leads to speculation, conjecture, and debate. As one late-twentieth-century physician noted: "When you find a number of different explanations coming from the medical profession, then you know that we don't know what we're talking about."[7] It was the experience of clinical medicine on which older practitioners depended to get them through such patient contacts. But it was not easy. The treatment methods available became increasingly sophisticated. Some of the old standbys continued, but over time, new ones such as radiation and hormone therapy gained acceptance by many. But as with so many treatments, a predictable pattern was followed: extravagant claims were made, use increased, criticisms emerged, and extravagant claims tempered. As we have seen with hormone therapy, however, tempering claims did not always lessen its attraction.

The Patient

Contacts with women patients were particularly problematic. The entire orientation of most physicians – to be clear and adamant about how the female body worked, how civilization and the changes it brought were hurting that body, and how the body destined women for a particular social role and woe betide the woman and her health if she rejected it – spoke to their unease with that body. The medical unease can be seen in how physicians assessed women's life cycle. Women's problems started with puberty, continued throughout their menstrual lives, became heightened through pregnancy and childbirth, and were evident in their sexual lives and then at the end of their reproductive lives with menopause. Practitioners' tendency was to list the problems that could occur with each even while knowing that most women wended their way through such life events just fine and that those who experienced difficulties did not experience all of them on the ever-growing list. Seeing women's bodies as problematic and inferior to men's was not unique to physicians. Their views reflected their own society's perceptions of women and their relationship vis-à-vis men. At the same time, both physicians and Canadians could live with the contradictions between that perception of women's bodies and the recognition of the biological advantage that women had over men. That they did so and emphasized the former more than the latter underscores societal values.

The cases where the husband was required to give consent to his wife's surgery revealed an attitude of woman not being responsible to give consent herself, as a being in need of protection by another. When the surgery involved ending her reproductive life, the agreement of the husband was understandable in that it clearly impinged on his role as a potential father. It is difficult, nevertheless, to imagine the reverse happening. Such reactions reveal a concern for the marital unit rather than the individual woman in it as did the unwillingness of some practitioners to inform a wife whose health and life was at risk from a husband with venereal disease. For Susan Bordo such situations would have reflected the lack of "subject-status" on the part of the woman.[8] The lack of "subject-status" occurred also when physicians presented a patient with a choice that did not take into account her personal life. The one clear exception to this was the willingness of doctors sometimes to take a more radical approach to treatment with women in the paid labour force than those not. They understood the pressures on working women and altered their "normal" assessment and advice accordingly. And class was not the only variable that shaped their treatment choices. They perceived differences between young and older women. Depending on the situation, the advantage went to one or the other. Differing approaches based on women's lived experiences reveal practitioners' ability to go beyond the binary of sex. Doing so was not always comfortable. The consensus about how the female body worked as opposed to the male body was clear, whereas that of the working-class body compared to the middle-class body was fraught with a tension caused by social beliefs and fears. The sympathy towards working-class women and the harshness of many aspects of their lives was offset by many practitioners' fears of what they saw as their heightened sexuality, immorality, and challenge to the normative standard of womanhood. As for middle-class women, at one level they represented the normative standard and were the model for the female body as described in the medical literature. But they, too, posed challenges to practitioners' desire for stability. The modern woman was too often frivolous, seeking gratification outside the home, and rejecting her central purpose in life – reproduction.

Adding to these tensions, there are hints in the research that women had, and probably still have, a different sense of their bodies than did physicians.[9] They did not keep track of their menstrual cycles to the degree that physicians wanted or expected them to. They did not acknowledge the medically perceived urgency to consult a physician early in an illness; they were more willing to cope until they could no cope no longer. Alexandria Dundas Todd has expressed those differences well: "Women ... bring their health concerns in the social matrix of family, work, finances, and so forth. Their health concerns are not strictly medical. They need doctors to hear of these concerns and to extend and apply their knowledge accordingly."[10] Doctors seemed to have a symptom definition of ill health whereas women (and perhaps men as well) had a performance-driven definition. Certainly the examples of women who waited a long time after they first noted problems before they sought out medical help would suggest that the symptom approach did not predominate. Case records reveal that some women tended to differentiate between a chronic illness and an acute one. As long as they could function reasonably well many women did not seek medical help. And the refusal of a few to have potential life-saving surgery suggests that being alive was not so much an issue as being able to live life in a manner they had chosen. Such reactions to their bodies revealed a strength that most medical commentators on women ignored.

Biological differences between men and women cannot be ignored, but the belief that they had to be placed in a hierarchical positioning reflected the wider view of women in society. That hierarchy underlay the medicalization of women's bodies – the expansion of aspects of women's bodies and indeed their lives coming under the examination of medicine. The more this happened, the more potential there was for medical intervention. Almost from birth, physicians made distinctions between males and females and more often than not saw in those differences confirmation of the inferiority of the latter. The medical attitudes towards puberty, sexuality, and menopause revealed a profession that was willing to proffer advice on a vast array of issues that were not inherently medical; that is, all were "normal" or average experiences. Certainly some women experienced problems with those normal experiences and the tendency of physicians was to generalize from those women to all women. For many practitioners, social destiny and biological destiny seemed as one. What we see in the foregoing chapters is that the tendency over time was not to pay as much attention to the patient's narrative of her own symptoms but rather to trust the clinical expertise of the physician to determine signs of a specific problem or, as became more common the closer we come to mid century, to trust diagnostic tests to "prove" the nature of the body's workings. Not all physicians, however, did so and we have seen how physicians such as H.B. Atlee acknowledged the lived lives of women as something physicians needed to recognize and not make part of their biological destiny.

Nature and Environment

Throughout the discourse on women patients, physicians alluded to what occurred in nature and what was natural. They went so far as to compare some of the specific functions of a woman's body to those of animals in order to understand women better. The idea of women being closer to nature than men stems from women's heightened awareness of their bodies, being reminded of their bodies every month in a very real way, going through the process of childbirth and lactation, and finally going through menopause. In the relationship of women's bodies to nature was a hierarchy based on race, culture, and class; the closer to nature the less civilized. If physicians saw the Anglo-Celtic, white, middle-class woman as the epitome of civilization, those not fitting that description became "others," unable because of class, culture, or race to partake in the niceties of civilized modernity. And while class and culture could "possibly" be overcome, race could not. Practitioners saw race as immutable, and in the abstract discussions of body, the bodies of "others" highlighted the "normality" and success of evolution in the white body. At a practical level, however, those distinctions did not always prove as significant or as clear as the above might suggest.

What brought the differences in women's bodies together was placing them in a different category than men. Not that men totally escaped nature or being seen as a biological being, but this perception was largely confined to the medical view of men's sexuality, which physicians deemed almost dominating and thus in need of control. In so many more ways, women were aligned with nature and in that alignment physicians seemed to be aligning them with something that was universal and presocial.[11] They would have ascribed to what Mary O'Brien has called "reproductive consciousness," the idea that, for women, reproduction is something that is part of their being whereas for men it is separated from it. Unable to challenge the notion of reproductive consciousness in women, to envision it instead as a given with consequences that were "natural" and thus difficult to change, Canadians continued to conceptualize both sexual and gender differences as though they were fixed rather than possibly contingent, at least in their consequences. In seeing woman's body as natural, as aligned with nature, Canadians, lay and medical, appealed to a concept of stability. As Leonore Tiefer has argued, using the word "nature" or "natural" is inherently an explanatory device, rhetorical in power. It convinces a reader that what is being referred to has "solidity and validity."[12] Of course such a view of nature and the natural denies nature's changeability, a concept that entered the debate with Darwin's writings in the nineteenth century.

While there are positive elements to being aligned with nature – such as being more intuitive – there are also negatives – such as being connected to the past, not as connected to the developments of civilization and the "man"-made world. When body seemed to support particular values of the society that physicians supported, they saw nature as immutable and difficult to change; if it did change, ramifications could be severe. At times, however, physicians saw nature as not up to date, as lacking regularity and being much too unpredictable. In such cases they believed they could or should improve on nature in "fixing" women's biological nature or at the very least adjusting it so that women could cope with the modern society that was Canada in the first half of the twentieth century. In their eyes, nature had limits and as practitioners they wanted to overcome the limits of the female body, especially its unpredictability.

All that being said, physicians also understood at one level that body was not fixed. They were aware of the pressures the specific lived body was under and recognized that the environment/society in which women lived worked against them. Some, such as H.B. Atlee, sympathized but did not see themselves in any position to change that society. All they could do was to try and help the body adjust to the pressures of living in a particular social/cultural environment. They also were aware that the interplay of the body and the environment could change the functioning of the body. The most obvious was the timing of menstruation, the age of which had lowered over time. They were mindful of the changes in the body that came with age. Thus while seeing bodies as unchanging and mechanistic, they were also aware of their fluidity and changeability. The tension for physicians was the theory of medicine, which often (not totally) stressed the unchanging nature of the body and the reality of a body that was constantly changing.

The striving of the profession and its practitioners to understand women's bodies and the problems they faced in their contact with women patients in their day-to-day practice reveals a growing maturity within the Canadian profession. It is evidenced by Canadian practitioners' increased willingness to publish their ideas on medicine, their case records for review, and their constant endeavours to keep up with the latest international advances. Canadian medicine was not parochial. In some areas, such as cancer studies, it could be on the forefront of treatment. The profession was a maturing one, at times willing to speak out against treatment it saw as dangerous and useless. The dynamic of medicine – its ebb and flow of treatment, its divisions between practitioners – was both part of its weakness and its strength. In generalizing medicine, however, I found myself becoming entranced by individual doctors whose work is open to criticism, but at the same time was often based on a deep-seated desire to help their women patients, seeing in them more than bodies that had failed.

Notes on Sources and Methodology

Primary sources are a historian's conduit to the past but they can never be a mirror.[1] The research sources used in this study fall into several categories. The first is the literature produced by the medical profession for its own adherents. The medical journals published in this country during 1900–1950 were especially numerous (over 100) and valuable.[2] Some were long running, others lasted less than a year; some were general, others specialized. Edited by many different individuals, it is doubtful that any significant approaches to "regular" medicine were overlooked in them and as such they are a tremendous resource for those interested in the history of medicine. In them, physicians from across the nation – from cities, towns, and rural areas – described their practices through patient histories and debated issues in medicine that concerned them. That being said, the urban medical elite, often attached to teaching hospitals, tended to dominate the editorships of the major journals and thus their content. The journals also contained reprints of the leading articles published outside Canada, suggesting that despite the isolation of some physicians in their practices, they could keep abreast of the latest medical discoveries. Editorials helped in this as did descriptions of conferences and what had taken place at them. While local, national, and international articles could exist side by side, the Canadian content held pride of place for these journals were the public forum for Canadian practitioners and teachers of medicine. Publishing in them offered the authors status but there was a similarity to many of the narratives, either describing an unusual case and emphasizing the degree of difficulty in bringing it to a successful conclusion or offering colleagues a different way of treating disease/illness modalities.

The textbooks in Canadian medical colleges for the training of medical students during this period were a second source of professional literature examined. Most were non-Canadian in origin, most often British or American with an urban vantage point. Textbooks focus on the most up-to-date medical practices and thinking on those practices; they represent the level of best practices and theory of medicine, and the procedures described are usually those on which physicians agree. They create and propagate the givens of medical practice and are in the words of Diana Scully and Pauline Bart "one of the primary professional socialization agents for practitioners."[3] They may have been the authoritative voice of the profession, but on reading them, the differing ways of practising medicine and perceiving the body emerge. Unlike the journal literature, the texts provided the student reader with the normative case and how to respond to it. Like the journal literature, however, once the normative was dealt with, the texts would trace the variety of problems that a practicing physician could face in treating a specific condition. In doing so, both the journals and the textbooks made the healthy body seem an aberration. The non-Canadian content within the medical journals and the textbooks themselves are significant to examine because they are part of the context of medical practice and ignoring such content would distort the world Canadian physicians inhabited. Canadian physicians lived and practised in Canada, but their intellectual world was not confined by national boundaries. Whether journals or textbooks, such sources reflect what Canadian practitioners were being taught and what they were reading, writing, and doing. They provide a glimpse of the wider Western perception and treatment of women as seen by practitioners in Canada.

Linked to the professional literature were popular medical writings – health manuals and advice appearing in the periodical press – providing a sense of what information was available to Canadians about their bodies. And the audiences for these writings could be significant. *Chatelaine*, for example, had a readership of 70,000 in its first year of publication and by the 1940s it was over 252,000.[4] Coupled with those to whom the magazine was passed on to read and those who were told about the health advice it contained, the numbers of people reached were impressive. Such publications are full of contradictions and tensions, with a multiplicity of meanings to appeal to different audiences. When the authors were practitioners, they had to both maintain their professional status and also seem to give the reader power. They addressed an audience who was ready to listen and so the literature often reinforced what the reader was willing to hear.[5] And readers were obviously willing to listen to physicians on a raft of topics including those not particularly medical in nature.

Hospital patient records were used, in part, to help offset the overwhelming voices of physicians. However, gaining access to these records was and is a hit-and-miss experience. I received various responses to queries about access, many of them negative, most from hospitals not set up for researchers and uncomfortable about patient privacy and confidentiality issues. Patient records in archives proved the most accessible and so I was able to access significant records in eastern and central and the far western part of Canada.[6] Condition of access was to maintain anonymity of the patients so none of the names used are real, although their initials are the same and names chosen reflect the specific ethnic group of the patient.[7] The way in which I examined the collections varied depending on their size. Because I was interested in women's experiences my focus was on their records. I did not include obstetrical cases for this book since I had already written on childbirth; I generally did not examine records of women with diseases/conditions that were not specifically gendered; for example, I would not have looked at certain diagnoses such as measles or broken limbs. For records in which a gendered aspect had been found in both sexes in the wider literature, such as neurasthenia and hysteria, I would look at records for women and for men. When there was a long run and many records I would chose every fifth patient every fifth year. For an overview of hospital care, reasons for all patients entering, etc., I also found the *Annual Reports* of specific hospitals helpful.[8]

The point of examining the patient records was to bring the patients to life. It was not to undertake a quantitative exercise similar to what I had done in parts of *The Nature of Their Bodies*. Quantitative history is incredibly labour intensive and for the questions I was asking not as valuable as a close reading of the patient records themselves, which in the twentieth century had become much larger and more complex compared to the late nineteenth century. While written by medical professionals, patient records give insight into the lives of the women who came to hospitals and underwent various procedures. The case records remind the researcher that these people were real and that their medical forays were only a part of their lives and, depending on the situation, only a very minor part. Over the years, I've come to appreciate their value and the ethical demands of working with them. Such records provide an entree into the individual patient's experience.[9] The patient records are, however, self-selected in that they reflect those individuals who sought out medical help. Those who felt marginalized in the society – whether through age, class, ethnicity, race, culture, or where they lived – would be underrepresented compared to those who accepted Western medical practices and felt comfortable doing so.[10] The records reveal a profession more diverse and at times more sympathetic than much of the literature on medical treatment of women has suggested and indicate practitioners' actions as opposed to what they discuss as best practices in the published literature. The latter often reveal a more radical treatment response (for example in breast cancer) than patient records suggest.

Several conclusions emerge from the kinds of material contained in these records. First is the sheer volume of information in the files and how over time that amount increased, as well as of what it consisted. Historians of medicine need to query the ability of any one physician to absorb and make sense of the information. Even when it is not clear why the physicians wanted or needed the information, it appeared that value existed in having it, that somehow treatment would be better if more information was available. Such data collection was and is the foundation of clinical research and part of scientific culture. Not all hospital records, however, are as generous as others in the amount of information offered. What often survives are the admission records and the history of the patient and a summary of treatment. In some hospitals surgical records were kept separate from the admission records and anaesthesia records could be separate as could detailed autopsy reports.[11] The second finding is that familiarity with patient records forces the historian to be aware of the peculiarities of record keeping and its fallibility. The former can sometimes be revealing. For example, the tendency to view a woman not as an individual in her own right but as part of a marital unit was reflected in many of the patient case files. The fallibility of records is found in discrepancies between the diagnosis given on the covering sheet of a file and the actual problems experienced by the patient described in the file. The third conclusion is the limitation of case records in providing a complete sense of women's health experience. After all, they describe women who chose to seek medical help because of some health or perceived health problem. Their experiences cannot be assumed to reflect those of the majority of women or even of women who experienced health problems. Case histories are narratives and stories of experience taken by medical personnel. They are summaries or a distillation of a life or part of a life and can never be assumed to represent that life. That being said, there is much to learn from the case records. For one, the difference between what physicians thought important compared to what women patients thought important was intriguing. How long a woman waited before seeking medical help suggested a specific way of looking at her body, one that a physician might not share when his perception was that she had waited too long. Any perusal of case records reveals the broad variety of women's experience. The harshness of some of their lives and their ability to cope with them can only remind us of their strength. The records illuminate the tension between the general compliance of most patients and the incidences that stand out as resistance. Women patients, in particular, have less agency than male patients. Nonetheless, they used what agency they had.

Interviews with women and some practitioners were the last major source used. Like patient records they were done to offset the dominance of the medical perspective. Altogether 22 interviews were done, 19 with women about their experiences with medicine and 3 with women practitioners who talked about both their experiences as women and as physicians. One of my research assistants did most of the interviews. In addition there was one other source of interviews, from an Ontario project called Traces, which interviewed the elderly about their lives during topically themed meetings, for example on first menstruation. There was no pretense of any systematic way of choosing individuals given the time period I was covering. I simply gathered names through what sociologists call a snowball effect. Old age homes were contact sources, mostly in Ontario, although given the long lives of these women, many had lived in different parts of Canada. Most of the interviews took place in 1993 while I was in research mode for this manuscript. Writing *Giving Birth in Canada, 1900–1950*, however, took me in a different direction and it was only in the last several years that I returned to the research for this book, including the interviews. The oldest woman interviewed was born in 1900 and the youngest in 1930. All would have reached adulthood by 1950. Those interviewed ran the gamut from being poor to wealthy, although most would have been middle class at some time. But given that they lived through the Depression even those who eventually were comfortable often had to make sacrifices to keep family together or struggled financially. Almost all were white Protestants although one was Jewish and another mixed Black and native. Most married and had children but some were single mothers due to early deaths of husbands or a husband's absence during war. Urban living dominated with only one farm woman among them.

Interviews have their own problems, specifically around the accuracy of memory of the person interviewed and the perspective of the interviewer.[12] But even if memories are diminished or refashioned with the passage of time, the interviews provide the clearest access to the experiences of women and how they saw them and despite Joan Scott's poststructuralist gaze on the flawed nature of experience, I agree with those who see individuals' memories of it as reflective of the society in which they lived.[13] Whether through interviews or patient records what emerges is a different perspective on health and body on the part of women from that of physicians. While health was significant to the individual woman, it was only one part of her life and we cannot assume that she gave it the same priority as the medical profession. What is also clear from some of the records is that women's knowledge of their bodies could be quite limited and even eccentric.

Notes

Acknowledgments

1 See "It's Not Society That's the Problem, It's Women's Bodies':
A Historical View of Medical Treatment of Women," in Kerry Petersen
(ed.), *Intersections: Women on Law, Medicine and Technology* (Aldershot:
Dartmouth Publishing, 1997), 25–48; "Problematic Bodies and Agency:
Women Patients in Canada, 1900–1950," in Franca Iacovetta and Wendy
Mitchinson (eds.), *On the Case: Explorations in Social History* (Toronto:
University of Toronto Press, 1998), 266–86; "Agency, Diversity, Constraints:
Women and Their Physicians, Canada, 1850–1950," in Susan Sherwin
et al., *The Politics of Women's Health: Exploring Agency and Autonomy*
(Philadelphia: Temple University Press, 1998), 122–49; "All Matter
Peculiar to Woman and Womanhood: The Medical Context for Women's
Education in Canada in the First Half of the Twentieth Century," in Paula
Bourne and Elizabeth Smyth (eds.), *Women Learning, Women Teaching:
Historical Perspectives* (Toronto: Ianna Publications and Education, 2006),
158–73; "Breast Cancer in Canada: Medical Response and Attitudes,
1900–1950," *Histoire Sociale* 76 (November 2005): 399–432; "No Longer the
Same Woman: Medical Perceptions of Menopause, 1900–1950," *Canadian
Bulletin of Medical History* 23, 1 (2006): 7–47; "H.B. Atlee on Obstetrics and
Gynaecology: A Representative and Singular Voice in 20thC Canadian
Medicine," *Acadiensis* 32, 2 (Spring 2003): 1–28. See also "Infertility:
Historical Overviews of Medical Perceptions in Canada, 1850–1950,"
report commissioned by the Royal Commission on New Reproductive
Technologies, 1991, in *The Prevalence of Infertility in Canada: Research Studies
of the Royal Commission on New Reproductive Technologies 6* (Ottawa: Minister
of Supply and Services, 1993), 1–59.

Introduction

1 See Wendy Mitchinson, *The Nature of Their Bodies: Women and Their Doctors in Victorian Canada* (Toronto: University of Toronto Press, 1991); Wendy Mitchinson, *Giving Birth in Canada, 1900–1950* (Toronto: University of Toronto Press, 2002).

2 E.H. Carr, *What Is History?* (Harmondsworth, Middlesex: Penguin Books, [1961] 1964), 7. For overviews of the "historiography" of theories historians have found useful see Mark T. Gilderhus, *History and Historians: A Historiographical Introduction* 5th ed. (Upper Saddle River, NJ: Prentice Hall, 2003); Patrick Fuery and Nick Mansfield, *Cultural Studies and Critical Theory* 2nd ed. (Melbourne and New York: Oxford University Press, 2000); Krishan Kumar, *From Post-Industrial to Post-Modern Society: New Theories of the Contemporary World* 2nd ed. (Oxford: Blackwell, 2005); Steven Seidman, *Contested Knowledge: Social Theory Today* 4th ed. (Oxford: Blackwell, 2008); Tim Woods, *Beginning Postmodernism* 2nd ed. (Manchester: Manchester University Press, 2009).

3 For this period see Gilderhus, *History and Historians*, 119, 123–4; for Canadian history see Carl Berger, *The Writing of Canadian History: Aspects of English-Canadian Historical Writing since 1900* 2nd ed. (Toronto: University of Toronto Press, 1986).

4 For structuralism see Steven Seidman, *Contested Knowledge: Social Theory Today* 4th ed. (Oxford: Blackwell, 2008), 156–7. For a significant use of structuralism in the analysis of science see Thomas Kuhn, *The Structure of Scientific Revolutions* 3rd ed. (Chicago: University of Chicago Press, 1996).

5 See Keith Jenkins, *Why History? Ethnics and Postmodernity* (New York: Routledge, 1999); Madan Sarup, *An Introductory Guide to Post-structualism and Postmodernism* (New York: Harvester Wheatsheaf, 1988).

6 Laura Lee Downs, *Writing Gender History* (London: Hodder Education, 2004), 73.

7 For criticisms of gender see Anne Fausto-Sterling, *Sexing the Body: Gender Politics and the Construction of Sexuality* (New York: Basic Books, 2000), 25; Elizabeth Grosz, *Volatile Bodies: Toward a Corporeal Feminism* (Bloomington & Indianapolis: Indiana University Press, 1994), xii; Elizabeth Grosz, *Space, Time, and Perversion: Essays on the Politics of Bodies* (New York: Routledge, 1995), xii.

8 Susan Bordo, *Unbearable Weight: Feminism, Western Culture, and the Body* (Berkeley: University of California Press, 1993), 288.

9 Denise Riley, *"Am I That Name?": Feminism and the Category of "Women" in History* (Basingstoke: Macmillan, 1988).

10 For a feminist approach to postcolonial theory see Reina Lewis and Sara Mills (eds.), *Feminist Postcolonial Theory: A Reader* (New York: Routledge, 2003). The word "postcolonial" has been deemed by some a misnomer. Meg Parsons, a historian of Aboriginals in Australia, contests its application in a context in which colonization is still ongoing. Conversation with Meg Parsons, *Gender and Health: Histories Workshop*, May 12–13, 2011, University of Waterloo. See also a critique of the concept of postcolonialism by Anne McClintock, "The Angel of Progress: Pitfalls of the Term 'Post-Colonialism,'" *Social Text* no. 31–2, Third World and Post-Colonial Issues (1992): 84–98

11 Cheryl Krasnick Warsh (ed.), *Gender, Health and Popular Culture: Historical Perspectives* (Waterloo: Wilfrid Laurier University Press, 2011), vii–viii.

12 See Annette Browne, Victoria L. Smye, and Colleen Varcoe, "Postcolonial Feminist Theoretical Perspectives and Women's Health," in Marina Morrow, Olena Hankivsky, and Colleen Varcoe (eds.), *Women's Health in Canada: Critical Perspectives on Theory and Policy* (Toronto: University of Toronto Press, 2007), 124–42; Katie Pickles and Myra Rutherdale (eds.), *Contact Zones: Aboriginal and Settler Women in Canada's Colonial Past* (Vancouver and Toronto: UBC Press, 2005); Patricia Jasen, "Race, Culture, and the Colonization of Childbirth in Northern Canada," *Social History of Medicine* 10, 3 (1997): 383–400; Maureen Lux, *Medicine That Walks: Disease, Medicine and Canadian Plains Native People, 1880–1940* (Toronto: University of Toronto Press, 2001); Kristen Burnett, "The Healing Work of Aboriginal Women in Indigenous and Newcomer Communities," in Jayne Elliott, Meryn Stuart, and Cynthia Toman (eds.), *Place and Practice in Canadian Nursing History* (Vancouver: UBC Press, 2008), 40–52; Mona Gleason, "Race, Class, and Health: School Medical Inspection and 'Healthy' Children in British Columbia, 1890–1950," and Myra Rutherdale, "Ordering the Bath: Children, Health and Hygiene in Northern Canadian Communities," in Cheryl Krasnick Warsh and Veronica Strong-Boag (eds.), *Children's Health Issues in Historical Perspective* (Waterloo: Wilfrid Laurier University Press, 2005), 287–304 and 305–24 respectively; Kim Anderson, *A Recognition of Being: Reconstructing Native Womanhood* (Toronto: Sumach Press, 2000); Mary-Ellen Kelm, *Colonizing Bodies: Aboriginal Health and Healing in British Columbia, 1900–50* (Vancouver: UBC Press, 1998).

13 James Waldram et al., quoted in Jennifer Poudrier, "The Geneticization of Aboriginal Diabetes and Obesity: Adding Another Scene to the Story of the Thrifty Gene," *The Canadian Review of Sociology and Anthropology (CRSA/ RCSA)* 44, 2 (2007): 241.

14 Kim Anderson, *Life Stages and Native Women: Memory, Teachings, and Story Medicine* (Winnipeg: University of Manitoba Press, 2011), 129–30.

15 The Annales school and the psychoanalytic approach to history can be seen as precursors of the affective turn. Areas in which the affective turn is evident are social, women's, family, body, commemoration, and oral history. Even topics that seem to attract anything but an affective approach such as political history and history of war have been illuminated by doing so. See C.P. Stacey, *A Very Double Life: The Private World of Mackenzie King* (Toronto: Macmillan of Canada, 1976); L.M. Grayson and Michael Bliss (eds.), *The Wretched of Canada: Letters to R.B. Bennett, 1930–1935* (Toronto: University of Toronto Press, 1971); Jonathan Vance, *Death So Noble: Memory, Meaning, and the First World War* (Vancouver: UBC, 1997). For a recent history using a form of the affective turn see Joy Parr, *Sensing Changes: Technologies, Environments, and the Everyday, 1953–2003* (Vancouver: UBC, 2010).

16 On the historiography of medicine see S.E.D. Shortt, "Antiquarians and Amateurs: Reflection on the Writing of Medical History in Canada," in S.E.D. Shortt (ed.), *Medicine in Canadian Society: Historical Perspectives* (Montreal: McGill-Queen's University Press, 1981), 1–17; Saul Jarcho, "Some Observations and Opinions on the Present State of American Medical Historiography," *Journal of the History of Medicine and Allied Sciences* 44 (1989): 288–90; A.M. Brandt, "Emerging Themes in the History of Medicine," *Milbank Quarterly* 69 (1991): 199–214; Wendy Mitchinson, "Medical Historiography in English Canada," *Health and Canadian Society/ Santé et Société Canadienne* 1, 1 (1993): 205–28; Jacques Bernier "La place de l'histoire de la médicine," *Health and Canadian Society/Santé et Société Canadienne* 1, 1 (1993): 19–49.

17 In translation see especially Michel Foucault, *Discipline and Punish: The Birth of the Prison* (New York: Pantheon Books, 1977), *The History of Sexuality* (New York: Pantheon Books, 1978), and *Mental Illness and Psychology* (New York: Harper & Row, 1976); see also Steven Seidman, *Contested Knowledge: Social Theory Today* 4th ed. (Oxford: Blackwell, 2008), Chapter 12, "Michel Foucault's Disciplinary Society," 171–83.

18 Joanne Entwistle, "Fashion and the Fleshy Body: Dress as Embodied Practice," *Fashion Theory* 4, 3 (2000): 329.

19 For further discussion of medicalization see Juanne Nancarrow Clarke in *Health, Illness and Medicine in Canada* 4th ed. (Don Mills: Oxford University Press, 2004), Chapter 10, "Medicalization: The Medical-Moral Mix," 220–8; Ivan Illich, *Limits to Medicine* (Toronto: McClelland and Stewart, 1976); Catherine Kohler, "Women and Medicalization: A New Perspective," in

Howard D. Schwartz (ed.), *Dominant Issues in Medical Sociology* 2nd ed. (New York: Random House, 1987), 101–21; Peter Conrad, *The Medicalization of Society: On the Transformation of Human Conditions into Treatable Disorders* (Baltimore: Johns Hopkins University Press, 2007).

20 Cheryl Krasnick Warsh's *Prescribed Norms: Women and Health in Canada and the United States since 1800* (Toronto: University of Toronto Press, 2010) is an excellent overview of the state of the literature on women's health. *Body Failure* overlaps with it primarily in the sections on puberty and menopause and expands on both for the 1900–50 period. See her Section 3 on Professions, 173–274. In 1911, only 2.79% of doctors were women; in 1921, 1.8%; and in 1941, 3.7%, (201). For that reason I refer to doctors in this study as male.

21 Karen Flynn, "'I'm Glad That Someone Is Telling the Nursing Story': Writing Black Women's History," *Journal of Black Studies* 38, 3 (January 2008): 443–60; Susan Smith, *Sick and Tired of Being Sick and Tired: Black Women's Health Activism in America, 1890–1950* (Philadelphia: University of Pennsylvania Press, 1995).

22 The literature on the medicalization of women's bodies is large. What follows is only a sample: Janice Delaney, M.J. Lupton and Emily Toth, *The Curse: A Cultural History of Menstruation* (New York: Mentor, 1976); Barbara Ehrenreich and Deirdre English, *For Her Own Good: 150 Years of the Experts' Advice to Women* (Garden City, NY: Anchor Press, 1978); Robert Mendelsohn, *Male Practice: How Doctors Manipulate Women* (Chicago: Contemporary Books, 1981); Barbara Rothman, *In Labour: Women and Power in the Birthplace* (London: Junction Books, 1982); Elaine Showalter, *The Female Malady: Women, Madness, and English Culture* (New York: Pantheon Books, 1985); Veronica Strong-Boag and Kathryn McPherson, "The Confinement of Women: Childbirth and Hospitalization in Vancouver, 1919–1939," *BC Studies* 69–70 (Spring–Summer 1986): 142–75; Frank Mort, *Dangerous Sexualities: Medico-Moral Politics in England since 1830* (London: Routledge and Kegan Paul, 1987); Sandra Coney, *The Unfortunate Experiment: The Full Story Behind the Inquiry into Cervical Cancer Treatment* (Auckland, NZ: Penguin Books, 1988); Dawn H. Currie and Valerie Raoul (eds.), *The Anatomy of Gender: Women's Struggle for the Body* (Ottawa: Carleton University Press, 1991); Emily Martin, "The Egg and the Sperm: How Science Has Constructed a Romance Based on Stereotypical Male-Female Roles," *Signs* 16, 3 (Spring 1991): 485–501; Nicole J. Grant, *The Selling of Contraception: The Dalkon Shield Case, Sexuality and Women's Anatomy* (Columbus, OH: Ohio State University Press, 1992).

23 Christopher E. Forth and Ivan Crozier (eds.), "Introduction," in their *Body Parts: Critical Explorations in Corporeality* (Lanham, MD: Lexington Books, 2005), 2–3.

24 McClintock, "The Angel of Progress," 97.

25 For an important regional study see Megan J. Davies, "Mapping 'Region' in Canadian Medical History: The Case of British Columbia," *Canadian Bulletin of Medical History* 17 (2000): 73–92.

26 To date there is little work in Canada to correspond to Susan Smith's *Sick and Tired of Being Sick and Tired*.

27 Quoted in Tony Judt, "Luck Breaks," *New York Review of Books*, 28 April 2010, 27.

28 See Margarete Sandelowski, *Women, Health and Choice* (Englewood, NJ: Prentice-Hall, 1981), 6; Janice Raymond, *Women as Wombs: Reproductive Technologies and the Battle over Women's Freedom* (San Francisco: Harper, 1993), 121.

29 Marc Berg and Paul Harterink, "Embodying the Patient: Records and Bodies in Early 20th-century US Medical Practice," *Body & Society* 10, 2–3 (2004): 28.

30 Alan Ryan, review of *The Ethics of Identity* by Kwame Anthony Appiah, "The Magic of 'I'," *New York Review of Books* 28 April 2005, 36; Walter Johnson, "On Agency," *Journal of Social History* 37, 1 (Fall 2003): 115.

31 Few registered physicians came from marginalized groups. Even nurses from such groups came to their profession late due to discrimination. See Karen Flynn, *Moving Beyond Borders: A History of Black Canadian and Caribbean Women in the Diaspora* (Toronto: University of Toronto Press, 2011). For the United States see Susan Smith, *Japanese American Midwives: Culture, Community, and Health Policy, 1880–1950* (Urbana: University of Illinois Press, 2005). For a discussion in accessing patient voices see Eberhard Wolff, "Perspectives on Patients' History: Methodological Considerations on the Example of Recent German-Speaking Literature," *Canadian Bulletin of Medical History* 15, 1 (1998): 207–28.

32 Linda Gordon in *Heroes of Their Own Lives: The Politics and History of Family Violence, Boston 1880–1960* (New York: Penguin Books, 1988), 18, maintains that although women as a group may be subordinate in power to men, this does not mean that an individual woman cannot have agency or that her life is predetermined.

33 Stephen Kern, *A Cultural History of Causality: Science, Murder Novels, and Systems of Thought* (Princeton and Oxford: Princeton University Press, 2004), 7, 13.

34 Paul Komesaroff, "Medicine and the Moral Space of the Menopausal Woman," in Paul Komesaroff, Phillipa Rothfeld, and Jeanne Daly (eds.), *Reinterpreting Menopause: Cultural and Philosophical Issues* (New York: Routledge, 1997), 5.

35 For a discussion of antimodernism see Donald A. Wright, "W.D. Lighthall and David Ross McCord: Antimodernism and English-Canadian Imperialism, 1880s–1918," *Journal of Canadian Studies* 32, 2 (Summer 1997): 135.

36 For a more detailed discussion of certainty versus uncertainty in medicine see Mitchinson, *Giving Birth in Canada*, Chapter 1, "The Uncertain World of Medicine and Medical Practitioners," 19–46, and Wendy Mitchinson, "The Uncertain World of Canadian Obstetrics, 1900 to 1950," *Canadian Bulletin for the History of Medicine* 17, 1–2 (2000): 193–208.

37 *Canadian Magazine* 21, 5 (September 1903): 407–9.

38 For the primitive cycle see *DMM* 21, 3 (September 1903): 187; for Drennan's present see *CJMS* 15, 2 (February 1904): 93.

39 Franz Boas, "The Eskimo of Baffin Island and Hudson Bay," *Bulletin of the American Museum of Natural History* XV (1901): 119; for reference to lack of gender differentiation in naming among Inuit groups see Kaj Birket-Smith, *The Caribou Eskimos: Material and Social Life and Their Cultural Position I Descriptive Part: Report of the Fifth Thule Expedition 1921–24 Volume 5* (Copenhagen, Gyldeddalske Boghandel, Nordisk, Forlag, 1929), 282; Vilhjalmus Stefansson, "The Stefansson-Anderson Arctic Expedition of the American Museum: Preliminary Ethnological Report" *Anthropological Papers of the American Museum of Natural History XIV, Part I* (New York: AMS Press, 1914), 367; Birket-Smith for bedarche see Jaarich G. Oosten, "Male and Female in Inuit Shamanism," *Etudes/Inuit/Studies* 10, 1–2 (1986): 115–31; for gender differentiation see Freda Ahenakeu and H.C. Wolfart (eds.), *Our Grandmothers' Lives: As Told in Their Own Words* (Saskatoon: Fifth House Publishers, 1992), 225.

40 For quote see Inez Houlihan, "The Image of Women in *Chatelaine* Editorials March 1928 to September 1977," MA thesis, University of Toronto, 1984, 38.

41 M.M. Kirkwood, *For College Women ... and Men* (Toronto: Oxford University Press, 1938), 36.

42 *Maclean's* 63 (15 August 1950): 7.

43 For Hutchinson see Cynthia R. Comacchio, *Nations Are Built of Babies: Saving Ontario's Mothers and Children 1900–1940* (Montreal and Kingston: McGill-Queen's University Press, 1993), 108-9; for Paquette see Andrée Lévesque, "Mères ou malades: Les Québécoises de l'entre-deux-guerres

vues par les médecins," *Revue d'histoire de l'Amérique française* 38, 1 (1984): 33.
44 Quoted in Harry Oxorn, *Harold Benge Atlee M.D.: A Biography* (Hantsport, Nova Scotia: Lancelot Press, 1983), 151–2.
45 *Saturday Night* 58 (31 October 1942): 22.

Chapter 1

1 *Canadian Magazine* 40, 3 (January 1913): 242.
2 Thomas Laqueur, *Making Sex: Body and Gender from the Greeks to Freud* (Cambridge: Harvard University Press, 1990), 195.
3 For a discussion of gender separation of chores among the Inuit see Asen Balickci, *The Netsilik Eskimo* (Garden City, NY: The Natural History Press, 1970, published for the American Museum of Natural History); Kaj Birket-Smith, *The Caribou Eskimos: Material and Social Life and Their Cultural Position I Descriptive Part. Report of the Fifth Thule Expedition 1921–1924 Volume 5* (Gyldeddalske Boghandel, Nordisk Forlag Copenhagen, 1929).
4 E.C. Dudley, *The Principles and Practice of Gynecology for Students and Practitioners* 5th ed. (Philadelphia and New York: Lea & Febiger, 1908), 511, 21.
5 *CL* 40, 7 (March 1907): 661.
6 For use of the phrase see Charles A.L. Reed (ed.), *A Text-Book of Gynecology* (New York: D. Appleton and Co., 1901), 5.
7 Nelly Oudshoorn, "On Measuring Sex Hormones: The Role of Biological Assays in Sexualizing Chemical Substances," *Bulletin of the History of Medicine* 64 (1990): 258.
8 J. Bland-Sutton and Arthur E. Giles, *The Diseases of Women: A Handbook for Students and Practitioners* (London and New York: Rebman, 1906), 35; *PHJ* 4, 4 (April 1913): 248; *CJMS* 35, 6 (June 1914): 321–2; *PHJ* 7, 4 (April 1916): 187.
9 *MMN* 18, 1 (January 1906): 5; Alfred Lewis Galabin and George Blacker, *The Practice of Midwifery* (London: J. & A. Churchill, 1910), 133. See Carol Tavris, *The Mismeasure of Women: Why Women Are Not the Better Sex, the Inferior Sex, or the Opposite Sex* (New York, London, Toronto: Touchstone Books, 1992), 55–6.
10 Galabin and Blacker, *The Practice of Midwifery*, 133.
11 For quickness of eye, etc., see *PHJ* 4, 4 (April 1913): 248; for baldness see Woods Hutchinson, *Common Diseases* (New York: Houghton Mifflin Co., 1913), 206.
12 See *CMAJ* 27, 3 (September 1932): 311; *CMAJ* 34, 3 (March 1936): 294.

13 For biological edge see *CMAJ* 17, 2 (February 1927): 208; P. Brooke Bland,
    Practical Obstetrics for Students and Practitioners (Philadelphia:
    F.A. Saunders, 1932), 62; *Saturday Night* 60 (16 December 1944): 28;
    Maclean's 59 (1December 1946): 12; *Chatelaine* 23, 5 (May 1950): 44. For
    President at Dalhousie see *CMAJ* 27, 5 (November 1932): 531.

14 For muscle strength see *MMB* 83 (July 1928): 12; *NSMB* 11, 3 (March 1932):
    149. For the quote see *CMAJ* 17, 2 (February 1927): 207. For problems of
    menstruation and menopause see also *NSMB* 10, 11 (November 1931): 798
    and *UTMJ* 7, 7 (May 1930): 236. For health problems see *CMAJ* 19, 2 (August
    1928): 231; *CPHJ* 25, 3 (March 1934): 107; *Saturday Night* 52 (17 April 1937):
    39; *Food for Thought* 6 (June 1940): 4; *CMAJ* 50, 4 (April 1944): 315.

15 For Atlee see Dalhousie University Archives, Harry Oxorn Fonds Ms-13-
    58, Letter from H.B. Atlee to Sarah January 8,1956; Harry Oxorn, *Harold
    Benge Atlee M.D.: A Biography* (Hantsport, Nova Scotia: Lancelot Press,
    1983), 152; *NSMB* 10, 11 (November 1931): 798. For a similar view see
    MMB 96 (August 1928): 12–13.

16 Mary-Ellen Kelm, *Colonizing Bodies: Aboriginal Health and Healing in British
    Columbia, 1900–50* (Vancouver: UBC Press, 1998), xxi.

17 *HW* 13, 5 (May 1918): 149.

18 For Sprague see *DMM* 38, 5 (May 1912): 148. For Hobbs see *CPMR* 26, 3
    (March 1901): 123.

19 *CMAJ* 17, 2 (February 1927): 208; *CMAJ* 34, 3 (March 1936): 294.

20 *Canadian Magazine* 67 (April 1927): 26; *MMB* 83 (July 1928): 12.

21 *NSMB* 11, 3 (March 1932): 149–50.

22 *MMJ* 29, 4 (April 1900): 269; *CPMR* 27, 5 (May 1902): 254; *DMM* 23, 5
    (November 1904): 322; *PHJ* 7, 6 (June 1916): 306. For a study of the impor-
    tance of motherhood see Veronica Strong-Boag, *Finding Families, Finding
    Ourselves: English Canada Encounters Adoption from the Nineteenth Century to
    the 1990s* (Toronto: Oxford University Press, 2006).

23 *DMM* 23, 5 (November 1904): 322.

24 See Angus McLaren, *Our Own Master Race: Eugenics in Canada, 1885–1945*
    (Toronto: McClelland and Stewart, 1990); also Stephen Jay Gould, *The
    Mismeasurement of Man* (New York: Norton, 1981) and Nancy Stepan,
    The Idea of Race in Science: Great Britain, 1800–1960 (Hamden, CT: Archon
    Books, 1982).

25 *CMAJ* 13, 11 (November 1923): 796.

26 *Health* 17 (September–October 1949): 10.

27 The pro-natalist stance and the status given to women as a result was even
    stronger among First Nations. Kelm, *Colonizing Bodies*, 6.

28 John McLeod, *Beginning Postcolonialism* (Manchester and New York:
    Manchester University Press, 2000), 22, 38.

29 Dudley, *The Principles and Practice of Gynecology*, 511.
30 For Drennan see *DMM* 21, 3 (September 1903): 187 and her quote in *CJMS* 15, 2 (February 1904): 91. For Smith see *DMM* 23, 5 (November 1904): 324.
31 Quoted in Emily Martin, "Medical Metaphors of Women's Bodies: Menstruation and Menopause," *International Journal of Health Services* 18, 2 (1988): 240.
32 For Chandler see *CMAJ* 17, 2 (February 1927): 208. For Watson see *CMAJ* 34, 3 (March 1936): 294–5.
33 *CMAJ* 34, 4 (April 1936): 425.
34 Deborah Findlay, "Professional Interests in Medicine's Construction of Women's Reproductive Health," paper presented to the Canadian Sociology and Anthropology Association, Winnipeg, 1986, 7.
35 See Myra Rutherdale, *Women and the White Man's God: Gender and Race in the Canadian Mission Field* (Vancouver: UBC Press, 2002), 98–112, and Kelm, *Colonizing Bodies*, 61–2. For non-Canadian literature see Anna Davin, "Imperialism and Motherhood," *History Workshop Journal* 5 (Spring 1978): 9–66, and Anne McClintock, *Imperial Leather: Race, Gender and Sexuality in the Colonial Context* (New York: Routledge, 1995).
36 *QMQ* 5, 4 (July 1908): 158; *Woman's Century* 3, 2 (August 1915): 3.
37 For bad mothers see *JPMS* 16, 3 (March 1914): 105–6; *PHJ* 3, 2 (February 1912): 64; Winfield Scott Hall, *Sexual Knowledge* (Philadelphia: The International Bible House, 1913), 30. On motherhood see Mariana Valverde, "'When the Mother of the Race Is Free': Race Reproduction and Sexuality in First-Wave Feminism," in Franca Iacovetta and Mariana Valverde (eds.), *Gender Conflicts: New Essays in Women's History* (Toronto: University of Toronto Press, 1992), 17.
38 *CMAJ* 55, 3 (September 1946): 293–4; see also *CN* 43, 5 (May 1947): 358. By the 1950s, some were discussing what they saw as the rights of such women being ignored in the push to provide adoptable babies to couples who could not have children of their own (*Saturday Night* 65 [15 August 1950]: 26). See Susan Crawford, "Public Attitudes in Canada toward Unmarried Mothers, 1950–1996," *Past Imperfect* 6 (1997): 111–32.
39 For childbirth trauma see McGill University Archives, Royal Victoria Hospital (Montreal Maternity Hospital), patient Mrs Roy, RG 95 vol. 888 obstetrical casebook, patient no. 321, admitted 25 March 1902, discharged 26 March 1902; Royal Victoria Hospital papers RG 95, vol. 5 gynaeco-logical case charts, 1903, patient no. 1459, Mrs Perle George, admitted 9 June 1903; Victoria General Hospital, Halifax, Archives, 650/05 Box 87 patient Mrs Terrance Moore, admitted 21 July 1905; McGill University Archives, Royal Victoria Hospital, RG 95, vol. 104, gynaecological case

charts, 1913, Mrs Ann Boulter, patient no. 6402, admitted 10 November 1913. For trauma of miscarriage and loss of babies see Margaret Blackman, *During My Time: Florence Edenshaw Davidson, A Haida Woman* (Vancouver: Douglas and McIntyre, 1982), 105; Mary Rubio and Elizabeth Waterson (eds.), *The Selected Journals of L.M. Montgomery, Volume 2: 1910–1921* (Toronto: Oxford University Press, 1987), 173. For accusations against mothers see Meryn Elisabeth Stuart, "'Let Not the People Perish for Lack of Knowledge': Public Health Nursing and the Ontario Rural Child Welfare Project, 1916–1930," PhD diss., University of Pennsylvania, 1987, 14; Penelope Stewart, "Infant Feeding in Canada: 1910–1940," MA thesis, Concordia University, 1982, 90. For maternal mortality see Wendy Mitchinson, *Giving Birth in Canada 1900–1950* (Toronto: University of Toronto Press, 2002), Chapter 8, 260–85.

40 For work of mothers see Roald Amundsen, *Roald Amundsen's "The Northwest Passage"; being the record of a voyage of exploration of the ship Gjoa 1903–1907* (London: A. Constable & Co., 1908), 312; for putting others first see *Annual Report of the Canadian Association for the Prevention of Tuberculosis, 1917,* 43.

41 Interview with Dorothy Atkinson, 15 June 1993.

42 For maternal mortality see *PHJ* 14, 6 (June 1923): 243; *PHJ* 14, 7 (July 1923): 322. For Lang see *CW* 16, 7 (January 1941): 13.

43 Oxorn, *Harold Benge Atlee M.D.,* 153; *NSMB* 10, 11 (November 1931): 798. For Menzies see *CMAJ* 26, 1 (January 1932): 60.

44 See Jean Cochrane, Abby Hoffman, and Pat Kincaid, *Sports: Women in Canadian Life Series* (Toronto: Fitzhenry & Whiteside, 1977); Helen Lenskyj, "Moral Physiology in Physical Education and Sport for Girls in Ontario, 1890–1930," *Proceedings,* 5th Canadian Symposium on the History of Sport and Physical Education (Toronto: University of Toronto Press, 1982), 139–50; Helen Lenskyj, *Out of Bounds: Women, Sport and Sexuality* (Toronto: The Women's Press, 1986). An excellent examination of women and sport is M. Ann Hall, *The Girl and the Game: A History of Women's Sport in Canada* (Peterborough: Broadview Press, 2002).

45 J. Clifton Edgar, *The Practice of Obstetrics ... for the Use of Students and Practitioners* (Philadelphia: P. Blakiston's Son & Co., 1907), 36; David Tod Gilliam, *A Text-book of Practical Gynecology* (Philadelphia: F.A. Davis C., 1907), 10–11.

46 Gilliam, *A Text-book of Practical Gynecology,* 10–11; *CJMS* 35, 6 (June 1914): 321–2; *CJMS* 38, 4 (April 1915): 111.

47 *CL* 34, 9 (May 1901): 460. For the nineteenth century see Wendy Mitchinson, *The Nature of Their Bodies: Women and Their Doctors in Victorian Canada* (Toronto: University of Toronto Press, 1991), see 64–6, 114.

48 *PHJ* 4, 4 (April 1913): 248.
49 *CJMS* 38, 4 (October 1915): 111.
50 Gilliam, *A Text-book of Practical Gynecology*, 10–11; Henry T. Byford, *Manual of Gynecology* (Philadelphia: P. Blakiston's Son & Co., 1895), 64; Jennette Winter Hall, *Life's Story – A Book for Girls* (Wisconsin: B.S. Steadwell, 1911), 58–9.
51 Quoted in *CMAJ* 30, 1 (January 1934): 102. See also Hall, *The Girl and the Game*, 68–9; Patrick Harrigan, "Women's Agency and the Development of Women's Intercollegiate Athletics, 1961–2001," *Historical Studies in Education* 15, 1 (Spring 2003): 37–78.
52 Harry Sturgeon Crossen and Robert James Crossen, *Diseases of Women* (St. Louis: The C.V. Mosby Company, 1930), 835, 231.
53 *CMAJ* 35, 5 (November 1936): 572; Fred L. Adair (ed.), *Obstetrics and Gynecology*, vol. 1 (Philadelphia: Lea & Febiger, 1940), 609. For lack of protection for the male body see Helen Lenskyj, "Femininity First: Sport and Physical Education for Ontario Girls, 1890–1930," *Canadian Journal of Sport* 13, 2 (1982): 13.
54 Edgar, *The Practice of Obstetrics*, 36. For general comments see *CL* 34, 5 (January 1901): 256.
55 *CPMR* 33, 3 (March 1908): 207–8. For anorexia see Queen's University Archives, Kingston General Hospital Fonds, death records, September 1903–December 26, 1919; Royal Jubilee Hospital, Victoria, BC, discharge books, 1891–1919.
56 For the Toronto study see *CPHJ* 30, 1 (January 1939): 6. Statistics point not to people having too little food to eat but too little of the right kind of food. For Halifax and Quebec City see Andrée Lévesque, "La Santé des femmes en période de dépression économique: l'exemple des patientes de l'Hôpital de la Miséricorde à Montréal pendant les années trente," *Bulletin du Regroupement des chercheurs-chercheures en histoire de travailleurs et travailleuses du Québec* 47/48 (Eté–Automne 1990): 12.
57 Lois Banner, *In Full Flower: Aging Women, Power, and Sexuality: A History* (New York: Alfred A. Knopf 1992), 50. For slender body image see *Canadian Magazine* 73 (May 1930): 21; *Chatelaine* 4, 6 (June 1931): 70; *Chatelaine* 7, 4 (April 1934): 44; *Canadian Magazine* 87 (April 1937): 63 *Chatelaine* (June 1946): 64; *Chatelaine* 23, 9 (September 1950): 75.
58 For ill health see *CH* 37, 5 (May 1930): 197–8; for women being "suckers" see *DMJ* 3, 3 (November 1938): 31.
59 *CMAJ* 30, 3 (March 1934): 311.
60 *CMAJ* 28, 6 (June 1933): 655.

61 For Snow see *CL* 34, 5 (January 1901): 256. For others see *CPMR* 27, 11
(November 1902): 662; *QMQ* 3, 1 (October 1905): 25; Edgar, *The Practice of
Obstetrics*, 36; Dudley, *The Principles and Practice of Gynecology*, 161; Gilliam,
A Text-book of Practical Gynecology, 8–9. On corsets see Valerie Steele, *The
Corset: A Cultural History* (New Haven: Yale University Press, 2004); Jill
Fields, "'Fighting the Corsetless Evil': Shaping Corsets and Culture,
1900–1930," *Journal of Social History* 33, 2 (Winter 1999): 355–84; Beatrice
Fontanel, *Support and Seduction: The History of Corsets and Bras* (New York:
Harry N. Abrams, 1997).

62 Dudley, *The Principles and Practice of Gynecology*, 161–62.

63 *PHJ* 1, 12 (December 1910): n.p.

64 *QMQ* 3, 1 (October 1905): 25.

65 For layering see Edgar, *The Practice of Obstetrics*, 36; Dudley, *The Principles
and Practice of Gynecology*, 159–60. For tight collars see Gilliam, *A Text-book
of Practical Gynecology*, 8. For high heels see Dudley, *The Principles and
Practice of Gynecology*, 159–60.

66 Edgar, *The Practice of Obstetrics*, 36.

67 *CPMR* 39, 5 (May 1914): 313–14.

68 *CC* 4, 9 (September/October 1923): 2–3; Carl Henry Davis (ed.),
Gynecology and Obstetrics, vol. 1 (Hagerstown, MD: W.F. Prior Company,
Inc., 1935), Chapter 5, 29; F.L. Adair (ed.), *Maternal Care and
Some Complications* (Chicago: The University of Chicago Press,
1939), 27.

69 *CMAJ* 40, 5 (May 1939): 478. For a history of brassieres see Marilyn Yalom,
A History of the Breast (New York: Alfred A. Knopf, 1997), 173.

70 For shoes see *HW* 22, 3 (September 1921): 64. For beauty contests see
CLP 67, 6 (December 1926): 222. For more history of beauty contests
in Canada see Patrizia Gentile, "'Queen of the Maple Leaf': A History
of Beauty Contests in Twentieth-Century Canada," PhD diss., Queen's
University, 2006, and Jane Nicholas, "Catching the Public Eye: The Body,
Space, and Social Order in 1920s Canadian Visual Culture," PhD diss.,
University of Waterloo, 2006, Chapter 2, 134–182. For cosmetics see
Saturday Night 42 (7 May 1927): 33; *CMAJ* 30, 3 (March 1934): 311; Mona
Gleason, "Size Matters: Medical Experts, Educators, and the Provision of
Health Services to Children in Early to Mid-Twentieth Century English
Canada," in Cynthia Comacchio, Janet Golden, and George Weisz (eds.),
*Healing the World's Children: Interdisciplinary Perspectives on Child Health in
the Twentieth Century* (Montreal and Kingson: McGill-Queen's University
Press, 2008), 187.

71 For lay attitudes see *Canadian Magazine* 18, 1 (November 1901): 80; *Canadian Magazine* 21, 5 (September 1903): 407; *Grain Grower's Guide*, 22 June 1910, 28; *Maclean's* 30, 4 (August 1910): 100–2; *Everywoman's World* (September 1914): 18.

72 Charles Harrington, *A Manual of Practical Hygiene for Students, Physicians, and Health Officers* (Philadelphia: Lea and Febiger, 1914), 677. See also *Report of the Royal Commission on a Dispute Respecting Hours of Employment between the Bell Telephone Company of Canada Ltd. and Operators at Toronto, Ont.* (Ottawa: Government Printing Bureau, 1907), 66, 71, 73; *PHJ* 7, 4 (April 1916): 189.

73 Henry Jellett, *A Manual of Midwifery for Students and Practitioners* (London: Billiere, Tindall and Cox, 1910), 253; Thomas Watts Eden, *A Manual of Gynaecology* (London: J. & A. Churchill, 1911), 76.

74 *CL* 40, 11 (July 1907): 974; *Report of the Royal Commission on a Dispute Respecting Hours of Employment between the Bell Telephone Company of Canada, Ltd. and Operators at Toronto, Ont.*, 66, 69, 72, 74; Carolyn E. Strange, "The Perils and Pleasures of the City: Single, Wage-Earning Women in Toronto, 1880–1930," PhD diss., Rutgers University, 1991, 41, 42.

75 Helen MacMurchy, *Report on Infant Mortality, Toronto 1910*, cited in Michael Piva, *Working Conditions of Working-Class Toronto* (Ottawa: University of Ottawa Press, 1979), 125; Harrington, *A Manual of Practical Hygiene*, 892.

76 *CL* 40, 11 (July 1907): 974. See also *CJMS* 35, 4 (April 1914): 222.

77 Henry J. Garrigues, *Gynecology, Medical and Surgical – Outlines for Students and Practitioners* (Philadelphia: J.B. Lippincott Company, 1905), 6; Reed (ed.), *A Text-Book of Gynecology*, 8.

78 For lead poisoning see Adam H. Wright, *A Textbook of Obstetrics* (New York: D. Appleton, 1908), 240; McGill University Archives, Royal Victoria Hospital, RG 95, gynaecology case charts, patient no. 1988, Audrey Goudre, admitted 3 February 1905.

79 *CJMS* 16 1 (July 1904): 48; Woods Hutchinson, *Common Diseases* (New York: Houghton Mifflin Co., 1913), 197; *PHJ* 4, 1 (January 1913): 30.

80 *CJMS* 21, 3 (March 1907): 170; *Report of the Royal Commission on a Dispute Respecting Hours of Employment between the Bell Telephone Company of Canada, Ltd. and Operators at Toronto, Ontario*, 69, 66–77.

81 *CJMS* 21, 3 (March 1907): 170. For women's reaction see Ruth A. Frager, *Sweatshop Strife: Class, Ethnicity and Gender in the Jewish Labour Movement of Toronto, 1900–1939* (Toronto: University of Toronto Press, 1992), 20.

82 *PHJ* 1, 8 (August 1910): 413.

83 W. Blair Bell, "Disorders of Function," in Thomas Watts Eden and Cuthbert Lockyer (eds.), *The New System of Gynaecology*, vol. 1 (Toronto: The

Macmillan Co. of Canada, 1917), 378. For concern about strength see *PHJ* 7, 6 (June 1916): 304; *PHJ* 7, 4 (April 1916): 187–8.

84 *CJMH* 3 (1921–22): 18–19.

85 J.S. Fairbairn, *Gynaecology with Obstetrics – A Text-Book for Students and Practitioners* (London: Humphrey Milford, Oxford University Press, 1924), 734.

86 Milton J. Rosenau, *Preventative Medicine and Hygiene* (New York: A. Appleton, 1927), 1224–5; Davis (ed.), *Gynecology and Obstetrics*, vol. 1, Chapter 5, 37; *Saturday Night* 58, (31 October 1942): 22. Modern studies have indicated that working with toxic substances also affects the health and reproductive abilities of male workers. Karen Messing, "Do Men and Women Have Different Jobs Because of Their Biological Differences?" in Elizabeth Fee (ed.), *Women and Health: The Politics of Sex in Medicine* (Farmingdale, NY: Baywood Publishing Co., 1982), 145–6.

87 Cynthia R. Comacchio, *"Nations Are Built of Babies": Saving Ontario's Mothers and Children 1900–1940* (Montreal and Kingston: McGill-Queen's University Press, 1993), 81–2; Rosenau, *Preventative Medicine and Hygiene*, 1224.

88 Fairbairn, *Gynaecology with Obstetrics*, 735.

89 For Atlee see Beth Light and Ruth Roach Pierson (eds.), *No Easy Road: Women in Canada 1920s to 1960s* (Toronto: New Hogtown Press, 1990), 187; Oxorn, *Harold Benge Atlee M.D.*, 155. That Atlee was ahead of his time is reflected in the work of Emily Martin, who notes that in the late twentieth century there was a great deal of opposition to making adjustments in the system that would make work more amenable to the needs of women. Martin, *The Woman in the Body*, 100. For Fleming see *CMAJ* 29, 2 (August 1933): 160.

90 Terry Copp, "The Health of the People: Montreal in the Depression Years," in D.A.E. Shephard and Andrée Lévesque (eds.), *Norman Bethune: His Times and His Legacy* (Ottawa: Canadian Public Health Association, 1982), 134.

91 *Saturday Night* 58 (31 October 1942): 22; *CJPH* 34, 6 (June 1943): 268–9.

92 *Canadian Hospital* 21, 9 (September 1944): 7.

93 *CW* 16, 7 (January 1941): 12; *CD* 9, 5 (May 1943): 25; *CJPH* 35, 11 (November 1944): 445.

Chapter 2

1 Mary Rubio and Elizabeth Waterson (eds.), *The Selected Journals of Lucy Maud Montgomery, Volume 2, 1910–1921* (Toronto: Oxford University Press, 1987), 96.

2 See Cynthia Comacchio, *The Dominion of Youth: Adolescence and the Making of Modern Canada, 1920–1950* (Waterloo: Wilfrid Laurier Press, 2006); Crista Deluzio, *Female Adolescence in American Scientific Thought, 1830–1930* (Baltimore: Johns Hopkins University Press, 2007).

3 Pediatrics was not developed significantly during the time period under study. Cynthia Comacchio, "'The Rising Generation': Laying Claim to the Health of Adolescents in English Canada, 1920–1970," *Canadian Bulletin of Medical History* 19, 1 (2002): 141. On raising children see Mona Gleason, *Normalizing the Ideal: Psychology, Schooling, and the Family in Postwar Canada* (Toronto: University of Toronto Press, 1999); Katherine Arnup, *Education for Motherhood: Advice for Mothers in Twentieth-Century Canada* (Toronto: University of Toronto Press, 1994); Jocelyn Raymond, *The Nursery World of Dr. Blatz* (Toronto: University of Toronto Press, 1991); Cynthia R. Comacchio, *"Nations Are Built of Babies": Saving Ontario's Mothers and Children, 1900–1940* (Montreal and Kingston: McGill-Queen's University Press, 1993); Denyse Baillargeon, "Care of Mothers and Infants in Montreal between the Wars: The Visiting Nurses of Metropolitan Life, les Gouttes de lait, and Assistance Maternelle," in Dianne Dodd and Deborah Gorham (eds.), *Caring and Curing: Historical Perspectives on Women and Healing in Canada* (Ottawa: University of Ottawa Press, 1994), 163–81; Norah L. Lewis, "Physical Perfection for Spiritual Welfare: Health Care for the Urban Child, 1900–1939," in Patricia T. Rooke and R.L. Schnell (eds.), *Studies in Childhood History: A Canadian Perspective* (Calgary: Detselig Enterprises, 1982), 135–66; Veronica Strong-Boag, "Intruders in the Nursery: Childcare Professionals Reshape the Years One to Five, 1920–1940," in Joy Parr (ed.), *Childhood and Family in Canadian History* (Toronto: McClelland and Stewart, 1982), 160–78. In recent years the focus of historians has changed to the health care of children. However, that care seldom is focused on the treatment proffered by physicians for specific medical problems. See Special Issue on Children's Health, Veronica Strong-Boag (ed.), *Canadian Bulletin of the History of Medicine* 19, 1 (2002), and the recent work of Mona Gleason: "Between Education and Memory: Health and Childhood in English Canada, 1900–1950," *Scientia Canadensis* 29, 1 (2006): 49–72; "From 'Disgraceful Carelessness' to 'Intelligent Precaution': Accidents and the Public Child in English Canada, 1900–1950," *Journal of Family History* 30, 2 (April 1995): 230–41; "Embodied Negotiations: Children's Bodies and Historical Change in Canada, 1930–1960," *Journal of Canadian Studies* 34, 1 (Spring 1999): 113–37. See also Cheryl Krasnick Warsh and Veronica Strong-Boag (eds.), *Children's Health Issues in Historical Perspective* (Waterloo: Wilfrid Laurier University Press, 2005).

4 On Hall see Comacchio, "'The Rising Generation,'" 143, and J.C. Connell, *The Book of a Life – From Generation to Generation* (Toronto: Ryerson Press, 1935), 13. On stages see also *Maclean's* 58 (1 January 1945): 37, and *Maclean's* 59 (15 November 1946): 63.

5 Joseph B. DeLee, *The Principles and Practice of Obstetrics* (Philadelphia: W.B. Saunders, 1913), 1.

6 Thomas Watts Eden and Cuthbert Lockyer, *Gynaecology for Students and Practitioners* (London: J. & A. Churchill, 1928), 78, and Ralph B. Winn (ed.), *Encyclopedia of Child Guidance* (New York: The Philosophical Library, 1943), 126.

7 David Tod Gilliam, *A Text-book of Practical Gynecology* 2nd ed. (Philadelphia: F.A. Davis, 1907), 79; E.E. Montgomery, *Practical Gynecology* (Philadelphia: Blakiston, 1912), 203. For a more extended look at hermaphrodites see Alice Domurat Dreger, *Hermaphrodites and the Medical Invention of Sex* (Cambridge, MA: Harvard University Press, 2000).

8 W.H.B. Stoddart, *Mind and Its Disorders: A Textbook for Students and Practitioners of Medicine* (Philadelphia: P. Blakiston's Son & Co., 1919), 70.

9 Howard A. Kelly et al., *Gynecology* (New York: D. Appleton, 1928), 1001; Dorothy Sangster, "The Spinster Who Lectures Wives on Love and Childbirth," *Maclean's* 70 (November 1957): 89.

10 Henry J. Garrigues, *Gynecology, Medical and Surgical: Outlines for Students and Practitioners* (Philadelphia: J.B. Lippincott, 1905), 182. For rape see Charles A.L. Reed (ed.), *A Text-Book of Gynecology* (New York: D. Appleton, 1901), 160–1; Maurice Craig, *Psychological Medicine – A Manual on Mental Diseases for Practitioners* (London: J. & A. Churchill, 1917), 34.

11 *CL* 34, 4 (December 1900): 175; Thomas Clifford Allbutt, W.S. Playfair, and Thomas Watts Eden (eds.), *A System of Gynaecology* (London: Macmillan, 1906), 76; Winfield Scott Hall, *Sexual Knowledge* (Philadelphia: The International Bible House, 1913), 106–7; Thomas Watts Eden and Cuthbert Lockyer (eds.), *The New System of Gynaecology*, vol. 1 (Toronto: Macmillan, 1917), 300.

12 Stoddart, *Mind and Its Disorders*, 74; for Wharton see *CMAJ* 36, 2 (February 1937): 155. For Blatz see *Maclean's* 59 (15 November 1946): 8, 63; Kelly et al., *Gynecology*, 1001.

13 Interview with Betsy Mackenzie, 19 July 1993; for tying hands see Kelly et al., *Gynecology*, 1004; for other interests see Percy E. Ryberg, *Health, Sex and Birth Control* (Toronto: The Anchor Press, 1942), 3–4.

14 *CPMR* 26, 5 (May 1901): 247; *CL* 38, 5 (1905): 431–2; E.C. Dudley, *The Principles and Practice of Gynecology for Students and Practitioners* 5th ed. (Philadelphia and New York: Lea & Febiger, 1908), 22; *PHJ* 4, 12

(December 1913): 649; *PHJ* 10, 11 (November 1919): 491; Carl Henry Davis (ed.), *Gynecology and Obstetrics*, vol. 1 (Hagerstown, MD: W.F. Prior Company, Inc., 1935) Chapter 2, 5.

15 For MacKenzie see *MMN* 14, 12 (December 1902), 437; J. Bland-Sutton and Arthur E. Giles, *The Diseases of Women: A Handbook for Students and Practitioners* (London and New York: Rebman, 1906), 14; Dudley, *The Principles and Practice of Gynecology*, 22.

16 Hall, *Sexual Knowledge*, 37. For a fascinating distinction between menstruation and wet dreams see Elizabeth Grosz, *Volatile Bodies: Toward a Corporeal Feminism* (Bloomington and Indianapolis: Indiana University Press, 1994), 205.

17 Luigi Luciani, *Human Physiology, vol. 5* (London: Macmillan, 1921), 261; Milton J. Rosenau, *Preventative Medicine and Hygiene* (New York: A. Appleton, 1927), 446; Fred Adair (ed.), *Obstetrics and Gynecology*, vol. 1 (Philadelphia: Lea & Febiger, 1940), 488; Winn (ed.), *Encyclopedia of Child Guidance*, 6.

18 Ten Teachers (ed.), *Diseases of Women* 5th ed. (London: Edward Arnold, 1935), 54; Adair (ed.), *Obstetrics and Gynecology*, vol. 1, 488.

19 See Wendy Mitchinson, *The Nature of Their Bodies: Women and Their Doctors in Victorian Canada* (Toronto: University of Toronto Press, 1991), Chapter 3.

20 J. Clifton Edgar, *The Practice of Obstetrics ... for the Use of Students and Practitioners* (Philadelphia: P. Blakiston's Son, 1907) 21; for MacKenzie see *MMN* 14, 12 (December 1902): 437; Davis (ed.), *Obstetrics and Gynecology*, vol. 1, Chapter 2, 3; for Canadian estimates see William Albert Scott and H. Brookfield Van Wyck, *The Essentials of Obstetrics and Gynecology* (Philadelphia: Lea & Febiger, 1946), 331.

21 J.S. Fairbairn, *Gynaecology with Obstetrics – A Text-Book for Students and Practitioners* (London: Humphrey Milford, Oxford University Press, 1924), 485; Davis (ed.), *Gynecology and Obstetrics*, vol. 3, Chapter 9, 32; Scott and Van Wyck, *The Essentials of Obstetrics and Gynecology*, 331.

22 Edgar, *The Practice of Obstetrics*, 22; Dudley, *The Principles and Practice of Gynecology*, 24; DeLee, *The Principles and Practice of Obstetrics*, 16.

23 J.M. Munro Kerr et al., *Combined Textbook of Obstetrics and Gynaecology for Students and Medical Practitioners* (Edinburgh: E. & S. Livinstone, 1933), 38; Ten Teachers (ed.), *Diseases of Women*, 54; Adair (ed.), *Obstetrics and Gynecology*, vol. 1, 489; Emil Novak, *Textbook of Gynecology* 2nd ed. (Baltimore: The Williams & Wilkins Co., 1944), 111.

24 *CPMR* 26, 5 (May 1901): 248; see also Edgar, *The Practice of Obstetrics*, 22; Barton Cooke Hirst, *A Text-Book of Obstetrics* (Philadelphia and London: W.B. Saunders Company, 1912), 74.

25 Reed (ed.), *A Text-Book of Gynecology*, 703.

26 R.W. Johnstone, *A Text-Book of Midwifery: For Students and Practitioners* (London: A. & C. Black, Ltd., 1934), 37; Adair (ed.), *Obstetrics and Gynecology*, vol. 1, 489; Novak, *Textbook of Gynecology*, 111; Archibald Donald Campbell and Mabel A. Shannon, *Gynaecology for Nurses* (Philadelphia: F.A. Davis Co., 1946), 23.

27 For race see Davis (ed.), *Gynecology and Obstetrics*, vol. 1, Chapter 2, 4; Adair (ed.), *Obstetrics and Gynecology*, vol. 1, 489; Winn (ed.), *Encyclopedia of Child Guidance*, 334. For climate see Johnstone, *A Text-Book of Midwifery*, 37.

28 See *CPMR* 27, 11 (November 1902): 663; Bland-Sutton and Giles, *The Diseases of Women*, 14; Hall, *Sexual Knowledge*, 179–80.

29 Hirst, *A Text-Book of Obstetrics*, 74.

30 Edgar, *The Practice of Obstetrics*, 22. On class see also DeLee, *The Principles and Practice of Obstetrics*, 16; W. Blair Bell, "Disorders of Function," in Eden and Lockyer (eds.), *The New System of Gynaecology*, vol. 1, 297. For ill health and/or exercise see DeLee, *The Principles and Practice of Obstetrics*, 16; Bell, "Disorders of Function," in Eden and Lockyer (eds.), *The New System of Gynaecology.* vol. 1, 297–8.

31 See Fairbairn, *Gynaecology with Obstetrics*, 61, 485; William P. Graves, *Gynecology* (Philadelphia and London: W.B. Saunders, 1929), 30; Harry Sturgeon Crossen and Robert James Crossen, *Diseases of Women* (St. Louis: The C.V. Mosby Company, 1930), 828; Johnstone, *A Text-Book of Midwifery*, 37; Adair (ed.), *Obstetrics and Gynecology*, vol. 1, 489; Winn (ed.), *Encyclopedia of Child Guidance*, 334; Novak, *Textbook of Gynecology*, 111.

32 Graves, *Gynecology*, 30; Davis (ed.), *Gynecology and Obstetrics*, vol. 1, Chapter 2, 4; Adair (ed.), *Obstetrics and Gynecology*, vol. 1, 489; Novak, *Textbook of Gynecology*, 111.

33 Explanations of age of puberty can vary with culture. In a study of Dene health care, several women agreed that the age of puberty had declined over time but they did not mention the issue of better health care accessibility. Rather, they focused on the changing nature of their society: "In the past girls had little contact with boys. Today, because boys and girls 'play around' with each other at an early age, menstruation happens earlier." In Marie Adele Rabesca, Diane Romie, Martha Johnson, and Joan Ryan, *Traditional Dene Medicine, Part 2: Database* (Lac La Martre, North West Territories: Traditional Dene Medicine Project, 1993), 317.

34 David Berry Hart, *Guide to Midwifery* (London: Rebman Ltd., 1912), 43; Gilliam, *A Text-book of Practical Gynecology*, 62.

35 For ill health and female puberty see *MMN* 14, 12 (December 1902): 439;
    MHR 9, 8 (August 1904): 3; *CL Lancet* 41, 1 (September 1907): 93–4; *PHJ* 4,
    12 (December 1913): 649; *CJMS* 37, 5 (May 1915): 138.

36 Ryberg, *Health, Sex and Birth Control*, 77; Francis H.A. Marshall, *The
    Physiology of Reproduction* (London: Longmans, Green and Co., 1922), 713.
    See also Crossen and Crossen, *Diseases of Women*, 828; P. Brooke Bland,
    Practical Obstetrics for Students and Practitioners (Philadelphia:
    F.A. Saunders, 1932), 37.

37 Ten Teachers (ed.), *Diseases of Women*, 55.

38 For Goldbloom see *CMAJ* 43, 4 (October 1940): 338, and McGill University
    Archives, Rare Books, Alton Goldbloom Papers, manuscript on *Teenagers*,
    chapter on "Growing Up," 13.

39 Kerr et al., *Combined Textbook of Obstetrics and Gynaecology*, 38. See
    description in Winn (ed.), *Encyclopedia of Child Guidance*, 335–6.

40 Campbell and Shannon, *Gynaecology for Nurses*, 25.

41 Hall, *Sexual Knowledge*, 106, 36–7; Ryberg, *Health, Sex and Birth Control*,
    76, 16.

42 Hall, *Sexual Knowledge*, 106, 36–7; Graves, *Gynecology*, 158.

43 Gilliam, *A Text-book of Practical Gynecology*, 62; W. Blair Bell, *The Principles
    of Gynaecology* (London: Longmans, Green and Co., 1910), 68; Hart, *Guide
    to Midwifery*, 43. In *Sexual Knowledge*, Winfield Scott Hall apparently goes
    against this norm when he says that young women become self-centred
    at puberty but he sees this as temporary and reappearing again only with
    menopause. See 205.

44 For a review of the international literature on this issue see *CL* 38, 5
    (1905): 432.

45 *MMN* 14, 12 (December 1902): 439–40; see also Bell, *The Principles of
    Gynaecology*, 192; DeLee, *The Principles and Practice of Obstetrics*, 2.

46 Dalhousie University Archives, Harry Oxorn Fonds MS-13-58, H.B. Atlee,
    "The Problem of Being a Woman," n.d. (circa 1950), 9.

47 Marni Elizabeth Davis, "Southern Kwakiutl Medicine," MA thesis,
    University of Victoria, 1977, 21–4; Margaret Blackman, *During My Time:
    Florence Edenshaw Davidson, A Haida Woman* (Vancouver, Toronto: Douglas
    and McIntyre, 1982), 48, 91–2; Margaret Blackburn, "The Changing Status
    of Haida Women: An Ethnohistorical and Life History Approach," in
    Donald A. Abbott (ed.), *The World as Sharp as a Knife: An Anthology in
    Honour of Wilson Duff* (Victoria: Provincial Museum, 1981), 67; see also
    Jo-Anne Fiske, "Gender and Politics in a Carrier Indian Community," PhD
    diss., University of British Columbia, 1989, 117; Rabesca, Romie, Johnson,
    and Ryan, *Traditional Dene Medicine, Part 2: Database*, 317; Kaj Birket-Smith,

The Caribou Eskimos: Maternal and Social Life and Their Cultural Position I Descriptive Part Report of the Fifth Thule Expedition 1921–1924 Volume 5 (Gyldeddalske Boghandel, Nordisk Forlag Copenhagen, 1929), 23, 292; Julie Cruickshank, *Life Lived Like a Story: Life Stories of Three Yukon Elders* (Vancouver: University of British Columbia Press, 1992), 99–100, 169–70; Julie Cruikshank, "Becoming a Woman in Athapaskan Society: Changing Tradition on the Upper Yukon River," *The Western Canadian Journal of Anthropology* 5, 2 (1975): 10; Kim Anderson, *Life Stages and Native Women: Memory, Teachings, and Story Medicine* (Winnipeg: University of Manitoba Press, 2011), 83–94, 118–21, 164. For a more modern example of loss of traditional customs in the residential schools see Jo-Anne Fiske and Rose Johnny, "The Nedut'en Family: Yesterday and Today," in Marion Lynn (ed.), *Voices: Essays on Canadian Families* (Toronto: Nelson Thomson Learning, 2003), 235; see also Kim Anderson, *A Recognition of Being: Reconstructing Native Womanhood* (Toronto: Second Story Press, 2000), 38–39.

48 *CPMR* 27, 11 (November 1902): 662; *CL* 41, 1 (September 1907): 93; *CL* 43, 5 (January 1910): 400; *PHJ* 4, 12 (December 1913): 649; Bell, "Disorders of Function," in Eden and Lockyer (eds.), *The New System of Gynaecology*, vol. 1, 198.

49 *CL* 33, 9 (May 1900): 518. See also *CJMS* 11, 1 (January 1902): 3; Charles Penrose, *A Text-book of Diseases of Women* 5th ed. (Philadelphia: W.B. Saunders & Co., 1905), 20; Hall, *Sexual Knowledge*, 203; Bell, "Disorders of Function," in Eden and Lockyer (eds.), *The New System of Gynaecology*, vol. 1, 297.

50 R.W. Garrett, *Textbook of Medical and Surgical Gynaecology* 2nd ed. (Kingston: R. Uglow & Co., 1910), 11. For blood to the brain see *CPMR* 27, 11 (November 1902): 662.

51 For quote see Garrett, *Textbook of Medical and Surgical Gynaecology*, 11, 43; for other problems see *CPMR* 27, 11 (November 1902): 662; *CL* 39, 11 (July 1906): 1051.

52 *DMM* 23, 5 (November 1904): 323–4, 326–7.

53 *CL* 41, 2 (October 1907): 98–9; Garrett, *Textbook of Medical and Surgical Gynaecology*, 43; Gilliam, *A Text-book of Practical Gynecology*, 4.

54 *CMAJ* 11, 9 (September 1921): 619.

55 *HW* 22, 5 (November 1922): 187; Crossen and Crossen, *Diseases of Women*, 834–5.

56 *NHPW* 28, 3 (March 1922): 139.

57 Reed (ed.), *A Text-Book of Gynecology*, 728–9. For others see *CJMS* 11, 1 (January 1902): 4; R.H. Cole, *Mental Diseases – A Textbook of Psychiatry for*

Medical Students and Practitioners (London: University of London Press, 1913), 96; Eden and Lockyer (eds.), *The New System of Gynaecology,* vol. 1, 300–1. For a different view see Thomas Laqueur, *Solitary Sex: A Cultural History of Masturbation* (New York: Zone Books, 2003), 45.

58 McGill University Archives, RG 96 vol. 168 Montreal General Hospital papers, patient casebook – medicine 1907, patient number 331, admitted 16 April 1907, discharged 17 April 1907.

59 For masturbation see Graves, *Gynecology,* 155; *CMAJ* 22, 2 (February 1930): 183; *CMAJ* 36, 2 (February 1937): 155; Adair (ed.), *Obstetrics and Gynecology,* vol. 1, 543; *Maclean's* 58 (1 January 1945): 37; Edwin H. Hirsch, *Sex Power in Marriage with Case Histories – A Realistic Analysis Concerning the Sexual and Emotional Problems of Marriage* (Toronto: McClelland and Stewart, 1948), 31. For Quebec see Gaston Desjardins, *L'Amour en patience: La sexualité adolescente au Québec – 1940–1960* (Sainte-Foy: Les Presses de l' Université du Québec, 1995), 34.

60 For aggressiveness see McGill University, Rare Books, Alton Goldbloom Manuscript, "Teenagers," chapter on sex, 5. See also *Maclean's* (January 1920), 28; *PHJ* 15, 6 (June 1924): 259; Graves, *Gynecology,* 158; *Maclean's* 59 (15 April 1946): 49; *Food for Thought* 9, 5 (February 1949): 46; *McMJ* 18, 4 (December 1949): 234.

61 Graves, *Gynecology,* 158; Novak, *Textbook of Gynecology,* 508. By focusing on the essentializing of female sexuality and ignoring that of male sexuality, historians seem to suggest that male sexuality was not essentialized. Kathy Peiss and Christina Simmons (eds.), "Introduction," *Passion and Power: Sexuality in History* (Philadelphia: Temple University Press, 1988), 9.

62 Interview with Gertrude Roswell, 16 July 1993.

63 *CPHJ* 23, 3 (March 1932): 118–9.

64 For loosening of morals see *Maclean's* 58 (1 January 1945): 38. See Comacchio, "The Rising Generation," 147, for a description of sexual concerns about both sexes and 157 for especial concerns during wartime about girls. For restraint on the part of girls' sexuality see *CC* 3, 7 (January 1923): 2; Graves, *Gynecology,* 158; *Maclean's* 59 (15 April 1946): 12.

65 See Victoria General Hospital, Halifax, Archives, patient records, register no. 1448, surgical department, patient no. 24, Amanda Peate, admitted 7 August 1921, discharged 7 October 1921; Victoria General Hospital, Halifax, Archives, patient records, register no. 1604, surgical department, patient no. 170, Maureen Cross, admitted 22 September 1921, discharged 11 November 1921; *CJMH* 3 (1921–2): 12–13; *HW* 17, 1 (January 1920): 15.

66 Joan Sangster, *Regulating Girls and Women: Sexuality, Family, and the Law in Ontario, 1920–1960* (Don Mills: Oxford University Press, 2001) and

"Domesticating Girls: The Sexual Regulation of Aboriginal and Working-Class Girls in Twentieth-Cantury Canada," in Katie Pickles and Myra Rutherdale (eds.), *Contact Zones: Aboriginal and Settler Women in Canada's Colonial Past* (Vancouver and Toronto: UBC Press, 2005), 179–201; see also Tamara Myers, *Caught: Montreal's Modern Girls and the Law, 1869–1945* (Toronto: University of Toronto Press, 2006).

67 For MacKenzie see *MMN* 14, 12 (December 1902): 439. R.H. Cole estimated that maturity was reached at age 25 for men and 23 for women. See Cole, *Mental Diseases*, 206.

68 Frederick Tracy, *The Psychology of Adolescence* (New York: Macmillan, 1920), 138–44; Marshall, *The Physiology of Reproduction*, 713; Connell, *The Book of a Life*, 33; *Maclean's* 59 (1 December 1946), 12; Desjardins, *L'Amour en patience*, 99.

69 *Saturday Night* 62 (8 March 1947): 16; see also *Chatelaine* 22, 7 (July 1949): 11; *Food for Thought* 9, 5 (February 1949): 46.

70 For Gardner see *CJMS* 8, 4 (October 1900): 244; see also Hall, *Sexual Knowledge*, 32; Hart, *Guide to Midwifery*, 52.

71 Correspondence with Dr Beth Richards, 9 August 1993; interview with Joan Carr, 22 July 1993; Interview with Wilma Hallman, 11 August 1993; Marion O. Robinson, *Give My Heart: The Dr. Marion Hilliard Story* (Garden City, NY: Doubleday, 1964), 33; Gérard Bouchard, "La sexualité comme pratique et rapport chez les couples paysans du Saguenay (1860–1930)," *Revue d'histoire de l'Amérique française* 54, 2 (Automne 2000): 191; Blackman, *During My Time*, 48, 91–2. For an American study of menarche see Joan Jacobs Brumberg, "'Something Happens to Girls': Menarche and the Emergence of the Modern American Hygiene Imperative," *Journal of the History of Sexuality* 4, 1 (July 1993): 99–127.

72 The WCTU distributed the Sex and Self series widely. See Michael Bliss, "Pure Books on Avoided Subjects," 105. For information on the Ukrainian community see Karen Dubinsky, *Improper Advances: Rape and Heterosexual Conflict in Ontario, 1880–1929* (Chicago: University of Chicago Press, 1993), 140.

73 Brumberg, "'Something Happens to Girls,'" 117–18.

74 *NHPW* 28, 5 (May 1922): 249–50; *Maclean's* 58 (1 January 1945): 38. For historical studies of sex education see Sharra L. Vostral, "Advice to Adolescents: Menstrual Health and Menstrual Education Films, 1946–1982," in Cheryl Krasnick Warsh (ed.), *Gender, Health, and Popular Culture: Historical Perspectives* (Waterloo: Wilfrid Laurier University Press, 2011), 47–64; Susan K. Freeman, *Sex Goes to School: Girls and Sex Education before the 1960s* (Urbana: University of Illinois Press, 2008); Christabelle Sethna,

"The Facts of Life: The Sex Instruction of Ontario Public School Children, 1900–1950," PhD diss., University of Toronto, 1995.

75 For Renaud see Beth Light and Ruth Roach Pierson (eds.), *No Easy Road: Women in Canada 1920s to 1960s* (Toronto: New Hogtown Press, 1990), 103–4. Translated from Thérèse Renaud, *Une Mémoire Déchirée: Recit* (Montreal: n.p., 1978), 65–6. For appendix story see Joan Sangster, "Incarcerating 'Bad Girls': The Regulation of Sexuality through the Female Refuges Act in Ontario, 1920–1945," *Journal of the History of Sexuality* 7, 2 (1996): 253. For male blandishments see Ryberg, *Health, Sex and Birth Control*, 54. For Hilliard see Sangster, "The Spinster who Lectures Wives on Love and Childbirth," 89.

76 Desjardins, *L'amour en patience*, 77, 115–19, 28–30, 98.

77 For morality of sex education see Sethna, "The Facts of Life," 3. For nurses see *Chatelaine* 10, 11 (November 1947): 14; for film see *CN* 43, 12 (December 1947): 968. Even in the twenty-first century, adolescents are not particularly knowledgeable about the details of sexual matters. See Canadian Population Health Initiative, *Women's Health Surveillance Report: A Multi-dimensional Look at the Health of Canadian Women* (Ottawa: Canadian Institute for Health Information, 2003), 49.

78 Cheryl Krasnick Warsh, "Wendy's Last Night in the Nursery: The 'Disease' of Menstruation and Its Treatment," in her *Prescribed Norms: Women and Health in Canada and the United States since 1800* (Toronto: University of Toronto Press, 2010), 31. Joan Jacobs Brumberg makes the point that most such instruction, at least in the advertisements, was "desexualized" (Brumberg, "Something Happens to Girls," 123).

79 "First Menstruation" in the project Traces, 24 April 1990, tape GRP26; interview with Jennie Graham, 29 June 1993.

80 Mona Gleason, "Disciplining the Student Body," *History of Education Quarterly* 41, 2 (Summer 2001): 211.

81 Interviews with Dorothy Atkinson, 15 June 1993; Betsy Lawrence, 30 August 1993; Faith Matthews, 21 October 1993; "First Menstruation," Traces, 24 April 1990, tape GRP #26; for fathers as educators see interviews with Eunice Jordan, 14 July 1993, and Bestsy Mackenzie, 19 August 1993. For others see Memorial University of Newfoundland, Folklore and Language Archive, No. 84-307A, John Burke, "Mrs. Annie LeMoine: A Profile of the Traditional Midwife in Port au Port," 10; "First Menstruation," Traces, 24 April 1990, tape GRP #26; interviews with Isme Southern, 24 August 1993; Eunice Jordan, 14 July 1993; Janice Yeomans, 3 June 1993; Joan Carr, 22 July 1993; Velma Messinger, 14 July 1992; and Gertrude Roswell, 16 August 1993; Bouchard, "La sexualité comme

pratique et rapport chez les couples paysans du Saguenay (1860–1930)," 193–94.

82 William Victor Johnston, *Before the Age of Miracles: Memoirs of a Country Doctor* (Toronto: Fitzhenry and Whiteside, 1972), 144.

83 See "First Menstruation," Traces, 24 April 1990, tape GRP #26 and interview with Ruth Howard, 25 August 1993; see also correspondence with Dr Beth Richards, 9 August 1993; interviews with Dorothy Atkinson, 15 June 1993; Betsy Lawrence, 30 August 1993; Dr Aurora Hespler, 29 October 1993; Esther Thomas, 21 July 1992.

84 Based on interview with Joan Carr, born 1918, 22 July 1993; interviews about "First Menstruation" in the project Traces, 24 April 1990, tape GRP #26.

85 Mary Rubio and Elizabeth Waterson (eds.), *The Selected Journals of Lucy Maud Montgomery, Volume 3, 1921–29* (Toronto: Oxford University Press, 1992), 157; Max Braithwaite, *Never Sleep Three in a Bed* (New York: Dodd, Mead and Co., 1970), 5, 143, 146–9; Charles Ritchie, *My Grandfather's House: Scenes of Childhood and Youth* (Toronto: Macmillan of Canada, 1987), 74. See also Lesley A. Hall, *Hidden Anxieties: Male Sexuality, 1900–1950* (Cambridge: Polity Press, 1991), 40–60, for the more unsavoury ways boys learned about sex in Britain and also the ignorance on the part of men in sexual matters (90–113).

86 Sethna, "The Facts of Life," 3.

Chapter 3

1 Archibald Donald Campbell and Mabel A. Shannon, *Gynaecology for Nurses* (Philadelphia: F.A. Davis Co., 1946), 25.

2 Janice Delaney, M.J. Lupton, and Emily Toth, *The Curse: A Cultural History of Menstruation* (New York: Mentor, 1976); Louise Lander, *Images of Bleeding: Menstruation as Ideology* (New York: Orlando Press, 1988); Etienne van de Walle and Elisha P. Renne (eds.), *Regulating Menstruation: Beliefs, Practices, Interpretations* (Chicago: University of Chicago Press, 2001); Lara Freidenfelds, *The Modern Period: Menstruation in Twentieth-Century America* (Baltimore: John Hopkins University Press, 2009); Cheryl Krasnick Warsh, *Prescribed Norms: Women and Health in Canadian and the United States since 1800* (Toronto: University of Toronto Press, 2010), Chapter 1, "Wendy's Last Night in the Nursery: The 'Disease' of Menstruation and Its Treatment," 3–46; Kim Anderson, "Algonquian Women: Life Stage, Gender and Identity, 1930–1960," PhD diss., University of Guelph, 2010, Chapter 4.

3 Harry Oxorn, *Harold Bengee Atlee M.D.: A Biography* (Hantsport, Nova Scotia: Lancelot Press, 1983), 122.

4 Margarete Sandelowski, *Women, Health, and Choice* (Englewood Cliffs, NJ: Prentice-Hall, 1981), 39.

5 For variation see Henry T. Byford et al., *An American Text-book of Gynaecology, Medical and Surgical, for Practitioners and Students* (Philadelphia: W.B. Saunders Co., 1896), 81; for Robinson see *CPMR* 27, 11 (November 1902): 621. For Drennan see *DMM* 21, 3 (September 1903): 188, and *CJMS* 15, 2 (February 1904): 90. W. Blair Bell, *The Principles of Gynaecology* (London: Longmans, Green and Co., 1910), 73; David Berry Hart, *Guide to Midwifery* (London: Rebman, 1912), 49.

6 Francis H.A. Marshall, *The Physiology of Reproduction* (London: Longmans, Green and Co., 1922), 59. For variability see *UTMJ* 2, 6 (April 1925): 193; R.W. Johnstone, *A Text-Book of Midwifery: For Students and Practitioners* (London: A.& C. Black, Ltd., 1934), 36; Henricus J. Stander, *Williams Obstetrics: A Textbook for the Use of Students and Practitioners* 8th ed. (New York: D. Appleton-Century Co., 1941), 72. For quote see Ten Teachers, *Midwifery* 5th ed. (London: Edward Arnold & Co., 1935), 55–6. For timing of ovulation see *UTMJ* 17, 5 (March 1940): 250; Stander, *Williams Obstetrics*, 81.

7 Interview with Betsy Lawrence, 30 August 1993; see also "First Menstruation," Traces, 24 April 1990, tape GRP #26.

8 Lois W. Banner, *In Full Flower: Aging Women, Power, and Sexuality: A History* (New York: Alfred A. Knopf, 1992), 277.

9 For variation see Byford et al., *An American Text-book of Gynaecology*, 81; for Robinson see *CPMR* 27, 11 (November 1902): 621. For Drennan see *DMM* 21, 3 (September 1903): 188 and *CJMS* 15, 2 (February 1904): 90. For animal analogy see Charles A.L. Reed (ed.), *A Text-Book of Gynecology* (New York: D. Appleton and Co., 1901), 700–1, 704–5; W. Blair Bell, *The Principles of Gynaecology* (London: Longmans, Green and Co., 1910), 73; David Berry Hart, *Guide to Midwifery* (London: Rebman, 1912), 49.

10 Henry J. Garrigues, *Gynecology, Medical and Surgical: Outlines for Students and Practitioners* (Philadelphia: J.B. Lippincott Co., 1905), 100.

11 CJMS 15, 2 (February 1904): 90–1; Thomas Watts Eden, *A Manual of Gynaecology* (London: J. & A. Churchill, 1911), 78; Hart, *Guide to Midwifery*, 51; for the unnamed author see *CPMR* 41, 3 (March 1916): 181.

12 William P. Graves, *Gynecology* (Philadelphia and London: W.B. Saunders, 1929), 34. For Collip see *CMAJ* 22, 2 (February 1930): 214; for Hanley see *UTMJ* 17, 5 (March 1940): 250.

13 For Marlow see *CN* 20, 3 (March 1924): 152. For Mitchell see *CMAJ* 22, 4 (April 1930): 587; for Atlee see Dalhousie University Archives, Oxorn Fonds MS-13-58, H.B. Atlee "Medical Lecture Notes – Gynaecology," 8.

14 *UTMJ* 14, 6 (April 1937): 224, 228.

15 *CMAJ* 41, 4 (October 1939): 426.

16 J. Bland-Sutton and Arthur E. Giles, *The Diseases of Women: A Handbook for Students and Practitioners* (London and New York: Rebman, 1906), 21; David Tod Gilliam, *A Text-book of Practical Gynecology* 2nd ed. (Philadelphia: F.A. Davis Co., 1907), 74; J. Clifton Edgar, *The Practice of Obstetrics ... for the Use of Students and Practitioners* 3rd ed. (Philadelphia: P. Blakiston's Son & Co., 1907), 23–4; Joseph B. DeLee, *The Principles and Practice of Obstetrics* (Philadelphia and London: W.B. Saunders Co., 1913), 17; for length and quantity of flow see Eden, *A Manual of Gynaecology*, 72.

17 *CMAJ* 13, 11 (November 1923): 781.

18 For amount of blood see Marshall, *The Physiology of Reproduction*, 60; J.S. Fairbairn, *Gynaecology with Obstetrics: A Text-Book for Students and Practitioners* (London: Humphrey Milford, Oxford University Press, 1924), 61. For length of flow see Fairbairn, *Gynaecology with Obstetrics*, 61. For years of activity see Ten Teachers, *Midwifery*, 7.

19 Marshall, *The Physiology of Reproduction*, 158; Stander, *Williams Obstetrics*, 73. For the power menstruation gave native women see Kim Anderson, *Life Stages and Native Women: Memory, Teaching, and Story Medicine* (Winnipeg: University of Manitoba Press, 2011), 88–90.

20 Anne Fausto-Sterling, "Hormonal Hurricane: Menstruation, Menopause and Female Behaviour," in Laurel Richardson and Verta Taylor (eds.), *Feminist Frontiers II: Rethinking Sex, Gender and Society* (New York: McGraw-Hill, 1989), 294. See also Susan Sherwin, *No Longer Patient: Feminist Ethics and Health Care* (Philadelphia: Temple University Press, 1992), 185.

21 For different terms see Byford et al., *An American Text-book of Gynaecology*, 81; Garrigues, *Gynecology, Medical and Surgical*, 100; Thomas Clifford Allbutt, W.S. Playfair, and Thomas Watts Eden (eds.), *A System of Gynaecology* (London: Macmillan and Co., 1906), 92.

22 For pain see *CL* 33, 9 (May 1900): 518; Edgar, *The Practice of Obstetrics*, 20; Eden, *A Manual of Gynaecology*, 137. For both mental and/or physical problems see *CJMS* 11, 1 (January 1902): 3; Allbutt, Playfair, and Eden (eds.), *A System of Gynaecology*, 92; Stewart Purves, "Nervous Diseases Associated with Morbid Conditions of the Pelvic Organs in Women," in Thomas Watts Eden and Cuthbert Lockyer (eds.), *The New System of Gynaecology*, vol. 1 (Toronto: the Macmillan Co. of Canada, 1917), 739.

23 Vilhjalmus Stefansson, "The Stefansson-Anderson Arctic Expedition of the American Museum: Preliminary Ethnological Report," *Anthropological Papers of the American Museum of Natural History XIV, Part 1* (New York: AMS Press, 1914), 182; Marni Elizabeth Davis, "Southern Kwakiutl Medicine," MA thesis, University of Victoria, 1977, 59–60; Jo-Anne Fiske, "Gender and Politics in a Carrier Indian Community," PhD diss., University of British Columbia, 1989, 117; Marie Adele Rabesca, Diane Romie, Martha Johnson, and Joan Ryan, *Traditional Dene Medicine, Part 2: Database* (Lac La Martre, North West Territories: Traditional Dene Medicine Project, 1993), 317; Margaret Blackman, *During My Time: Florence Edenshaw Davidson, A Haida Woman* (Vancouver and Toronto: Douglas and McIntyre, 1982), 91; Asen Balickci, *The Netsilik Eskimo* (Garden City, NY: The Natural History Press, 1970, published for the American Museum of Natural History), 222, 224; Naomi Griffen, *The Roles of Men and Women in Eskimo Culture* (Chicago: Chicago University Press, 1930), 62. For limitations see Anderson, *Life Stages and Native Women*, 102–3.

24 For various symptoms see Marshall, *The Physiology of Reproduction*, 158; Frank A. Craig, *Diseases of Middle Life: The Prevention, Recognition and Treatment of the Morbid Processes of Special Significance in This Critical Life Period, vol. 2* (Philadelphia: F.A. Davis Co., 1924), 479; *CJMS* 59, 5 (May 1926): 138; Graves, *Gynecology*, 31, 148; Harry Sturgeon Crossen and Robert James Crossen, *Diseases of Women* 7th ed. (St. Louis: The C.V. Mosby Co., 1930), 830; Johnstone, *A Text-Book of Midwifery*, 41; Stander, *Williams Obstetrics*, 73; Percy E. Ryberg, *Health, Sex and Birth Control* (Toronto: The Anchor Press, 1942), 34.

25 *CJMS* 59, 5 (May 1926): 140.

26 For more on PMS see Warsh, *Prescribed Norms*, 33–7.

27 Ryberg, *Health, Sex and Birth Control*, 33–34. For insignia of their sex and benefits see Howard A. Kelly and Collaborators, *Gynecology* (New York and London: D. Appleton and Company, 1928), 654; Graves, *Gynecology*, 148; Ten Teachers, *Diseases of Women* 5th ed. (London: Edward Arnold & Co., 1935), 81. For Baragar see *CPHJ* 23, 3 (March 1932): 120; J.M. Munro Kerr et al., *Combined Textbook of Obstetrics and Gynaecology for Students and Medical Practitioners* (Edinburgh: E. & S. Livinstone, 1933), 720.

28 *Chatelaine* 16, 11 (November 1943): 13; see *CMAJ* 49, 2 (August 1943): 151, advertisement.

29 Sally Shuttleworth, "Female Circulation: Medical Discourse and Popular Advertising in the Mid-Victorian Era," in Mary Jacobus, Evelyn Fox Keller, and Sally Shuttleworth (eds.), *Body/Politics: Women and the Discourses of Science* (New York and London: Routledge, 1990), 47.

30 Interview with Dr Hespler, 29 October 1993.
31 Davis, "Southern Kwakiutl Medicine," 59. For use of algae Betty Anne
    Daviss-Putt, "Rights of Passage in the North: From Evacuation to the
    Birth of a Culture," in Mary Crnkovich (ed.), *"Gossip": A Spoken History
    of Women in the North* (Ottawa: Canadian Arctic Resources Committee,
    1990), 93. For other items see Northwest Territories Archives, Northen Life
    Museum Archives, 87-01-13.11.0, Elizabeth Cass Collection, tape 1, 11–12.
32 Interview with Wilma Hallman, 11 August 1993.
33 For napkins see Jane Farrell-Beck and Laura Klosterman Kidd, "The
    Role of Health Professionals in the Development and Dissemination of
    Women's Sanitary Products, 1880–1940," *Journal of the History of Medicine*
    51 (July 1996): 325–52; Laura Klosterman Kidd, "Menstrual Technology
    in the United States: 1854 to 1921," PhD diss., Iowa State University, 1994;
    Joan Jacob Brumberg, "'Something Happens to Girls': Menarche and the
    Emergence of the Modern American Hygiene Movement," *Journal of the
    History of Sexuality* 4, 1 (July 1993): 99–127; Irene Heywood Jones, " The
    History of Sanitary Protection," *Nursing Times* 76, 10 (6 March 1980): 407–8;
    Vern Bullough, "Merchandising the Sanitary Napkin: Lillian Gilbreth's
    1927 Survey," 10, 3 (1985): 615–23.
34 Interviews with Betty Mackenzie, 19 August 1993; Dr Eleanor Mackay, 29
    October 1993; Joan Carr, 22 July 1993.
35 Interview with Ruth Howard, 25 August 1993 and Jane Rutherford, 28 July
    1993.
36 For Noonan see *CJMS* 59, 5 (May 1926): 138–9.
37 For Church see Jones, " The History of Sanitary Protection," 408; Emil
    Novak, *Textbook of Gynecology* 2nd ed. (Baltimore: The Williams & Wilkins
    Co., 1944), 113; Arthur Hale Curtis and John William Huffman, *A Textbook
    of Gynecology* (Philadelphia and London: W.B. Saunders Co., [1950] 1951),
    129; interview with Dr Hespler, 29 October 1993.
38 She remembered telling him about a little cup to catch the blood that you
    inserted, made out of rubber. She wore it for four to five years but couldn't
    find another one. Interview with Dr Mackay, 29 October 1993. Ryberg,
    Health, Sex and Birth Control, 46.
39 For quotes see *Chatelaine* 2, 5 (May 1929): 44 and *Chatelaine* 2, 8 (August
    1929): 43; *Chatelaine* 8, 7 (July 1935): 3. See also *Chatelaine* 5, 5 (May 1932):
    41; *Chatelaine* 15, 5 (May 1942): 40.
40 For various advertisements for tampons see *Chatelaine* 19, 7 (July 1936): 34;
    Chatelaine 11, 7 (July 1938): 30; *Chatelaine* 12, 8 (August 1939): 30; *Chatelaine*
    12, 8 (August 1939): 30; *Chatelaine* 15, 2 (February 1942): 28; *Chatelaine* 15, 4
    (April 1942): 27; *Chatelaine* 18, 2 (February 1945): 29.

41 *CMAJ* 55, 3 (September 1946): ciii.
42 Annette Scambler and Graham Scambler, *Menstrual Disorders* (London and New York: Tavistock/Routledge, 1993), 24.
43 Scambler and Scambler, *Menstrual Disorders*, 6.
44 Ten Teachers, *Diseases of Women*, 78.
45 For underdevelopment see Bland-Sutton and Giles, *The Diseases of Women*, 397. For ill health see *CPMR* 26, 5 (May 1901): 251; Bland-Sutton and Giles, *The Diseases of Women*, 397; E.C. Dudley, *The Principles and Practice of Gynecology for Students and Practitioners* 5th ed. (Philadelphia and New York: Lea & Febiger, 1908), 748; *CPMR* 39, 4 (April 1914): 225; For emotional or mental causation see Maurice Craig, *Psychological Medicine: A Manual on Mental Diseases for Practitioners and Students* 3rd ed. (London: J. &. A. Churchill, 1917), 87; W. Blair Bell, "Disorders of Function," in Eden and Lockyer (eds.), *The New System of Gynaecology*, vol. 1, 327.
46 Bell, "Disorders of Function," in Eden and Lockyer (eds.), *The New System of Gynaecology*, vol. 1, 323–4, 297; *CPMR* 27, 8 (August 1902): 478.
47 For poor health and living habits see Crossen and Crossen, *Diseases of Women*, 832, 834. For anorexia nervosa see Ten Teachers, *Diseases of Women*, 87. For Cantor see *CMAJ* 47, 1 (July 1942): 18. For endocrine cause see *CMAJ* 53, 1 (July 1945): 67. Hyperthryoidism was also an issue in this. See *UTMJ* 27, 6 (March 1950): 239.
48 *CMAJ* 44, 1 (July 1941): 69.
49 For marriage see *CPMR* 26, 5 (May 1901): 251; Bland-Sutton and Giles, *The Diseases of Women*, 397; Dudley, *The Principles and Practice of Gynecology*, 748. For anaemia see Bell, "Disorders of Function," in Eden and Lockyer (eds.), *The New System of Gynaecology*, vol. 1, 323.
50 For Campbell and Collip see *CMAJ* 22, 2 (February 1930): 219–30. For Chapple see *CMAJ* 44, 4 (April 1941): 402.
51 *CMAJ* 42, 6 (June 1940): 585.
52 For Cantor see *CMAJ* 47, 1 (July 1942): 19; Novak, *Textbook of Gynecology*, 559.
53 Crossen and Crossen, *Diseases of Women*, 837.
54 Eden, *A Manual of Gynaecology*, 137.
55 *CL* 34, 9 (May 1901): 460–1. For habits and neurasthenia see *CPMR* 30, 2 (February 1905): 92.
56 Bland-Sutton and Giles, *The Diseases of Women*, 410; Gilliam, *A Text-book of Practical Gynecology*, 74; Bell, *The Principles of Gynaeology*, 209.
57 Allbutt, Playfair and Eden (eds.), *A System of Gynaecology*, 94.
58 Joan Kerik, compiler, *Living with the Land: Use of Plants by the Native People of Alberta* (Edmonton: Alberta Culture, Youth and Recreation, Provincial

Museum of Alberta, 1975), 16; Rabesca, Romie, Johnson, and Ryan, *Traditional Dene Medicine, Part 1,* 48, 55; Daviss-Putt, "Rights of Passage in the North," 93.

59 For whiskey, etc., see *CL* 34, 9 (May 1901): 459, 461. For various surgical procedures see *CPMR* 29, 5 (May 1914): 327; *CL* 33, 9 (May 1900): 521; Fairbairn, *Gynaecology with Obstetrics,* 710; *CL* 34, 9 (May 1901): 460–1. McGill University Archives, Royal Victoria Hospital, RG 95, vol. 35, gynaecological case charts, patient no. 29913, Mrs Susan Doane, admitted 19 July 1907.

60 Victoria General Hospital Archives, Halifax, patient number 75, register no. 58, medical department, Mrs Deborah Feist, admitted 23 November 1920, discharged 9 December 1920.

61 Fairbairn, *Gynaecology with Obstetrics,* 488, 734; Harry Beckman, *Treatment in General Practice* (Philadelphia: W.B. Saunders Co., 1931), 795; Ten Teachers, *Diseases of Women,* 105. For statistical estimates of pain see *UTMJ* 16, 3 (January 1939): 144.

62 *UTMJ* 16, 3 (January 1939): 144; Campbell and Shannon, *Gynaecology for Nurses,* 29.

63 Kerr et al., *Combined Textbook of Obstetrics and Gynaecology,* 720. For a similar dichotomy see Ten Teachers, *Diseases of Women,* 107.

64 For TB see *UTMJ* 16, 3 (January 1939): 144. For bad environments see Fairbairn, *Gynaecology with Obstetrics,* 734; Crossen and Crossen, *Diseases of Women,* 851 Ten Teachers, *Diseases of Women,* 110; *CN* 39, 5 (May 1943): 336. For lack of development see *CMAJ* 14, 12 (December 1924): 1218; Fairbairn, *Gynaecology with Obstetrics,* 489; Crossen and Crossen, *Diseases of Women,* 851.

65 Fairbairn, *Gynaecology with Obstetrics,* 489.

66 Thomas Watts Eden and Cuthbert Lockyer, *Gynaecology for Students and Practitioners* 3rd ed. (London: J. & A. Churchill, 1928), 160.

67 Interview with Dorothy Atkinson, 15 June 1993; Memorial University of Newfoundland, Folklore and Language Archive, 84-3071: John Burke, "Mrs. Annie LeMoine: A Profile of the Traditional Midwife in Port au Port," 10; interview with Betsy Lawrence, 30 August 1993; interview with Irma Avery, 15 June 1993; interview with Jennie Graham, 29 June 1993.

68 For Pinkam's tablets see *Chatelaine* 15, 10 (October 1942): 74. For Midol see *Chatelaine* 7, 4 (April 1934): 54; *Chatelaine* 11, 12 (December 1938): 28; *Chatelaine* 15, 3 (March 1942): 26; *Chatelaine* 19, 7 (July 1946): 36.

69 For commonsense advice see *CMAJ* 14, 12 (December 1924): 1219; Ten Teachers, *Diseases of Women,* 1101; *CMAJ* 38, 4 (April 1938): 377; *CN* 39, 5 (May 1943): 336; *CMAJ* 53, 5 (November 1945): 509. For peppermint essence see Ten Teachers, *Diseases of Women,* 110. For alcohol see Beckman,

Treatment in General Practice, 797. For opposition to alcohol see Ten Teachers, *Diseases of Women*, 110. For sedatives see *CN* 39, 5 (May 1943): 336. For pessaries see Beckman, *Treatment in General Practice*, 795.

70 Fairbairn, *Gynaecology with Obstetrics*, 491. For childbirth see also Crossen and Crossen, *Diseases of Women*, 859; *CMAJ* 32, 6 (June 1935): 610; *UTMJ* 16, 3 (January 1939): 144.

71 For Shute see *CMAJ* 42, 2 (February 1940): 149. Interview with Jennie Graham, 29 June 1993.

72 For Whitehouse see *CMAJ* 29, 6 (December 1933): 592; *Annual Report of the Superintendent*, Victoria General Hospital, 64, Appendix 4, 18–19; for Atlee see *CMAJ* 32,.1 (January 1935): 55–6. For criticism of the surgery see *CMAJ* 42, 4 (April 1940): 354.

73 W.G. Cosbie, *The Toronto General Hospital, 1819–1965: A Chronicle* (Toronto: Macmillan of Canada, 1975), 202–3.

74 For using hormone treatment see *CMAJ* 32, 1 (January 1935): 55; *CMAJ* 40, 1 (January 1939): 41; *CMAJ* 47, 2 (August 1942): 125; *CN* 39, 5 (May 1943): 336; Novak, *Textbook of Gynecology*, 573.

75 *MMC* 2, 5 (May 1947): n.p.

76 *CPMR* 27, 11 (November 1902): 664; Edgar, *The Practice of Obstetrics*, 23; Bell, "Disorders of Function," in Eden and Lockyer (eds.), *The New System of Gynaecology*, vol. 1, 336.

77 For VanWart see *MMN* 19, 10 (October 1907): 397. For other treatments see *CPMR* 34, 9 (September 1909): 549.

78 *CMAJ* 35, 6 (December 1936): 622.

79 For Goldbloom see *CMAJ* 43, 4 (October 1940): 338. Interview with Gertrude Roswell, 16 August 1993. For radiation see Kelly and Collaborators, *Gynecology*, 951. For Kirkland see *CN* 26, 5 (May 1930): 246.

80 *CMAJ* 47, 2 (August 1942): 125.

81 *CMAJ* 58, 2 (February 1948): 151.

Chapter 4

1 W.H.B. Stoddart, *Mind and Its Disorders: A Textbook for Students and Practitioners* (Philadelphia: P. Blakiston's Son & Co., 1919), 78.

2 Michel Foucault, *The History of Sexuality* (New York: Pantheon Books, 1978). For emphasis on the other "experts" see "Introduction," Kathy Peiss and Christina Simmons (eds.), *Passion and Power: Sexuality in History* (Philadelphia: Temple University Press, 1989), 9. For a recent and detailed discussion of the historiography on sexuality see Christopher O'Shea, "Visions of Masculinity: Home-health Advice Literature, Medical

Discourse and Male Sexuality in English Canada, 1870–1914," PhD diss., University of Guelph, 2003. For an overview of sexuality see John D'Emilio and Estelle B. Freedman, *Intimate Matters: A History of Sexuality in America* (New York: Harper and Row, 1989); Janice M. Irvine, *Disorders of Desire: Sex and Gender in Modern American Sexology* (Philadelphia: Temple University Press, 1990); Jeffrey Weeks, *Sex and Politics: The Regulation of Sexuality since 1800* 2nd ed. (London: Longman, 1989); Christina Simmons, *Making Marriage Modern: Women's Sexuality from the Progressive Era to World War II* (New York: Oxford University Press, 2009); Lesley Erickson, *Westward Bound: Sex Violence, the Law, and the Making of a Settler Society* (Vancouver: UBC Press, 2011).

3 As Adele E. Clarke has determined, "Not a single English-language book on the reproductive sciences was published until agricultural scientist F.H.A. Marshall's *Physiology of Reproduction* appeared in Britain in 1910." See Adele E. Clarke, *Disciplining Reproduction: Modernity, American Life Sciences, and "the Problems of Sex"* (Berkeley and Los Angeles: University of California Press, 1998), 5.

4 *CJMS* 9, 5 (May 1901): 364.

5 Interview with Drs Mackay and Hespler, 29 October 1993; letter to author from Dr Beth Richards, 9 August 1993. See also William R. Houston, *The Art of Treatment* (New York: Macmillan, 1936), 467; William Victor Johnston, *Before the Art of Miracles: Memoirs of a Country Doctor* (Toronto: Fitzhenry and Whiteside, 1972), 144.

6 See *NHPW* 28, 5 (May 1922): 249–50; Milton J. Rosenau, *Preventive Medicine and Hygiene* (New York: D. Appleton, 1927), 69, 83; *CH* 37, 6 (June 1930): 256; *CPHJ* 24, 7 (July 1933): 317–18; Carl Henry Davis (ed.), *Gynecology and Obstetrics*, vol. 1 (Hagerstown, MD: W.F. Prior Company, 1935), Chapter 2, 12; *CMAJ* 36, 2 (February 1937): 155.

7 Percy Ryberg, *Health, Sex and Birth Control* (Toronto: The Anchor Press, 1942), 64–5, 48. For a similar concern in Quebec see Gaston Desjardins, *L'Amour en patience: La sexualité adolescente au Québec – 1940–1960* (Sainte-Foy: Les Presses de l' Université du Québec, 1995), 26, 59–61.

8 For increasing focus on sexuality see *DMM* 17, 1 (January 1920): 16; Ryberg, *Health, Sex and Birth Control*, 48; M.M. Kirkwood, *For College Women ... and Men* (Toronto: Oxford University Press, 1938), 23; Library and Archives of Canada, Canadian Youth Commission Papers, MG 28I, II, vol. 63, file 9, the Christian Social Council of Canada, "Venereal Disease and Moral Conditions," 4; *CW* 17, 5 (October 1941): 26.

9 For impact of war see McGill University Archives, *Annual Report of the Royal Victoria Hospital, Montreal, Year ending December 1942*, 44; Alfred

Henry Tyrer, *Sex, Marriage and Birth Control* 10th ed. (Toronto: Marriage Welfare Bureau, 1943), 126; *CW* 20, 5 (15 October 1944): 6; *UTMJ* 25, 2 (November 1947): 54; Catherine Gidney, "Under the President's Gaze: Sexuality and Morality at a Canadian University during the Second World War," *Canadian Historical Review* 82, 1 (2001): 36–54.

10 Wendy Mitchinson, *The Nature of Their Bodies: Women and Their Doctors in Victorian Canada* (Toronto: University of Toronto Press, 1991), 243.

11 *CPMR* 27, 4 (April 1902): 223; for Jones's story see Alan Parkin, *A History of Psychoanalysis in Canada* (Toronto: The Toronto Psychoanalytic Society, 1987), 23; Barton Cooke Hirst, *A Text-Book of Obstetrics* (Philadelphia: W.B. Saunders Company, 1912), 69, 85. For concern about women's sexual arousal under anaesthesia see John J. Reese, *Text-Book of Medical Jurisprudence and Toxicology* 8th ed. (Philadelphia: P. Blakiston's Son & Co., 1912), 275 and *CPMR* 29, 5 (May 1914): 327.

12 Interview with Drs Mackay and Hespler, 29 October 1993, Halifax. For more on Atlee see Wendy Mitchinson, "H.B. Atlee on Obstetrics and Gynaecology: A Representative and Singular Voice in 20thC Canadian Medicine," *Acadiensis* 32, 2 (Spring 2002): 1–28.

13 Interview with Dorothy Atkinson, 15 June 1993.

14 Charles A.L. Reed (ed.), *A Text-Book of Gynecology* (New York: D. Appleton, 1901), 588; *JPMS* 15, 5 (November 1913): 266; Thomas Watts Eden and Cuthbert Lockyer (eds.), *The New System of Gynaecology,* vol. 1 (Toronto: Macmillan Co. of Canada, 1917), 402. For Canada see Michael Bliss, "Pure Books on Avoided Subjects," Canadian Historical Association *Papers* 1970, 94–5; Gérard Bouchard, "La sexualité comme pratique et rapport chez les couples paysans du Saguenay (1860–1930)," *Revue d'histoire de l'Amérique française* 56, 2 (Automne 2000): 196. Gail Bederman argues self-restraint for men declined by the end of the nineteenth century. See Bederman, *Manliness and Civilization: A Cultural History of Gender and Race in the United States, 1880–1917* (Chicago: University of Chicago Press, 1995), 11–14.

15 Winfield Scott Hall, *Sexual Knowledge* (Philadelphia: The International Bible House, 1913), 82–3.

16 For health see *PHJ* 4, 3 (March 1913): 129; Alice Stockham, *Tokology: A Book for Every Woman* (Toronto: McClelland, Goodchild and Stewart, 1916), 152; "The Double Standard," *Manhood Series Number Five* (Toronto: YMCA, 1918), 6; YMCA, "Facts for Fighters," *Manhood Series Number Three* (Toronto: YMCA,1918), 4. For its naturalness see Reed (ed.), *A Text-Book of Gynecology,* 588. See also Cecilia Benoit, "Mothering in a Newfoundland Community: 1900–1940," in Katherine Arnup, Andrée Lévesque, and Ruth Roach Pierson (eds.), *Delivering Motherhood: Maternal Ideologies and Practices*

in the 19th and 20th Centuries (London and New York: Routledge, 1990),
178. See chapter on menopause for further discussion of male sexuality in
old age.

17 For first quote see *CPHJ* 24, 7 (July 1933): 317–18; for the centrality of
the male sex urge see also *PHJ* 14, 11 (November 1923): 516; *CH* 37,
6 (June 1930): 256; Ryberg, *Health, Sex and Birth Control*, 115; *Maclean's* 59
(15 April 1946): 49; *Canadian Home Journal* 42 (February 1946): 24; *Food for
Thought* 9, 5 (February 1949): 46. For quote from 1940s text see Fred. L.
Adair (ed.), *Obstetrics and Gynecology*, vol. 1 (Philadelphia: Lea & Febiger,
1940), 539.

18 *CPHJ* 24, 7 (July 1933): 317.

19 *CLNH* 60, 1 (January 1923): 23.

20 *CH* 37, 6 (June 1930): 256.

21 *Woman's Century* (March 1920); 22; National Council of Women, *Yearbook*,
1922, 132; National Health Publication No. 24, *Information for Men: Syphilis
and Gonorrhoea* (Ottawa: Department of Pensions and National Health,
1935), 5; Ryberg, *Health, Sex and Birth Control*, 187–8, 22; Tyrer, *Sex, Marriage
and Birth Control*, 44. See also Carolyn E. Strange, "The Perils and Pleasures
of the City: Single, Wage-earning Women in Toronto, 1880–1930," PhD
diss., Rutgers University, 1991, 346.

22 Bederman, *Manliness and Civilization*, 19.

23 Christina Simmons, "Modern Sexuality and the Myth of Victorian
Repression," in Peiss and Simmons (eds.), *Passion and Power*, 157–77.

24 On impotence see Henry C. Chapman, *A Manual of Medical Jurisprudence
and Toxicology* 2nd ed. (Philadelphia: W.B. Saunders, 1896), 141–2; Henry
H. Morton, *Genito-Urinary Diseases and Syphilis* (Philadelphia: F.A. Davis,
1906), 93, 467; Henry Jellett, *A Manual of Midwifery for Students and
Practitioners* (London: Bailliere, Tindall and Cox, 1910), 587. See also Angus
McLaren, *Impotence: A Cultural History* (Chicago: University of Chicago
Press, 2007).

25 Morton, *Genito-Urinary Diseases and Syphilis*, 467, 470.

26 *CMAJ* 14, 2 (February 1924): 138; Houston, *The Art of Treatment*, 474;
Ryberg, *Health, Sex and Birth Control*, 137; *UTMJ* 21, 1 (October 1943): 24.

27 *CMAJ* 14, 2 (February 1924): 138–9; Rosenau, *Preventative Medicine and
Hygiene*, 86; *CMAJ* 36, 2 (February 1937): 155; *CPHJ* 31, 7 (July 1940):
469; *CMAJ* 48, 3 (March 1943): 231–2; *CMAJ* 55, 2 (August 1946): 138;
Edwin H. Hirsch, *Sex Power in Marriage with Case Histories: A Realistic
Analysis Concerning the Sexual and Emotional Problems of Marriage* (Toronto:
McClelland and Stewart, 1948), xiv; *CMAJ* 60, 1 (January 1949): 32; *McMJ*
18, 4 (December 1949): 234.

28 For transfer problems see *OJNP* 1, 4 (March 1924): 8; Hirsch, *Sex Power in Marriage with Case Histories*, xiv.

29 Morton, *Genito-Urinary Diseases and Syphilis*, 90; J. Clifton Edgar, *The Practice of Obstetrics ... for the Use of Students and Practitioners* 3rd ed. (Philadelphia: P. Blakiston's & Son, 1907), 35.

30 Daniel Clark, *Mental Diseases. A Synopsis of Twelve Lectures Delivered at the Hospital for the Insane, Toronto, to the Graduating Medical Classes* (Toronto: William Briggs n.d.), 154–5; Hall, *Sexual Knowledge*, 145, 106–7.

31 Frank Winthrop Draper, *A Text-book of Legal Medicine* (Philadelphia: W.B. Saunders, 1905), 122. See also Chapman, *A Manual of Medical Jurisprudence and Toxicology*, 97; Henry J. Garrigues, *Gynecology, Medical and Surgical: Outlines for Students and Practitioners* (Philadelphia: J.B. Lippincott, 1905), 182.

32 Charles C. Norris, *Gonorrhea in Women: Its Pathology, Symptomology, Diagnosis, and Treatment: Together with a Review of the Rare Varieties of the Disease Which Occur in Men, Women and Children* (Philadelphia and London: W.B. Saunders, 1913), 142; *CJMS* 40, 3 (September 1916): 87.

33 William Brend, *A Handbook of Medical Jurisprudence and Toxicology* (London: Griffin, 1941), 100.

34 Rosenau, *Preventive Medicine and Hygiene*, 86.

35 *McMJ* 18, 4 (December 1949): 234.

36 Stoddart, *Mind and Its Disorders*, 187; Rosenau, *Preventive Medicine and Hygiene*, 81; *CMAJ* 36, 2 (February 1937): 155; Adair (ed.), *Obstetrics and Gynecology*, vol. 1, 547–8; Houston, *The Art of Treatment*, 478; *CMAJ* 36, 2 (February 1937): 155; Ryberg, *Health, Sex and Birth Control*, 74–7.

37 Stoddart, *Mind and Its Disorders*, 196; Sir James Purves-Stewart, *The Diagnosis of Nervous Diseases* 8th ed. (London: Edward Arnold, 1937), 602.

38 Ryberg, *Health, Sex and Birth Control*, 79. For Laycock see *CMAJ* 63, 3 (September 1950): 246–8. For a discussion of homosexuality and identity see Anna Clark, *Desire: A History of European Sexuality* (New York: Routledge, 2008), 6, 11.

39 For recognition of homosexuality and gender flexibility in some native cultures see Kim Anderson, *A Recognition of Being: Reconstructing Native Womanhood* (Toronto: Second Story Press, 2000), 88–91; Sabine Lang, "Various Kinds of Two Spirit People: Gender Variance and Homosexuality in Native American Communities," in Sue Ellen Jacobs, Wesley Thomas, and Sabine Lang (eds.), *Two Spirit People: Native American Gender Identity, Sexuality and Spirituality* (Chicago: University of Illinois Press, 1997), 100–118.

40 Reed (ed.), *A Text-Book of Gynecology*, 700–1.

41 *CJMS* 15, 2 (February 1904): 92.
42 Angus McLaren, *A History of Contraception from Antiquity to the Present Day* (Oxford: Basil Blackwell, 1990), 49. See also Edgar, *The Practice of Obstetrics*, 26–7; Hirst, *A Text-Book of Obstetrics*, 86. Others denied its necessity. See J. Bland-Sutton and Arthur E. Giles, *The Diseases of Women: A Handbook for Students and Practitioners* (London and New York: Rebman, 1906), 69. Thomas Laqueur argues the end of the association in "In Parenthesis: Immaculate Conceptions and Feminine Desire," in Mary Jacobus, Evelyn Fox Keller, and Sally Shuttleworth (eds.), *Body/Politics: Women and the Discourses of Science* (New York and London: Routledge, 1990), 11.
43 Norris, *Gonorrhea in Women*, 388; W. Blair Bell, "Disorders of Function," in Eden and Lockyer (eds.), *The New System of Gynaecology*, vol. 1, 385.
44 Chapman, *A Manual of Medical Jurisprudence and Toxicology*, 149; Charles Jewett (ed.), American Authors, *The Practice of Obstetrics* 2nd ed. (New York: Lea Brothers, 1901), 24. See also Lisa Jean Moore and Adele E. Clarke, "Genital Conventions and Transgressions: Graphic Representations in Anatomy Text, c 1900–1991," *Feminist Studies* 22, 1 (1996): 255–301.
45 Hirst, *A Text-Book of Obstetrics*, 85.
46 Bell, "Disorders of Function," in Eden and Lockyer (eds.), *The New System of Gynaecology*, vol. 1, 402. See also *CPMR* 42, 8 (August 1918): 241.
47 *CH* 37, 6 (June 1930): 256; Ryberg, *Health, Sex and Birth Control*, 122; Adair (ed.), *Obstetrics and Gynecology*, vol. 1, 524, 539; Emil Novak, *Textbook of Gynecology* 2nd ed. (Baltimore: The Williams & Wilkins Co., 1944), 508.
48 *CMAJ* 32, 5 (May 1935): 511.
49 On the clitoris see William P. Graves, *Gynecology* (Philadelphia and London: W.B. Saunders, 1929), 159; Davis (ed.), *Gynecology and Obstetrics*, vol. 3, Chapter 8, 17; Ryberg, *Health, Sex and Birth Control*, 24, 25; Hirsch, *Sex Power in Marriage with Case Histories*, 48–9. For the importance of the vagina see *Popular Sex Science* 2 (August 1940), 18; Adair (ed.), *Obstetrics and Gynecology*, vol. 1, 539. Patricia Jasen has argued that by the 1940s the view of the vagina as being the "adult" sexual organ was widely accepted by psychoanalysts. See Patricia Jasen, "Malignant Histories: Psychosomatic Medicine and the Female Cancer Patient in Postwar America," *Canadian Bulletin of Medical History* 20, 2 (2003): 273.
50 See chapter in this volume on menopause.
51 Francis H.A. Marshall, *The Physiology of Reproduction* (London: Longmans, Green and Co., 1922), 64; Harry Sturgeon Crossen and Robert James Crossen, *Diseases of Women* 7th ed. (St. Louis: The C.V. Mosby Co., 1930), 869; Davis (ed.), *Gynecology and Obstetrics*, vol. 3, Chapter 8, 17; Adair (ed.), *Obstetrics and Gynecology*, *vol. 1*, 524; Arthur Hale Curtis and John

William Huffman, *A Textbook of Gynecology* (Philadelphia and London: W.B. Saunders, [1950] 1951), 563.

52 Eden and Lockyer (eds.), *The New System of Gynaecology*, vol. 1, 299, 396; see also Garrigues, *Gynecology, Medical and Surgical*, 378.

53 Bland-Sutton and Giles, *The Diseases of Women*, 69.

54 For mention of frigidity see *CMAJ* 36, 2 (February 1937): 155; *UTMJ* 21, 1 (October 1943): 24; Hirsch, *Sex Power in Marriage with Case Histories*, 59. For different treatments see *NSMB* 10, 7 (July 1931): 437; Ten Teachers, *Diseases of Women* (London: Edward Arnold, 1935), 122; Curtis and Huffman, *A Textbook of Gynecology*, 97.

55 For focus on the husband see Adair (ed.), *Obstetrics and Gynecology*, vol. 1, 547; Ryberg, *Health, Sex and Birth Control*, 140; Novak, *Textbook of Gynecology*, 509; Curtis and Huffman, *A Textbook of Gynecology*, 97. For focus on education see Hirsch, *Sex Power in Marriage with Case Histories*, 71.

56 *NHPW* 28, 5 (May 1922): 249–50; *CMAJ* 25, 2 (August 1931): 142; *CMAJ* 36, 2 (February 1937): 155; Adair (ed.), *Obstetrics and Gynecology*, vol. 1, 543; *Maclean's* 59 (15 November 1946): 8.

57 Kitchener-Waterloo Hospital records, patient number 97, Mrs Emily Lauts, admitted 10 January 1943; for Mrs H. see *CMAJ* 25, 2 (August 1931): 199.

58 *CL* 35, 2 (October 1901): 98.

59 R.W. Garrett, *Textbook of Medical and Surgical Gynaecology* (Kingston, 1897), 129.

60 Angus McLaren, *Our Own Master Race: Eugenics in Canada, 1885–1945* (Toronto: McClelland and Stewart, 1990), 73; *PHJ* 4, 3 (March 1913): 126; *PHJ* (March 1918): 99.

61 *PHJ* 9, 8 (August 1918): 355.

62 *HW* 17, 1 (January 1920): 15; *CJMH* 3 (1921–22): 11–12; *PHJ* 14, 1 (January 1923): 6; Andrée Lévesque, "Mères ou malades: Les Québecoises de l'entre-deux-guerres vues par les médecins," *Revue d'histoire de l'Amérique française* 38, 1 (1984): 35.

63 Heagarty quoted in Joan Sangster, *Regulating Girls and Women: Sexuality, Family, and the Law in Ontario, 1920–1960* (Don Mills: Oxford University Press, 2001), 90; Victoria General Hospital, Halifax, Archives, patient records, register no., 1448, surgical department, patient no. 24, Amanda Peate, admitted 7 August 1921, discharged 7 October 1921. For Clarke quote see *CJMH* 3 (1921–2): 12–13.

64 Quotes by Dr K.J. Blackman, director of Disease Control for Manitoba in Cynthia Comacchio, "'The Rising Generation': Laying Claim to the Health of Adolescents in English Canada, 1920–1970," *Canadian Bulletin for the History of Medicine* 19, 1 (2002): 157.

65 *CW* 17, 5 (October 1941): 28–9.

66 *CMAJ* 51, 5 (November 1944): 399.

67 Ryberg, *Health, Sex and Birth Control*, xv; *Health* 16 (January–February 1948): 28. For a more in-depth look at prostitution see Danielle Lacasse, *La prostitution feminine à Montreal, 1945–1970* (Montreal: Boreal Press, 1994).

68 Chapman, *A Manual of Medical Jurisprudence and Toxicology*, 98, 103; Edgar, *The Practice of Obstetrics*, 35; Reese, *Text-Book of Medical Jurisprudence and Toxicology*, 282; *Woman's Century* (October 1917): 9.

69 Graves, *Gynecology*, 159; Ryberg, *Health, Sex and Birth Control*, 61–2; *CFW* 11, 5 (January 1936): 19.

70 For rape dreams see *OJNP* 1, 4 (March 1924): 14; Brend, *A Handbook of Medical Jurisprudence and Toxicology*, 99.

71 Memorial University of Newfoundland, Folklore and Language Archive, 75-21 Mary Harriet Doyle, "Midwifery in the Community of Calvert on the Southern Shore of Newfoundland," 4–5; Johnston, *Before the Age of Miracles*, 156.

72 For illegitimacy see Lori Chambers, *Misconceptions: Unmarried Motherhood and the Ontario Children of Unmarried Parents Act, 1921–1969* (Toronto: University of Toronto Press, 2007); for natives see Anderson, *A Recognition of Being*, 86–7.

73 Clark, *Mental Diseases*, 154–5; Garrigues, *Gynecology, Medical and Surgical*, 12; *CL* 43, 12 (August 1910): 912; R.H. Cole, *Mental Diseases – A Textbook of Psychiatry for Medical Students and Practitioners* (London: University of London Press, 1913), 96; Eden and Lockyer (eds.), *The New System of Gynaecology*, vol. 1, 300–1. For a study of the history of masturbation see Thomas Laqueur, *Solitary Sex: A Cultural History of Masturbation* (New York: Zone Books, 2003), 66–73, 222.

74 *CL* 44, 2 (October 1910): 128.

75 Clark, *Mental Diseases*, 154–5.

76 H. MacNaughton-Jones, *Practical Points in Gynaecology* (London: Wood, 1901), 88–9.

77 Eden and Lockyer (eds.), *The New System of Gynaecology*, vol. 1, 300–1.

78 Jennette Winter Hall, *Life's Story – A Book for Girls* (Wisconsin: B.S. Steadwell, 1911), 44–5; Eden and Lockyer (eds.), *The New System of Gynaecology*, vol. 1, 300.

79 Garrigues, *Gynecology, Medical and Surgical*, 12.

80 For tremors see Maurice Craig, *Psychological Medicine – A Manual on Mental Disease for Practitioners and Students* (London: J. & A. Churchill, 1917), 34. For the appearance of the clitoris see Reed (ed.), *A Text-Book of Gynecology*, 160–1.

81 *CL* 34, 4 (December 1900): 175; *MMN* 14, 12 (December 1902): 442; *CL* 43, 12 (August 1910): 912; Cole, *Mental Diseases*, 96; Craig, *Psychological Medicine*, 34. For quote on indulgence see Hall, *Sexual Knowledge*, 125, 108.

82 Houston, *The Art of Treatment*, 472. See also Rosenau, *Preventative Medicine and Hygiene*, 86; *CMAJ* 22, 2 (February 1930): 185; *CMAJ* 30, 3 (March 1934): 288.

83 Rosenau, *Preventive Medicine and Hygiene*, 83; Graves, *Gynecology*, 159.

84 Davis (ed.), *Gynecology and Obstetrics*, vol. 3, Chapter 8, 13–14.

85 Graves, *Gynecology*, 123, 125, 157, 159, 162; John Glaister, *Medical Jurisprudence and Toxicology* 7th ed. (Edinburgh: E. & A. Livinstone, 1942), 354.

86 *PHJ* 17, 11 (November 1926): 530; Graves, *Gynecology*, 160; *CMAJ* 28, 6 (June 1933): 626; Davis (ed.), *Gynecology and Obstetrics*, vol. 3, Chapter 8, 13.

87 Rosenau, *Preventive Medicine and Hygiene*, 83; Adair (ed.), *Obstetrics and Gynecology*, vol. 1, 543; Hirsch, *Sex Power in Marriage with Case Histories*, 95.

88 Rosenau, *Preventive Medicine and Hygiene*, 83; see also Stoddart, *Mind and Its Disorders*, 187; Howard A. Kelly et al., *Gynecology* (New York: D. Appleton, 1928), 1002; *CMAJ* 30, 3 (March 1934): 287; *CMAJ* 36, 2 (February 1937): 155; Hirsch, *Sex Power in Marriage with Case Histories*, 64–5.

89 *CMAJ* 30, 3 (March 1934): 288.

90 Jeffrey Weeks, "Movements of Affirmation: Sexual Meanings and Homosexual Identities," in Peiss and Simmons (eds.), *Passion and Power*, 73; George Chauncey, Jr., "From Sexual Inversion to Homosexuality: The Changing Medical Conceptions of Female 'Deviance,'" in Peiss and Simmons (eds.), *Passion and Power*, 87–8; Lillian Faderman, *Odd Girls and Twilight Lovers: A History of Lesbian Life in Twentieth-Century America* (New York: Columbia University Press, 1991). For an overview of lesbianism in Canada see Cameron Duder, *Awfully Devoted Women: Lesbian Lives in Canada, 1900–1965* (Vancouver: UBC, 2010).

91 Rosenau, *Preventive Medicine and Hygiene*, 81; James Winfred Bridges, *Psychology Normal and Abnormal with Special Reference to the Needs of Medical Students and Practitioners* (New York and London: D. Appleton, 1930), 168.

92 For Mitchell see *CMAJ* 22, 2 (February 1930): 184. Ryberg, *Health, Sex and Birth Control*, 78–9. Ryberg's view goes against the intolerance of such friendships as described by Patricia E. Stevenson and Joanne Hall in "A Critical Historical Analysis of the Medical Construction of Lesbianism," *International Journal of Health Services* 21, 2 (1991): 294.

93 *Canadian Forum* 9 (April 1929): 243–4; *CFW* 11, 5 (January 1936): 19; Houston, *The Art of Treatment*, 478; *CMAJ* 36, 2 (February 1937): 155; Purves-Stewart, *The Diagnosis of Nervous Diseases*, 602; Adair (ed.),

Obstetrics and Gynecology, vol. 1, 547–8; Glaister, *Medical Jurisprudence and Toxicology,* 387; Ryberg, *Health, Sex and Birth Control,* 74–5; *ManMR* 30, 5 (May 1950): 289; *CJP* 4, 2 (1950): 63–74.

94 Interviews with Becki Crawford, 9 July 1993; Eunice Jordan, 14 July 1993; Drs Mackay and Hespler, Halifax, 29 October 1993; Isme Southern, 24 August 1993.

95 Interviews with Betsy Lawrence, 30 July 1993; Dorothy Atkinson, 15 June 1993; Betty Mackenzie, 19 August 1993; Wilma Hallman, 11 August 1993; Geraldine Mitchell, 6 August 1993.

96 *PHJ* 14, 11 (November 1923): 516.

97 See Joan Sangster, "Domesticating Girls: The Sexual Regulation of Aboriginal and Working-Class Girls in Twentieth-Century Canada," in Katie Pickles and Myra Rutherdale (eds.), *Contact Zones: Aboriginal and Settler Women in Canada's Colonial Past* (Vancouver: UBC Press, 2005), 179–201; Tamara Adilman, "A Preliminary Sketch of Chinese Women and Work in British Columbia, 1858–1950," in Gillian Creese and Veronica Strong-Boag (eds.), *British Columbia Reconsidered* (Vancouver: Press Gang Publishers, 1992), 309–39; Robin Jarvis Bownlee, "Intimate Surveillance: Indian Affairs, Colonization and the Regulation of Aboriginal Woman's Sexuality," in Pickles and Rutherdale (eds.), *Contact Zones,* 160–178; Jean Barman, "Taming Aboriginal Sexuality: Gender, Power, and Race in British Columbia, 1850–1900," *BC Studies: The British Columbian Quarterly* (Fall–Winter, 1997–98): 237–66. Even having a relationship with a man from a distrusted group placed a woman at risk from society. See the autobiography of Velma Demerson, *Incorrigible* (Waterloo: Wilfrid Laurier Press, 2004) who was incarcerated because of her relationship with a Chinese man.

Chapter 5

1 OMA quoted in John Ferguson, compiler, *History of the Ontario Medical Association* (Toronto: Murray Publishing Company, 1930), 41.

2 Quoted in Meryn Elizabeth Stuart, "'Let Not the People Perish for Lack of Knowledge': Public Health Nursing and the Ontario Rural Child Welfare Project, 1916–1930," PhD diss., University of Pennsylvania, 1987, 14.

3 See Karen Lystra, *Searching the Heart: Women, Men, and Romantic Love in Nineteenth-Century America* (New York: Oxford University Press, 1989), 20, 117; John D'Emilio and Estelle B. Freedman, *Intimate Matters: A History of Sexuality in America* (New York: Harper & Row, 1988), 274; Christina Simmons, *Making Marriage Modern: Women's Sexuality from the Progressive Era to World War II* (New York: Oxford University Press, 2009); Kristin

Celello, *Making Marriage Work: A History of Marriage and Divorce in the Twentieth-Century United States* (Chapel Hill: The University of North Carolina Press, 2009).

4 For influence of the Western marriage see Adele Perry, "Metropolitan Knowledge, Colonial Practice, and Indigenous Womanhood: Missions in Nineteenth-Century British Columbia," in Katie Pickles and Myra Rutherdale (eds.), *Contact Zones: Aboriginal and Settler Women in Canada's Colonial Past* (Vancouver and Toronto: UBC Press, 2005), 109–130; Myra Rutherdale, *Women and the White Man's God: Gender and Race in the Mission Field* (Vancouver: UBC Press, 2002), 108, 112.

5 Sir Comyns Berkeley and Victor Bonney, *A Textbook of Gynaecological Surgery* (New York: Cassell, 1942), 392–3. For the purpose of marriage see *DMM* 23, 5 (November 1904): 324; Henry Jellett, *A Manual of Midwifery for Students and Practitioners* (London: Bailliere, Tindall and Cox, 1910), 597; *CPMR* 41, 2 (February 1916): 90; *PHJ* 16, 11 (November 1925): 524–5; *UTMJ* 11, 4 (February 1934): 116; Fred Adair (ed.), *Obstetrics and Gynecology*, vol. 1 (Philadelphia: Lea & Febiger, 1940), 538.

6 For age of marriage see James Snell, *In the Shadow of the Law: Divorce in Canada 1900–1939* (Toronto: University of Toronto Press, 1991), 133.

7 For Smith see *DMM* 23, 5 (November 1904): 323–4. For materialistic reasons see *PHJ* 1, 8 (August 1910): 413.

8 For physiological reasons see *CJMS* 37, 5 (May 1915): 138–40; for concern about early marriages see Henry J. Garrigues, *Gynecology, Medical and Surgical: Outlines for Students and Practitioners* (Philadelphia: J.B. Lippincott, 1905), 2; David Berry Hart, *Guide to Midwifery* (London: Rebman Ltd., 1912), 52; Charles Harrington, *Manual of Practical Hygiene for Students, Physicians, and Health Officers* 5th ed. (Philadelphia and New York: Lea and Febiger, 1914), 892.

9 *CPMR* 41, 2 (February 1916): 90.

10 W. Blair Bell, "Disorders of Function," in Thomas Watts Eden and Cuthbert Lockyer (eds.), *The New System of Gynaecology*, vol. 1 (Toronto: Macmillan, 1917), 336.

11 For marriage as a cure see *CPMR* 26, 5 (May 1901): 251; J. Bland-Sutton and Arthur E. Giles, *The Diseases of Women: A Handbook for Students and Practitioners* (London: Rebman, 1906), 397; E.C. Dudley, *The Principles and Practice of Gynecology for Students and Practitioners* 5th ed. (Philadelphia: Lea & Febiger, 1908), 748; W. Blair Bell, "Disorders of Function," in Eden and Lockyer (eds.), *The New System of Gynaecology*, vol. 1, 300–1, 336. As a preventative against insanity see "Report of the Superintendent 1904–5," The Provincial Hospital, St John, N.B., *Journals of the House of Assembly*

of N.B., 1906, 13. For curing gleet see *MMJ* 29, 4 (April 1900): 263; Henry H. Morton, *Genito-Urinary Diseases and Syphilis* (Philadelphia: F.A. Davis, 1906), 115; W. Blair Bell, *The Principles of Gynaecology* (London: Longmans, Green and Co., 1910), 244.

12 Interview with Becki Crawford, 9 July 1993; Harry Sturgeon Crossen and Robert James Crossen, *Diseases of Women* 7th ed. (St. Louis: The C.V. Mosby Co., 1930), 837, 859; *CMAJ* 42, 4 (February 1940): 149; *UTMJ* 23, 3 (December 1945): 110; *CMAJ* 56, 3 (March 1947): 345.

13 Vilhjalmus Stefansson, "The Sefansson-Anderson Arctic Expedition of the American Museum: Preliminary Ethnological Report," *Anthropological Papers of the American Museum of Natural History XIV, Part I* (New York: AMS Press, 1914), 184, 319, 379–80.

14 See Asen Balickci, *The Netsilik Eskimo* (Garden City, NY: The Natural History Press, 1970, published for the American Museum of Natural History), 55; for gendered roles see also Kaj Birket-Smith, *The Caribou Eskimos: Maternal and Social Life and Their Cultural Position I Descriptive Part Report of the Fifth Thule Expedition 1921–1924 Volume 5* (Copenhagen, Gyldeddalske Boghandel, Nordisk, Forlag, 1929); Richard C. Condon, *Inuit Behavior and Seasonal Change in the Canadian Arctic* (Ann Arbor, MI: UMI Research Press [1981] 1983), 83.

15 For working class see Joan Sangster, "Incarcerating 'Bad Girls': The Regulation of Sexuality through the Female Refuges Act in Ontario, 1920–1945," *Journal of the History of Sexuality* 7, 2 (1996): 255.

16 For the OMA see Ferguson (compiler), *History of the Ontario Medical Association,* 43.

17 Barton Cooke Hirst, *A Text-Book of Obstetrics* (Philadelphia and London: W.B. Saunders, 1912), 697.

18 Milton J. Rosenau, *Preventive Medicine and Hygiene* (New York: D. Appleton, 1927), 53; *DMJ* 2, 2 (April 1937): 45; Heagerty quoted in Joan Sangster, *Regulating Girls and Women: Sexuality, Family, and the Law in Ontario, 1920–1960* (Don Mills: Oxford University Press, 2001), 90.

19 James Winfred Bridges, *Psychology Normal and Abnormal with Special Reference to the Needs of Medical Students and Practitioners* (New York and London: D. Appleton and Co., 1930), 351; Samuel S. Peikoff, *Yesterday's Doctor: An Autobiography* (Winnipeg: Prairie Publishing Company, 1980), 33.

20 Angus McLaren, *Our Own Master Race: Eugenics in Canada, 1885–1945* (Toronto: McClelland & Stewart, 1990).

21 For Kendall see McGill University Archives, Royal Victoria Hospital Papers, RG 95, vol. 112, gynaecology case charts, patient number 19276,

Mrs Ginette Kendall, admitted 25 August 1921. For the Sidney story see Julie Cruickshank, *Life Lived Like a Story: Life Stories of Three Yukon Elders* (Vancouver: University of British Columbia, 1992), 35; for consent form see McGill University Archives, Montreal General Hospital, RG 96, vol. 200, patient cases 45–95 1950. Patient no. 69, Mrs G., admitted 3 January 1950, discharged 12 January 1950.

22 *CL* 43, 9 (May 1910): 658; see also Hart, *Guide to Midwifery*, 343.

23 *PHJ* 15, 5 (May 1924): 201–2; Andrée Lévesque, "Mères ou malades," *Revue d'histoire de l'Amérique française* 38 (1984–5): 37. For concern on the part of the British Medical Association see Angus McLaren, "Privileged Communication: Medical Confidentiality in Late Victorian Britain," *Medical History* 37 (1993): 129. In his article, McLaren refers to the 1920 meeting of the association in which there was a debate on keeping silent.

24 See Christabelle Sethna, "The New Heaven Needs a She-Devil: The Ideal Canadian Wife in Alfred Henry Tyrer's *Sex, Marriage and Birth Control (1936)*," paper given at the Ottawa Conference on the History of Marriage and Sexuality, 1991, 19.

25 Charles A.L. Reed (ed.), *A Text-Book of Gynecology* (New York: D. Appleton, 1901), 9.

26 J. Clifton Edgar, *The Practice of Obstretrics ... for the Use of Students and Practitioners* 3rd ed. (Philadelphia: P. Blakiston's Son & Co, 1907), 26–7; see also Hirst, *A Text-Book of Obstetrics*, 86.

27 Wendy Mitchinson, *Giving Birth in Canada, 1900–1950* (Toronto: University of Toronto Press, 2002), 139.

28 Franz Boas, "The Eskimo of Baffin Island and Hudson Bay," *Bulletin of the American Museum of Natural History* History XV (1901): 160.

29 Paula S. Fass, *The Damned and the Beautiful: American Youth in the 1920s* (New York: Oxford University Press, 1977), 278; Mike Featherstone and Mike Hepworth, "The History of the Male Menopause 1848–1936," *Maturitas* 7 (1985): 255; D'Emilio and Freedman, *Intimate Matters*, 266.

30 William Victor Johnston, *Before the Age of Miracles: Memoirs of a Country Doctor* (Toronto: Fitzhenry and Whiteside, 1972), 144; for linkage between sexual and marital incompatibility see Milton J. Rosenau, *Preventative Medcine and Hygiene* (New York: D. Appleton and Company, 1927), 449.

31 Hirst, *A Text-Book of Obstetrics*, 86; Carl Henry Davis (ed.), *Gynecology and Obstetrics*, vol. 3 (Hagerstown, MD: W.F. Prior, 1935), Chapter 8, 17; William R. Houston, *The Art of Treatment* (New York: Macmillan, 1936), 470; Percy Ryberg, *Health, Sex and Birth Control* (Toronto: The Anchor Press, 1942), 25, 136.

32 *CN* 16, 6 (June 1920): 334–5; *NSMB* 12, 4 (April 1933): 243; Ryberg, *Health, Sex and Birth Control,* 127, 121.

33 For women needing time see William P. Graves, *Gynecology* (Philadelphia and London: W.B. Saunders, 1929), 159; Crossen and Crossen, *Diseases of Women,* 869; *NSMB* 12, 4 (April 1933): 243; Ryberg, *Health, Sex and Birth Control,* 115.

34 Interviews with Irma Avery, 15 June 1993; Becki Crawford, 9 August 1993; Betty Mackenzie, 19 August 1993; Jane Rutherford, 28 July 1993; Dorothy Atkinson, 15 June 1993.

35 Adair (ed.), *Obstetrics and Gynecology,* vol. 1, 545.

36 Ryberg, *Health, Sex and Birth Control,* 25.

37 Ryberg, *Health, Sex and Birth Control,* 116–17; Edwin H. Hirsch, *Sex Power in Marriage with Case Histories: A Realistic Analysis Concerning the Sexual and Emotional Problems of Marriage* (Toronto: McClelland and Stewart, 1948), 216; Arthur Hale Curtis and John William Huffman, *A Textbook of Gynecology* (Philadelphia and London: W.B. Saunders [1950] 1951), 129.

38 Ryberg, *Health, Sex and Birth Control,* 44.

39 Interview with Dorothy Atkinson, 15 June 1993.

40 Beth Light and Ruth Roach Pierson (eds.), *No Easy Road: Women in Canada 1920s to 1960s* (Toronto: New Hogtown Press, 1990), 18; Sethna, "The New Heaven Needs a She-Devil," 5, 16.

41 J.G. Snell and C.C. Abeele, "Regulating Nuptiality: Restricting Access to Marriage in Early Twentieth-Century English-Speaking Canada," *Canadian Historical Review* 69, 4 (December 1988), 469–70; *MMJ* 29, 4 (April 1900): 264.

42 For Smith see *CL* 40, 11 (July 1907): 978; *CJMS* 37, 5 (May 1915): 140; for Siegel see McLaren, *Our Own Master Race,* 75–6.

43 *CL* 32, 6 (February 1900): 304; *DMM* 23, 5 (November 1904): 321; *CL* 40, 7 (March 1907): 635; Hart, *Guide to Midwifery,* 341; Arthur Shillitoe, "Syphilis in Women," in Eden and Lockyer (eds.), *The New System of Gynaecology,* vol. 1, 685. The promiscuous women were seen as coming from the various groups noted in the previous chapter – the working class, natives, and non-European immigrant groups. For example, see Mary-Ellen Kelm, *Colonizing Bodies: Aboriginal Health and Healing in British Columbia, 1900–50* (Vancouver: UBC Press, 1998).

44 For advice to infected men about marriage see Morton, *Genito-Urinary Diseases and Syphilis,* 115; Dudley, *The Principles and Practice of Gynecology,* 168. For Toronto General Hospital Report see Charles K. Clarke, "The Social Diseases" (Toronto: The National Committee for the Suppression of the White Slave Traffic, 1917), 9.

45 For Cassidy see *CJMS* 36, 1 (July 1914): 10. For certificates see *CJMS* 11, 1 (January 1902): 9; *CL* 39, 1 (September 1905): 74; *CN* 13, 4 (April 1917): 183.

46 Charles C. Norris, *Gonorrhea in Women: Its Pathology, Symptomology, Diagnosis, and Treatment* (Philadelphia and London: W.B. Saunders Company, 1913), 165, 171–2.

47 See *PHJ* 15, 5 (May 1924): 199; Crossen and Crossen, *Diseases of Women*, 252; *NSMB* 16, 10 (October 1937): 568; *CMAJ* 38, 5 (May 1938): 448; Alfred C. Beck, *Obstetrical Practice* 4th ed. (Baltimore: The Williams & Wilkins Co., 1947), 602.

48 Snell and Abeele, "Regulating Nuptiality," 475, 484.

49 For support of certificates see *PHJ* 15, 5 (May 1924): 201; Thomas Watts Eden and Cuthbert Lockyer, *Gynaecology for Students and Practitioners* (London: J. & A. Churchill, 1928), 288; *CMAJ* 23, 1 (July 1930), 48; *CMAJ* 32, 5 (May 1935): 515; *ManMR* 17, 7 (July 1937): 132; *CMAJ* 55, 1 (July 1946): 70; *CJPH* 38, 5 (May 1947): 233–4; *CJPH* 405 (May 1949): 201; *Health* 16 (January–February 1948): 12. For Ross see *PHJ* 15, 5 (May 1924): 200–2. For jurisdictions see *CMAJ* 55, 1 (July 1946): 70.

50 *CJPH* 40, 5 (May 1949): 201, 203.

51 For transmission of characteristics see *CN* 13, 4 (April 1917): 181. For numbers see McLaren, *Our Own Master Race*, 182, no. 102.

52 *CL* 41, 2 (October 1907): 102; see also *CL* 41, 9 (May 1908): 710.

53 *PHJ* 4, 3 (March 1913): 125.

54 *CN* 13, 4 (April 1917): 181.

55 *CMAJ* 33, 2 (August 1935): 192; *Maclean's* 59 (15 February 1946): 39; McLaren, *Our Own Master Race* and Harvey Simmons, *From Asylum to Welfare: The Evolution of Mental Retardation Policy in Ontario from 1831 to 1980* (Toronto: National Institute on Mental Retardation, 1982). For an examination of feeblemindedness in the United States see Allison C. Carey, "Beyond the Medical Model: A Reconsideration of 'Feeblemindedness,' Citizenship and Eugenic Restriction," *Disability and Society* 18 (2003): 411–30 and Mark A. Largent, *Breeding Contempt: the History of Coerced Sterilization in the United States* (New Brunswick, NJ: Rutgers University Press, 2008).

56 For Clarke see *CJMH* 3 (1921–2): 17. For Benvie see *NSMB* 11, 1 (January 1932): 72.

57 Alfred Lewis Galabin and George Blacker, *The Practice of Midwifery* (London: J. & A. Churchill, 1910), 1077.

58 For various prohibitive conditions see *CJMS* 11, 1 (January 1902): 9; Jellett, *A Manual of Midwifery*, 597; *CJMS* 35, 4 (April 1914): 22; *JPMS* 16, 3 (March 1914): 114; *CN* 13, 4 (April 1917): 181–3. The wider society also

disapproved of racially mixed marriages. That concern did not appear in the mainstream medical literature, but as Angus McLaren has noted, many physicians were supportive of eugenics. See McLaren, *Our Own Master Race*.

59 *CLP* 71, 4 (October 1928): 123; Davis (ed.), *Gynecology and Obstetrics*, vol. 3, Chapter 8, 16.

60 *NSMB* 16, 5 (May 1938): 374.

61 Dianne Dodd, "Advice to Parents: The Blue Books, Helen MacMurchy, MD and the Federal Department of Health, 1920–1934," *Canadian Bulletin of Medical History* 8, 2 (1991): 203–30; Denyse Baillargeon, *Babies for the Nation: The Medicalization of Motherhood in Quebec, 1910–1970*, trans. W. Donald Wilson, (Waterloo: Wilfrid University Press, 2009); Cynthia R. Comacchio, *"Nations Are Built of Babies": Saving Ontario's Mothers and Children 1900–1941* (Montreal and Kingston: McGill-Queen's University Press, 1993). For the application of such an ideal to native women see Myra Rutherdale, *Women and the White Man's God: Gender and Race in the Mission Field* (Vancouver: UBC Press, 2002), 98–112; Kelm, *Colonizing Bodies*, 61–2. Midge Ayukawa describes a different reality for Japanese families in Canada when children were often sent back to Japan for the grandparents to raise. This was not cultural but reflected the disadvantaged position of the Japanese in Canada. See "Pioneer Japanese Women: Fighting Racism and Rearing the Next Generation," in Marlene Epp, Franca Iacovetta, and Frances Swripa (eds.), *Sisters or Strangers? Immigrant, Ethnic and Racialized Women in Canadian History* (Toronto: University of Toronto Press, 2004), 233–47.

62 Rima D. Apple, "Constructing Mothers: Scientific Motherhood in the Nineteenth and Twentieth Centuries," in Rima D. Apple and Janet Golden (eds.), *Mothers and Motherhood: Readings in American History* (Columbus, OH: Ohio State University Press, 1997), 91; see also Marion Royce, *Eunice Dyke: Health Care Pioneer – From Pioneer Health Nurse to Advocate for the Ages* (Toronto: Dundurn Press, 1983), 59; Kari Dehli, "'Health Scouts' for the State? School and Public Health Nurses in Early Twentieth-Century Toronto," *Historical Studies in Education* 2, 2 (1990): 253.

63 *CC* 7, 8 (August 1926): 4; Comacchio, *"Nations Are Built of Babies,"* 93.

64 For McCullough see *Chatelaine* 7, 3 (March 1934): 51. For bathing see McGill University Archives, Montreal General Hospital RG 96, vol. 9421, file 00635, "Notes on Nursing Obstetrics," n.p.; *CMAJ* 37, supplement (1937): 66; *CN* 41, 5 (May 1945): 357. For clinics see McGill University Archives, *Annual Report of the Montreal General Hospital 1931*, 58.

65 *Annual Report, Kingston General Hospital, 1936,* 10–11. For advertisement see *ManMR* 14, 9 (September 1934): 2.

66 For poor see Dianne Dodd, "Advice to Parents: The Blue Books, Helen MacMurchy, MD and the Federal Department of Health, 1920–1934," *Canadian Bulletin of Medical History* 8, 2 (1991): 224. For turning to other women see Denyse Baillargeon, "L'encadrement de la maternité au Quebec entre les deux guerres: Les gardes de La Metropolitaine, les Gouttes de lait et L'Assistance maternelle," *Bulletin du Regroupement des chercheurs-chercheures en histoire des travailleurs et travailleuses du Québec,* 47–8 (Eté–Automne, 1990): 41. For Brinkley see *Chatelaine* 4, 12 (December 1931): 39.

67 McGill University, Osler Library, Alton Goldbloom Papers, letter from Alton Goldbloom to Mrs H.V. Banford, 13 January 1925; Alton Goldbloom Papers, unpublished manuscripts, Speech to Symposium, n.p., 2–3.

68 *UTMJ* 10, 1 (November 1932): 49; Comacchio, *"Nations Are Built of Babies,"* 118; Penelope Stewart, "Infant Feeding in Canada: 1910–1940," MA thesis, Concordia University, 1982, 134.

69 *Chatelaine* 13, 6 (June 1940): 43.

70 For historiography on infant feeding see Valerie Fildes, *Breasts, Bottles and Babies: A History of Infant Feeding* (Edinburgh: Edinburgh University Press, 1989); Janet Golden, *A Social History of Wet Nursing in America: From Breast to Bottle* (Cambridge: Cambridge University Press, 1996); Jacqueline H. Wolf, *Don't Kill Your Baby: Public Health and the Decline of Breastfeeding in the 19th and 20th Centuries* (Columbus, OH: Ohio State University Press, 2001); Stephanie Knaak, "Breast-feeding, Bottle-feeding and Dr. Spock: The Shifting Context of Choice," *Canadian Review of Sociology and Anthropology* 42, 2 (May 2005): 197–216; Stewart, "Infant Feeding in Canada"; Tasmin Nathoo and Aleck Ostry, *The One Best Way?: Breastfeeding History, Politics, and Policy in Canada* (Waterloo: Wilfrid University Press, 2009).

71 The Provincial Board of Health, Ontario, *A Little Talk about Baby* (Toronto: King's Printer, 1913), 6; MacMurchy quoted in Stewart, "Infant Feeding in Canada," 125.

72 For Brown see *CN* 14, 7 (July 1918): 1158–9 and *CPHJ* 29, 7 (July 1938): 341. For the idea of breast feeding and the primitive see Nancy Shoemaker, "The Natural History of Gender," *Gender & History* 6, 3 (November 1994): 324.

73 *CL* 40, 5 (January 1907): 402; Egbert H. Grandin and George W. Jarman, *A Textbook on Practical Obstetrics* (Philadelphia: F.A. Davis Company, 1901), 253.

74 *PHJ* 9, 4 (April 1918): 165.

75 For Hill see *CMAJ* 11, 9 (September 1921): 618. For MacMurchy and
    Montreal Health Booklet see Stewart, "Infant Feeding in Canada," 27,
    124–5. For concern about infant mortality and artificial feeding see
    Aleck William Bourne, *Synopsis of Midwifery and Gynaecology* (Toronto:
    The Macmillan Co. of Canada Ltd., 1925), 194; P. Brooke Bland, *Practical
    Obstetrics for Students and Practitioners* (Philadelphia: F.A. Saunders
    Company, 1932), 637; Ten Teachers, *Diseases of Women* (London: Edward
    Arnold & Co., 1935), 79.

76 For the quotes see Grandin and Jarman, *A Textbook on Practical Obstetrics*,
    253; American Authors, Charles Jewett (ed.), *The Practice of Obstetrics* (New
    York: Lea Brothers & Co., 1901), 273; Edgar, *The Practice of Obstetrics*, 787.
    On milk see E. Melanie Dupuis, *Nature's Perfect Food: How Milk Became
    America's Drink* (New York: New York University Press, 2002).

77 Jellett, *A Manual of Midwifery*, 469, 1153–4; for Strathy see *CJMS* 32, 3
    (September 1912): 190, 192.

78 Edgar, *The Practice of Obstetrics*, 787; Jellett, *A Manual of Midwifery*, 1151;
    Galabin and Blacker, *The Practice of Midwifery*, 406; Joseph B. DeLee, *The
    Principles and Practice of Obstetrics* (Philadelphia: W.B. Saunders Co., 1913),
    323.

79 For use of "primitive" see *DMM* 21, 3 (September 1903): 187; J. Clarence
    Webster, *A Textbook of Obstetrics* (Philadelphia: W.B. Saunders & Co., 1903),
    615.

80 As birth control see Ten Teachers, *Diseases of Women*, 79. As a drain on
    women's energy see *CMAJ* 39, 1 (July 1939): 77; as uncivilized see *CMAJ* 39,
    1 (July 1938): 77.

81 Quoted in *CPHJ* 27, 3 (March 1936): 120; see also *CMAJ* 40, 5 (May 1939):
    477–8.

82 For early nursing see Webster, *A Textbook of Obstetrics*, 274; Edgar, *The
    Practice of Obstetrics*, 787; *CPMR* 37, 4 (April 1912): 234; *CC* 4, 9 (September/
    October 1923): 2; Bland, *Practical Obstetrics*, 637; Ten Teachers, *Midwifery*,
    567–8; *CMAJ* 47, 5 (November 1942): 413.

83 Hart, *Guide to Midwifery*, 590; Thomas Watts Eden, *A Manual of Midwifery*
    (Toronto: The Macmillan Co. of Canada, 1915), 561; McGill University
    Archives, Montreal General Hospital, RG 96, vol. 0421, file 00635, "Notes
    on Nursing Obstetrics," n.d.

84 For scheduling see David James Evans, *Obstetrics: A Manual for Students
    and Practitioners* (Philadelphia: Lea Brothers & Co., 1900), 151; Grandin and
    Jarman, *A Textbook on Practical Obstetrics*, 235; Jellett, *A Manual of Midwifery*,
    469; *CPMR* 37, 4 (April 1912): 234; *CL* 48, 7 (March 1915): 425.

85 *CL* 40, 3 (November 1906): 220.

86 See Bourne, *Synopsis of Midwifery and Gynaecology,* 194; *CMAJ* 17, 7 (July 1927): 774.

87 Galabin and Blacker, *The Practice of Midwifery,* 406; American Authors, *The Practice of Obstetrics,* 273; Hart, *Guide to Midwifery,* 591; *CJMS* 32, 3 (September 1912): 190.

88 For 1916 study and Montreal study see Stewart, "Infant Feeding in Canada," 19–20; see also *CN* 13, 6 (June 1917): 311; *PHJ* 9, 7 (July 1918): 297. For 1930s and 1940s see Alfred Henry Tyrer, *Sex, Marriage and Birth Control* (Toronto: Marriage Welfare Bureau, 1943), 113.

89 On length of breast feeding see Aleck Samuel Ostry, *Nutrition Policy in Canada, 1870–1939* (Vancouver: University of British Columbia Press, 2006), 3, 51; *CN* 17, 1 (January 1921): 30; *CN* 22, 3 (March 1926): 142; *Health* 3, 2 (June 1935): 34.

90 Grandin and Jarman, *A Textbook on Practical Obstetrics,* 253; *CMAJ* 7, 3 (March 1917): 246; *CMAJ* 7, 3 (March 1917): 245; Rosemary R. Gagan, "Mortality Patterns and Public Health in Hamilton, Canada, 1900–14," *Urban History Review* 17, 3 (February 1989): 168.

91 Chandler quoted in Stewart, "Infant Feeding in Canada," 29. For civilization see Edgar, *The Practice of Obstetrics,* 787.

92 For Brown see *CN* 13, 6 (June 1917): 312–13 and *CMAJ* 7, 3 (March 1917): 246. For others see *PHJ* 9, 4 (April 1918): 165.

93 Gagan, "Mortality Patterns and Public Health in Hamilton, Canada, 1900–14," 168.

94 *PHJ* 9, 7 (July 1918): 297 and *CN* 14, 7 (July 1918): 1158–9.

95 For references to wet nurses see *Annual Report of the Montreal Maternity Hospital, 1901,* 7; see also *CJMS* 32, 3 (September 1912): 193; DeLee, *The Principles and Practice of Obstetrics,* 216; Comacchio, "Nations Are Built of Babies," 119.

96 American Authors, *The Practice of Obstetrics,* 278; see also Adam H. Wright, *A Textbook of Obstetrics* (New York: D. Appleton and Co., 1908), 162; Jellett, *A Manual of Midwifery,* 1154.

97 Stewart, "Infant Feeding in Canada," 66, 29, 90, 106.

98 See Dupuis, *Nature's Perfect Food.*

99 Interview with Betsy Mackenzie, 19 August 1993.

100 *ManMR* 14, 9 (September 1934): 2, advertisement.

101 On breast feeding and physicians' lack of training see *PHJ* 9, 4 (April 1918): 150; *CJMS* 51, 4 (April 1922): 159; *CLP* 68, 1 (January 1927): 29; and Ten Teachers, *Midwifery,* 564, 569.

102 *CMAJ* 47, 5 (November 1942): 413.

103 Interviews with Irma Avery, 15 June 1993; Jane Rutherford, 28 July 1993; Betsy Mackenzie, 19 August 1993; Becki Crawford, 9 August 1993.
104 Interview with Dr Warren, 29 October 1993, Halifax. Patient records at the Royal Victoria, Montreal Maternity Hospital, indicate the it followed the mixed feeding regimen as well, as did the Montreal General. McGill University Archives, Montreal General Hospital, RG 96, vol. 0421, file 00635, "Notes on Nursing Obstetrics."
105 For lessening of blame see Davis (ed.), *Gynecology and Obstetrics, Volume II*, Chapter 5, 15.
106 Ten Teachers, *Midwifery*, 571.
107 Condon, *Inuit Behavior and Seasonal Change in the Canadian Arctic*, 71.

Chapter 6

1 James William Kennedy and Archibald Donald Campbell, *Vaginal Hysterectomy* (Philadelphia: F.A. Davis, 1944), 133.
2 Little research has been done on the history of infertility in Canada. For American literature see Margarete Sandelowski, "Failures of Volition: Female Agency and Infertility in Historical Perspective," *Signs* 15, 3 (1990): 475–99; Margaret Marsh, "Motherhood Denied: Women and Infertility in Historical Perspective," in Rima D. Apple and Janet Golden (eds.), *Mothers & Motherhood: Reading in American History* (Columbus, OH: Ohio State University Press 1997), 216–41. The most detailed study is Margaret Marsh and Wanda Ronner, *The Empty Cradle: Infertility in America from Colonial Times to the Present* (Baltimore: Johns Hopkins University Press 1996). Two recent books illustrate the consequences of infertility, that is, making the decision to adopt a child and the lengths people go to do so. Veronica Strong-Boag, *Finding Families, Finding Ourselves: English Canada Encounters Adoption from the Nineteenth Century to the 1990s* (Toronto: Oxford University Press, 2006) and Karen Balcom, *The Traffic in Babies: Cross-Border Adoption and Baby-Selling between the United States and Canada, 1930–1972* (Toronto: University of Toronto Press, 2011).
3 *MMR* 29, 3 (1949): 125.
4 Harry Sturgeon Crossen and Robert James Crossen, *Diseases of Women* (St. Louis: The C.V. Mosby Co., 1930), 878; Fred L. Adair (ed.), *Obstetrics and Gynecology*, vol. I (Philadelphia: Lea & Febiger, 1940), 59; *MMC* 3, 6 (1948): 44; *AMB* 13, 1 (1948): 64; *MMC* 4, 10 (1949): 49. For five weeks see E.C. Dudley, *The Principles and Practice of Gynecology for Students and Practitioners* (Philadelphia: Lea & Febiger, 1908), 765.

5 Queen's University Archives, Faculty of Medicine, Examination Papers 1900–1926 and Examination Papers 1921–42; for literature see *CMAJ* 23, 1 (1930): 17. For Royal Victoria Hospital see D. Sclater Lewis, *Royal Victoria Hospital, 1887–1947* (Montreal: McGill University Press, 1969): 207; for statistics on 1936 and 1937 see McGill University Archives, *Annual Report, Royal Victoria Hospital, Montreal, 1937*, 59.

6 *CMAJ* 43, 4 (1940): 404.

7 For three years see *CPMR* 29, 3 (1904): 141; Thomas Watts Eden, *A Manual of Gynaecology* (London: J. & A. Churchill, 1911): 124. Henry J. Garrigues, *Gynecology, Medical and Surgical: Outlines for Students and Practitioners* (Philadelphia: J.B. Lippincott, 1905), 377. For 18 months see Barton Cook Hirst, *A Text-Book of Obstetrics* (Philadelphia: W.B. Saunders Co., 1912), 89.

8 McGill University Archives, Royal Victoria Hospital, Montreal, RG 95, vol. 112, gynaecology case charts, Mrs Mary Donohue, admitted 24 August 1921; J.S. Fairbairn, *Gynaecology with Obstetrics: A Text-Book for Students and Practitioners* (London: Humphrey Milford, Oxford University Press, 1924), 501.

9 For various times see Aleck Bourne, *Synopsis of Midwifery and Gynaecology* (Toronto: The Macmillan Co. of Canada Ltd., 1925), 415; Howard A. Kelly et al., *Gynecology* (New York: D. Appleton and Co., 1928), 158; William P. Graves, *Gynecology* (Philadelphia: W.B. Saunders, 1929), 655; Ten Teachers, *Diseases of Women* (London: Edward Arnold and Co., 1935), 125; *CMAJ* 37, 3 (1937): 232; *CMAJ* 42, 3 (1940): 243; *CMAJ* 49, 3 (1943): 172; *ManMR* 29, 3 (1949): 125.

10 Thomas Watts Eden and Cuthbert Lockyer (eds.), *The New System of Gynaecology*, vol. 1 (Toronto: The Macmillan Company of Canada, 1917), 404.

11 For various terms see *MMJ* 29, 3 (1900): 182; *CLt* 40, 1 (1906): 8–9; J. Bland-Sutton and Arthur Giles, *The Diseases of Women: A Handbook for Students and Practitioners* (London: Rebman, 1906), 420–1; David Tod Gilliam, *A Text-book of Practical Gynecology* (Philadelphia: F.A. Davis Co., 1907), 79; *CL* 43, 9 (1910): 658; Hirst, *A Text-Book of Obstetrics*, 91; *CMAJ* 5, 1 (1915): 13; Bourne, *Synopsis of Midwifery and Gynaecology*, 413; Kelly et al., *Gynecology*, 158; *CJMS* 78, 4 (1935): 106; *Saturday Night* 60 (10 March 1945), 12; *McMJ* 16, 1 (February 1947): 59; *ManMR* 29, 3 (1949): 122; *CMAJ* 62, 1 (1950): 51.

12 For estimates see *CL* 37, 10 (1904): 922; Dudley, *The Principles and Practice of Gynecology*, 763; *DMM* 33, 3 (1909): 90; Crossen and Crossen, *Diseases of Women*, 870; Carl Davis (ed.), *Gynecology and Obstetrics*, vol. 3 (Hagerstown, MD: W.F. Prior Co. Ltd., 1935), Chapter 9, 3; *CMAJ* 40, 2 (1939): 117;

Emil Novak, *Textbook of Gynecology* (Baltimore: The Williams & Wilkins Co., 1944), 588; *ManMR* 29, 3 (1949): 121.

13 Garrigues, *Gynecology, Medical and Surgical*, 375; Archibald Donald Campbell and Mabel A. Shannon, *Gynaecology for Nurses* (Philadelphia: F.A. Davis Co., 1946), 56; for recent figures see Royal Commission on New Reproductive Technologies, *Newsletter*, December 1993, 8.

14 *CMAJ* 40, 2 (1939): 117.

15 Eden and Lockyer (eds.), *The New System of Gynaecology*, vol. 1, 413. See also *CL* 37, 10 (1904): 922; W. Blair Bell, *The Principles of Gynaecology* (London: Longmans, Green and Co., 1910), 217; Thomas Watts Eden and Cuthbert Lockyer, *Gynaecology for Students and Practitioners* (London: J. & A. Churchill, 1928), 128; Davis (ed.), *Gynecology and Obstetrics*, vol. 3, Chapter 9, 13; Adair (ed.), *Obstetrics and Gynecology*, vol. 1, 523–4; *ManMR* 29, 3 (1949): 122.

16 Bell quoted in Eden and Lockyer (eds.), *The New System of Gynaecology*, vol. 1, 413. For Tew see *CMAJ* 40, 2 (1939): 116; for mid century see *McMJ* 18, 4 (December 1949): 233; Dalhousie University Archives, Oxorn Fonds MS-13-58, H.B. Atlee, *The Problems of Being a Woman* (manuscript n.d.), 59.

17 Garrigues, *Gynecology, Medical and Surgical*, 375; William Albert Scott and H. Brookfield Van Wyck, *The Essentials of Obstetrics and Gynecology* (Philadelphia: Lea & Febiger, 1946), 338.

18 For early years see Garrigues, *Gynecology, Medical and Surgical*, 376. For later years see *ManMR* 29, 3 (1949): 122; see also *CMAJ* 24, 5 (1931): 660 and *ManMR* 30, 5 (1950): 290.

19 For MacMurchy see Carolyn E. Strange, "The Perils and Pleasures of the City: Single, Wage-Earning Women in Toronto, 1880–1930," PhD diss., Rutgers University, 1991, 201, note 63. On gonorrhoea see *CL* 40, 1 (September 1906): 8–9; R.W. Garrett, *Textbook of Medical and Surgical Gynaecology* (Kingston, 1897), 11; *MMJ* 29, 3 (March 1900): 182; *CN* 13, 4 (April 1917): 183; *PHJ* 10, 9 (September 1919): 414. For mid century see Arthur Hale Curtis and John William Huffman, *A Textbook of Gynecology* 6th ed. (Philadelphia: W.B. Saunders Co., [1950] 1951), 562.

20 For statistics see *CL* 32, 6 (1900): 304; *CPHJ* 14, 6 (1923): 245. For syphilis and sterility see American Authors, *The Practice of Obstetrics* (New York: Lea Brothers & Co., 1901), 342; *MMJ* 32, 3 (1903): 101–2; *CL* 401 (1906): 8; *CMAJ* 11, 9 (1921): 616; *CMAJ* 12, 3 (1922): 163; *PHJ* 14, 6 (1923): 245; *CMAJ* 17, 12 (1927): 1473; *CH* 37, 6 (1930): 257; *CMAJ* 42, 5 (1940): 477.

21 For birth control use and sterility see J. Clifton Edgar, *The Practice of Obstetrics ... for Use of Students and Practitioners* (Philadelphia: P. Blakiston's Son & Co., 1907), 38–9; E.E. Montgomery, *Practical Gynecology*

(Philadelphia: Blakiston, 1912), 23; Eden and Lockyer (eds.), *The New System of Gynaecology*, vol. 2, 76–7; Campbell and Shannon, *Gynaecology for Nurses*, 59; *McMJ* 17, 3 (October 1948): 309.

22 For abortion and sterility see Henry J. Garrigues, *A Text-book of the Diseases of Women* (Philadelphia: W.B. Saunders, 1894), 128–9; Charles A.L. Reed (ed.), *A Text-Book of Gynecology* (New York: D. Appleton and Co., 1901), 10; *PHJ* 7, 3 (1916): 139; Bourne, *Synopsis of Midwifery and Gynaecology*, 414; *NSMB* 11, 4 (April 1932): 462; *CMAJ* 37, 3 (1937): 236–7. For self-induced abortion see Dafoe in *CMAJ* 22, 6 (1930): 794; see also *CMAJ* 53, 3 (1945): 298; Scott and Van Wyck, *The Essentials of Obstetrics and Gynecology*, 339. For an excellent examination of the medical discourse on abortion see Tracy Penny Light, "Shifting Interests: The Medical Discourse on Abortion in English Canada, 1850–1969," PhD diss., University of Waterloo, 2003.

23 *CPMR* 25, 1 (1900): 48; *CMAJ* 37, 3 (1937): 236–7; *Maclean's* 60 (1 April 1947), 62; Curtis and Huffman, *A Textbook of Gynecology*, 562.

24 For women and work and sterility see *PHJ* 7, 7 (1916): 349; *PHJ* 7, 4 (1916): 189; American Authors, *The Practice of Obstetrics*, 342; Davis (ed.), *Gynecology and Obstetrics*, vol. 1, Chapter 5, 7; *CMAJ* 37, 3 (1937): 235; *Saturday Night* 58 (31 October 1942), 22; Adair (ed.), *Obstetrics and Gynecology* vol. 1, 513.

25 *CPMR* 27, 11 (1902): 662; see also *CPMR* 30, 2 (1905): 92; Alice Stockham, *Tokology: A Book for Every Woman* (Toronto: McClelland, Goodchild and Stewart, 1916), 105.

26 For nutrition see Eden and Lockyer (eds.), *The New System of Gynaecology*, vol. 1, 412; see also Dudley, *The Principles and Practice of Gynecology*, 217. For vitamin E see *CMAJ* 11, 9 (1921): 616; *CLP* 74, 2 (1930): 41–2; *CJMS* 75, 2 (1934): 41; *CPHJ* 30, 1 (1939): 9; *CMAJ* 47, 1 (1942): 18; *MMC* 4, 10 (1949): 49.

27 *CLP* 74, 2 (1930): 41–2; see also *CMAJ* 55, 4 (1946): lxxv.

28 For obesity see *CL* 40, 1 (1906): 8; Dudley, *The Principles and Practice of Gynecology*, 217; *CMAJ* 5, 8 (1915): 667; *CMAJ* 14, 11 (1924): 1052; *PHJ* 18, 2 (1927): 95–6; Graves, *Gynecology*, 69; Adair (ed.), *Obstetrics and Gynecology* vol. 1, 508–12.

29 *CPMR* 27, 8 (1902): 478; *CMAJ* 40, 2 (1939): 117.

30 *CL* 37, 10 (1904): 922; *CL* 37, 10 (1904): 922; Eden and Lockyer (eds.), *The New System of Gynaecology*, vol. 1, 414; *CLNH* 63, 1 (1924): 2; J. Munro Kerr et al., *Combined Textbook of Obstetrics and Gynecology for Students and Medical Practitioners* (Edinburgh: E. & S. Livinstone, 1933), 730; *CMAJ* 40, 2 (1939): 116; Percy E. Ryberg, *Health, Sex and Birth Control* (Toronto: The Anchor Press, 1942), 174; *Canadian Home Journal* 40 (August 1943), 11; Scott and

Van Wyck, *The Essentials of Obstetrics and Gynecology*, 339; *ManMR* 29, 3 (1949): 125.

31 *ManMR* 30, 5 (1950): 290.

32 *CL* 34, 1 (1900): 20; *CMAJ* 14, 9 (1924): 797; *CMAJ* 14, 2 (1924): 139; Crossen and Crossen, *Diseases of Women*, 870–2; Adair (ed.), *Obstetrics and Gynecology* vol. 1, 514.

33 For childbirth practices see *MMJ* 31, 4 (1904): 277; *CMAJ* 1, 2 (1911): 131–2; *CMAJ* 10, 10 (1920): 901; *PHJ* 14, 6 (1923): 243; *CMAJ* 19, 2 (1928): 228; *CJMS* 66, 3 (1929): 71; *NSMB* 14, 3 (March 1935): 172. For c-sections see *CPHJ* 23, 12 (1932): 566; *CMAJ* 56, 2 (1947): 170.

34 Graves, *Gynecology*, 679; *CMAJ* 25, 5 (1931): 584; *CMAJ* 48, 6 (1943): 546.

35 For various ailments and sterility see American Authors, *The Practice of Obstetrics*, 342; Gilliam, *A Text-book of Practical Gynecology*, 81; Dudley, *The Principles and Practice of Gynecology*, 217; Garrigues, *Gynecology, Medical and Surgical*, 376; R.M. Franks, "A Genetic and Comparative Study of Depressed Female Patients in the Toronto Psychiatric Hospital," MA thesis, University of Toronto, 1929, n.p.

36 Ten Teachers, *Diseases of Women*, 122.

37 *CL* 34, 1 (1900): 21; see also *CL* 40, 1 (1906): 7; *CPMR* 33, 12 (1908): 758–9; *CL* 45, 10 (1912): 781; *CL* 48, 2 (1914): 79; Bourne, *Synopsis of Midwifery and Gynaecology*, 415; *PHJ* 18, 2 (1927): 95–6; *CMAJ* 23, 1 (1930): 20; *CMAJ* 31, 5 (1934): 526; *CJMS* 79, 1 (1936): 17; Adair (ed.), *Obstetrics and Gynecology* vol. 1, 523–4; *CMAJ* 49, 3 (1943): 168; *ManMR* 26, 1 (1946): 14; *ManMR* 39, 3 (1949): 122.

38 Kerr et al., *Combined Textbook of Obstetrics and Gynecology*, 735.

39 Garrett, *Textbook of Medical and Surgical Gynaecology*, 128; *CL* 34, 1 (1900): 20; *CL* 40, 1 (1906): 7; Dudley, *The Principles and Practice of Gynecology*, 766; Montgomery, *Practical Gynecology*, 23; *CMAJ* 5, 8 (1915): 668; *PHJ* 18,2 (1927): 95–6; Graves, *Gynecology*, 655; *CMAJ* 30, 4 (1934): 400; *CMAJ* 44, 1 (1941): 69; *CMAJ* 49, 3 (1943): 167.

40 Allbutt, Playfair, and Eden (eds.), *A System Of Gynaecology*, 114; For uterine displacements see Reed (ed.), *A Text-Book of Gynecology*, 289; *DMM* 20, 2 (1903): 82; *CPMR* 33, 12 (1908): 758; *CL* 45, 10 (1912): 781; *DMM* 48, 3 (1917): 63; *DMM* LVI, 6 (June 1921): 9; *CMAJ* 14, 9 (1924): 797; Kelly et al., *Gynecology*, 160; *CMAJ* 23, 6 (1930): 763; *CMAJ* 41, 2 (1939): 117; Adair (ed.), *Obstetrics and Gynecology* vol. 1, 508–12; *CMAJ* 48, 6 (1943): 515–16; Scott and Van Wyck, *The Essentials of Obstetrics and Gynecology*, 339. For challenges to displacements see Allbutt, Playfair, and Eden (eds.), *A System of Gynaecology*, 114; *DMM* LVI, 6 (June 1921): 5; *CMAJ* 48, 6 (June 1943): 515–16; *NSMB* 28, 10 (October 1949): 237.

41 *McMJ* 17, 3 (October 1948): 307.

42 *ManMR* 30, 5 (1950): 290. For growths and fibromyomata see *CL* 34, 1 (1900): 20; *CPMR* 33, 12 (1908): 758–9; *CL* 50, 6 (1917): 265; Kelly et al., *Gynecology*, 160; *CMAJ* 26, 6 (1932): 749; *CMAJ* 30, 4 (1934): 400; Adair (ed.), *Obstetrics and Gynecology* vol. 1, 508–12; *CMAJ* 53, 4 (1945): 366.

43 *MMC* 2, 8 (1947): 31; see also Graves, *Gynecology*, 685; *CJMS* 78, 4 (1935): 106; *CMAJ* 40, 1 (1939): 36; Novak, *Textbook of Gynecology*, 610; *CMAJ* 56, 3 (1947): 345; *ManMR* 30, 2 (1950): 74–5.

44 Quoted in *Canada Lancet* 34, 1 (1900): 20; see also Garrett, *Textbook of Medical and Surgical Gynaecology*, 128; Eden and Lockyer (eds.), *The New System of Gynaecology*, vol. 1, 405; Crossen and Crossen, *Diseases of Women*, 879; Davis (ed.), *Gynecology and Obstetrics*, vol. 3, Chapter 9, 27; *CMAJ* 40, 2 (1939): 118; Novak, *Textbook of Gynecology*, 600. Such a view existed in the nineteenth century and never really disappeared, apparently re-emerging in the 1950s in a major way. See Marsh and Ronner, *The Empty Cradle*, 197.

45 *CMAJ* 5, 8 (1915): 667; *CMAJ* 30, 4 (1934): 400; *CMAJ* 40, 2 (1939): 117. See also *CMAJ* 14, 9 (1924): 797; Crossen and Crossen, *Diseases of Women*, 894; *CMAJ* 24, 5 (1931): 660; *CMAJ* 40, 1 (1939): 41; *CMAJ* 49, 3 (1943): 167; *AMB* 13, 1 (1948): 67; *ManMR* 29, 3 (1949): 122.

46 Cheryl Krasnick Warsh, *Prescribed Norms: Women's Health in Canada and the United States since 1800* (Toronto: University of Toronto Press, 2010), 165–6. For changes see Henry C. Chapman, *A Manual of Medical Jurisprudence and Toxicology* (Philadelphia: W.B. Saunders, 1896), 142; Eden, *A Manual of Gynaecology*, 125; John J. Reese, *Text-Book of Medical Jurisprudence and Toxicology* (Philadelphia: P. Blakiston's Son & Co., 1912), 262. For a history of impotence see Angus McLaren, *Impotence: A Cultural History* (Chicago: University of Chicago Press, 2007).

47 For the 7–40 percent estimated see Dudley, *The Principles and Practice of Gynecology*, 763; for the 20–50 percent see Kelly et al., *Gynecology*, 158; for other estimates see *CL* 34, 1 (1900): 20; *CL* 33, 12 (1900): 679; *CL* 37, 10 (1904): 922; *CL* 40, 1 (1906): 7; *DMM* 33, 3 (1909): 92; J.W. Thomson Walker, *Surgical Diseases and Injuries to the Genito-Urinary Organs* (Toronto: Cassell and Co. Ltd., 1914), 798; *CMAJ* 14, 2 (1924): 139; Bourne, *Synopsis of Midwifery and Gynaecology*, 413; *CMAJ* 23, 1 (1930): 21; Kerr et al., *Combined Textbook of Obstetrics and Gynecology*, 729; *MMAR* 14, 7 (1934): 8; *CMAJ* 37, 3 (1937): 232; Adair (ed.), *Obstetrics and Gynecology* vol. 2, 673; *CMAJ* 49, 3 (1943): 167; Novak, *Textbook of Gynecology*, 589; *Saturday Night* 60 (10 March 1945), 13; *ManMR* 29, 3 (1949): 124; *CMAJ* 63, 4 (1950): 344–5.

48 *CL* 33, 12 (1900): 679; *CL* 40, 1 (1906): 7; *DMM* 35, 2 (1910): 48; *CL* 48, 2 (1914): 79; Eden and Lockyer (eds.), *The New System of Gynaecology*, vol. 1,

124–5; *CMAJ* 14, 2 (1924): 137; *CMAJ* 23, 1 (1930): 21; *CMAJ* 30, 4 (1934): 402; *CMAJ* 40, 2 (1939): 118; *CMAJ* 49, 3 (1943): 167; *Saturday Night* 60 (19 March 1945), 13; *AMB* 14, 4 (1949): 13; *NSMB* 28, 10 (October 1949): 237.

49 Quote in *CMAJ* 30, 4 (1934): 400. See also *DMM* 33, 3 (1909): 92; Campbell and Shannon, *Gynaecology for Nurses*, 57; *McMJ* 17, 3 (October 1948): 310; *ManMR* 29, 3 (1949): 125.

50 For Ross see *MMJ* 32, 2 (1903): 101; Allbutt, Playfair, and Eden (eds.), *A System of Gynaecology*, 111. For excess see also American Authors, *The Practice of Obstetrics*, 343; Edgar, *The Practice of Obstetrics*, 28; *CMAJ* 14, 2 (1924): 139; *CMAJ* 24, 5 (1931): 660; Adair (ed.), *Obstetrics and Gynecology* vol. 1, 529; Ryberg, *Health, Sex and Birth Control*, 15; Scott and Van Wyck, *The Essentials of Obstetrics and Gynecology*, 338–9; *ManMR* 29, 3 (1949): 125.

51 Curtis and Huffman, *A Textbook of Gynecology*, 562; see also Novak, *Textbook of Gynecology*, 609, 577; Scott and Van Wyck, *The Essentials of Obstetrics and Gynecology*, 338–9; *ManMR* 29, 3 (1949): 125.

52 For masturbation see Henry H. Morton, *Genito-Urinary Diseases and Syphilis* (Philadelphia: F.A. Davis Co., 1906), 467; *CMAJ* 14, 2 (1924): 138–9. For birth control see Edgar, *The Practice of Obstetrics*, 38–9; Stockham, *Tokology: A Book for Every Woman*, 325; *CMAJ* 17, 12 (1927): 1473.

53 Eden, *A Manual of Gynaecology*, 124; see also *CJMS* 15, 2 (February 1904): 92; Davis (ed.), *Gynecology and Obstetrics*, vol. 3, Chapter 9, 6; *CMAJ* 40, 2 (1939): 117; Adair (ed.), *Obstetrics and Gynecology* vol. 1, 506; Novak, *Textbook of Gynecology*, 590; *ManMR* 29, 3 (1949): 125; Curtis and Huffman, *A Textbook of Gynecology*, 563.

54 Morton, *Genito-Urinary Diseases and Syphilis*, 473; *CMAJ* 17, 12 (1927): 1473; Davis (ed.), *Gynecology and Obstetrics* vol. 3, Chapter 9, 6; *CMAJ* 37, 3 (1937): 235; Adair (ed.), *Obstetrics and Gynecology* vol. 1, 513; Henricus J. Stander, *Williams Obstetrics* (New York: Appleton-Century, 1941), 813.

55 For diet see Graves, *Gynecology*, 673; *CMAJ* 24, 5 (1931): 660; Davis (ed.), *Gynecology and Obstetrics* vol. 3, Chapter 9, 6; *CMAJ* 40, 2 (1939): 117; Novak, *Textbook of Gynecology*, 590; Curtis and Huffman, *A Textbook of Gynecology*, 563. For expressions of concern about obesity see *CL* 40, 1 (1906): 8; *PHJ* 18, 2 (1927): 95; *CMAJ* 40, 2 (1939): 117. For expressions of the value of vitamin E in diet see *CMAJ* 38, 6 (1938): 615; *CMAJ* 40, 2 (1939): 117; Adair (ed.), *Obstetrics and Gynecology* vol. 1, 57; *AMB* 14, 2 (1949): 28.

56 *CL* 40, 1 (1906): 8; Morton, *Genito-Urinary Diseases and Syphilis*, 473; *CMAJ* 17, 12 (1927): 1473; Crossen and Crossen, *Diseases of Women*, 878; *CMAJ* 24, 5 (1931): 660; *CMAJ* 40, 2 (1939): 117; Scott and Van Wyck, *The Essentials of Obstetrics and Gynecology*, 338–9; *ManMR* 29, 3 (1949): 125.

57 Chapman, *A Manual of Medical Jurisprudence and Toxicology*, 142; *CL* 33, 12
    (1900): 679; Allbutt, Playfair, and Eden (eds.), *A System of Gynaecology*, 109;
    CL 40, 1 (1906): 12; Francis H.A. Marshall, *The Physiology of Reproduction*
    (London: Longmans, Green and Co., 1922), 644–5; *McMJ* 18, 4 (December
    1949): 234; *CMAJ* 47, 1 (1942): 51; *CMAJ* 48, 3 (1943): 231–2.
58 For diseases see Morton, *Genito-Urinary Diseases and Syphilis*, 477; Dudley,
    The Principles and Practice of Gynecology, 765; Eden, *A Manual of Gynaecology*,
    125; Milton J. Rosenau, *Preventive Medicine and Hygiene* (New York: D.
    Appleton and Co., 1927), 64; *CMAJ* 37, 3 (1937): 235; *CMAJ* 47, 1 (1942):
    51; *AMB* 14, 2 (1949): 28. For developmental problems see Dudley, *The
    Principles and Practice of Gynecology*, 765; *CMAJ* 14, 2 (1924): 139; *CMAJ* 30,
    4 (1934): 400; *CMAJ* 37, 3 (1937): 234; Ryberg, *Health, Sex and Birth Control*,
    181; Novak, *Textbook of Gynecology*, 590, 609; *ManMR* 29, 3 (1949): 125.
59 Davis (ed.), *Gynecology and Obstetrics* vol. 3, Chapter 9, 1; Novak, *Textbook
    of Gynecology*, 590; *ManMR* 29, 3 (1949): 125; *DMJ* 6, 1 (November 1940):
    14–15.
60 *MMJ* 32, 2 (1903): 101; Morton, *Genito-Urinary Diseases and Syphilis*,
    477; Edgar, *The Practice of Obstetrics*, 28; Kerr et al., *Combined Textbook of
    Obstetrics and Gynecology*, 730; Ten Teachers, *Diseases of Women*, 125.
61 Walker, *Surgical Diseases*, 799; *CMAJ* 14, 2 (1924): 139; *ManMR* 29, 3 (1949):
    125.
62 Marni Elizabeth Davis, "Southern Kwakiutl Medicine," MA thesis,
    University of Victoria, 1977, 25; Lee Guemple, "Men and Women,
    Husbands and Wives: The Role of Gender in Traditional Inuit Society,"
    Etudes/Inuit/Studies 10, 1–2 (1986): 20.
63 Morton, *Genito-Urinary Diseases and Syphilis*, 470.
64 *CL* 34, 1 (1900): 23; *DMM* 20, 2 (1903): 82; *CL* 45, 3 (1911): 211; *CMAJ* 11, 11
    (1921): 831; *CMAJ* 14, 2 (1924): 139; Kelly et al., *Gynecology*, 103; Davis (ed.),
    Gynecology and Obstetrics vol. 3, Chapter 9, 28; Sir Comyns Berkeley and
    Victor Bonney, *A Textbook of Gynaecological Surgery* (London: Cassell and
    Co. Ltd., 1942), 76; Curtis and Huffman, *A Textbook of Gynecology*, 563.
65 Hirst, *A Text-Book of Obstetrics*, 90; Kelly et al., *Gynecology*, 103; Davis (ed.),
    Gynecology and Obstetrics vol. 3, Chapter 9, 28.
66 *CMAJ* 24, 5 (1931): 660; *CMAJ* 37, 3 (1937): 234; *CMAJ* 40, 6 (1939): 542;
    Adair (ed.), *Obstetrics and Gynecology* vol. 2, 673; Novak, *Textbook of
    Gynecology*, 600; Interview with Becki Crawford, 9 August 1993.
67 *McMJ* 17, 3 (October 1948): 310. Margaret Marsh claims that outside of elite
    practices not until mid century did semen analysis become routine in diag-
    nosing infertility in the United States. See Marsh, "Motherhood Denied,"
    in Apple and Golden (eds.), *Motherhood: Reading in American History*, 231.

68 McGill University Archives, *Annual Report, Royal Victoria Hospital, 1930, Montreal*, 127–31, RG 95, file 287, gynaecological reports, 1933, n.p.
69 *CMAJ* 23, 1 (1930): 20.
70 Bourne, *Synopsis of Midwifery and Gynaecology*, 415; Crossen and Crossen, *Diseases of Women*, 879; Adair (ed.), *Obstetrics and Gynecology* vol. 1, 527; Scott and Van Wyck, *The Essentials of Obstetrics and Gynecology*, 340.
71 Quoted in *MMC* 3, 6 (1948): 44. See also *AMB* 13, 1 (1948): 64; *MMC* 4, 10 (1949): 49.
72 For Cutts see *CL* 34, 1 (September 1900): 23. For Smith see *CMR* 30, 8 (August 1902): 340.
73 *DMM* 33, 3 (1909) 92; see also *DMM* 35, 2 (1910): 48.
74 For Polak see *CMAJ* 14, 9 (1924): 798; Graves, *Gynecology*, 680; Ten Teachers, *Diseases of Women*, 125.
75 *CL* 3, 2 (1870): 46–7; Dudley, *The Principles and Practice of Gynecology*, 770; see also Garrigues, *Gynecology, Medical and Surgical*, 378; J. Clarence Webster, *A Text-Book of Diseases of Women* (Philadelphia: W.B. Saunders Co., 1907), 700; Eden and Lockyer, *Gynaecology for Students and Practitioners*, 131; Crossen and Crossen, *Diseases of Women*, 880; Ten Teachers, *Diseases of Women*, 127; Davis (ed.), *Gynecology and Obstetrics*, vol. 3, Chapter 9, 27.
76 Rona Achilles, "Donor Insemination: The Future of a Public Secret," in Christine Overall (ed.), *The Future of Human Reproduction* (Toronto: The Women's Press, 1989), 116.
77 Alfred Henry Tyrer, *Sex, Marriage and Birth Control* (Toronto: Marriage Welfare Bureau, 1943), 238–9; Curtis and Huffman, *A Textbook of Gynecology*, 573.
78 *CMAJ* 23, 1 (1930): 20.
79 *CMAJ* 5, 8 (1915): 668; *CMAJ* 11, 11 (1921): 831; Thomas H. Cherry, *Surgical and Medical Gynecologic Technic* (Philadelphia: F.A. Davis Co., 1929), 635.
80 *CMAJ* 23, 1 (1930): 21; *CMAJ* 37, 3 (1937): 236; see also *CMAJ* 34, 3 (1936): 297; Novak, *Textbook of Gynecology*, 612; *CMAJ* 63, 4 (1950): 346.
81 *CMAJ* 42, 6 (1940): 583.
82 *ManMR* 29, 3 (1949): 124.
83 *DMJ* 6, 1 (November 1940): 14–15.
84 *CMAJ* 57, 4 (1947): 354. On diethylstilboestrol see *CMAJ* 42, 6 (1940): 583, 585; Novak, *Textbook of Gynecology*, 559; *AMB* 13, 1 (1948): 67; *AMB* 14, 2 (1949): 27.
85 Davis (ed.), *Gynecology and Obstetrics*, vol. 3, Chapter 9, 28.
86 *ManMR* 29, 3 (1949): 125. See also Marsh and Ronner, *The Empty Cradle*, 111.
87 *Chatelaine* 20, 6 (June 1947): 6.

88 Novak, *Textbook of Gynecology*, 589–90.
89 Barbara Ehrenreich, *Complaints and Disorders: The Sexual Politics of Sickness* (New York: Old Westbury, 1973), 5.

Chapter 7

1 Angus McLaren and Arlene Tigar McLaren, *The Bedroom and the State: The Changing Practices and Politics of Contraception and Abortion in Canada, 1880–1980* (Toronto: McClelland and Stewart, 1986), 9.
2 The historical literature is extensive. On birth control see Angus McLaren, *A History of Contraception from Antiquity to the Present Day* (Oxford: Basil Blackford, 1990); Andrea Tone, *Devices and Desires: A History of Contraceptives in America* (New York: Hill and Wang, 2001); McLaren and McLaren, *The Bedroom and the State*; Dianne Dodd, "The Canadian Birth Control Movement: 1929–1939," MA thesis, University of Toronto, 1982; Thomas Melville Bailey, *For the Public Good: A History of the Birth Control Clinic and the Planned Parenthood Society of Hamilton, Ontario, Canada* (Hamilton: The Planned Parenthood Society of Hamilton, 1974). On abortion see James Mohr, *Abortion in America: The Origins and Evolution of National Policy, 1800–1900* (New York: Oxford University Press, 1978); Kristen Luker, *Abortion and the Politics of Motherhood* (Berkeley: University of California Press, 1984); Barbara Brookes, *Abortion in England 1900–1967* (Kent: Croom Helm Ltd., 1988); Rickie Solinger (ed.), *Abortion Wars: A Half Century of Struggle, 1950–2000* (Berkeley: University of California Press, 1998); Leslie J. Reagan, *When Abortion Was a Crime: Women, Medicine, and Law in the United States, 1817–1973* (Berkeley: University of California Press, 1997); Gail Kellough, *Aborting Law: An Exploration of the Politics of Motherhood and Abortion* (Toronto: University of Toronto Press, 1996); William Beahen, "Abortion and Infanticide in Western Canada, 1874–1916: A Criminal Study," *The Canadian Catholic Historical Association, Historical Studies* 53 (1986): 53–70; McLaren and McLaren, *The Bedroom and the State*; Susanne Klaussen, "Doctors and Dying Declarations: The Role of the State in Abortion Regulation in British Columbia, 1917–33," *Canadian Bulletin of Medical History* 13, 1 (1996): 53–82; Gerald Stortz and Murray Eaton, "Pro Bono Publico: The 1936 Eastview Birth Control Trial," Atlantis 8 (1983): 51–60; Catherine Annau, "Eager Eugenicists: A Reappraisal of the Birth Control Society of Hamilton," *Histoire Sociale/Social History* 27, 53 (May 1984): 111–34; Tracy Penny Light, "Shifting Interests: The Medical Discourse on Abortion in English Canada, 1850–1969," PhD diss., University of Waterloo, 2003.

3 Foucault quoted in Adele E. Clarke, *Disciplining Reproduction: Modernity, American Life Sciences, and "the Problems of Sex"* (Berkeley: University of California Press, 1998), 205. For a feminist view see Mary A. Halas, "Sexism in Women's Medical Care," *Frontiers* 4, 2 (1979) 12; Alexandria Dundas Todd, *Intimate Adversaries: Cultural Conflict between Doctors and Their Women Patients* (Philadelphia: University of Pennsylvania Press, 1989), 31; Nikki Colodny, "The Politics of Birth Control in a Reproductive Rights Context," in Christine Overall (ed.), *The Future of Human Reproduction* (Toronto: The Women's Press, 1989) 30; Nora Kizeer Bell, "Women and AIDS: Too Little, Too Late," in Helen Bequaert Holmes and Laura M. Purdy, *Feminist Perspectives in Medical Ethics* (Bloomington and Indianapolis: Indiana University Press, 1992), 52.

4 See Victoria General Hospital, Halifax, Archives, Halifax, Martha Hesse, patient no. 3882, register 3742, surgical department, admitted 5 September 921, died 14 September 1921; Angus McLaren, "Illegal Operations: Women, Doctors, and Abortion, 1886–1939," *Journal of Social History* 26, 4 (Summer 1993): 804–9; Klaussen, "Doctors and Dying Declarations," 53–82.

5 Jacques Henripin, *Trends and Factors of Fertility in Canada* (Ottawa: Statistics Canada, 1972), 44–5; Robert Choiniere and Norbert Robitaille, "The Fertility of Inuit of Northern Quebec: A Half-Century of Fluctuations," *Acta Borealia* 4, 1–2 (1987): 53, 55.

6 For decline in morality see *Saturday Night* 14 (2 March 1901): 4; Terry Chapman, "Women, Sex and Marriage in Western Canada 1890–1920," *Alberta History* 33, 4 (Fall 1985): 6; Norah L. Lewis, "Goose Grease and Turpentine: Mother Treats the Family's Illnesses," *Prairie Forum* 15, 1 (Spring 1990): 79. For women's selfishness see *Saturday Night* 14 (1 March 1901): 4; *Hansard* (11 April 1918): 638; Angus McLaren, "Policing Pregnancies: Sexuality and the Family, 1900–1940," *Transactions of the Royal Society of Canada* Vol. III Sixth Series 1992, 18.

7 For Irwin see *Woman's Century* (March 1920) 33, 22. For Catholics see *Social Welfare* 17 (June 1938) 97; *Maclean's* 63 (15 August 1950): 7; McLaren, *A History of Contraception from Antiquity to the Present Day*, 234; Diane Gervais and Danielle Gauvreau, "Women, Priests, and Physicians: Family Limitations in Quebec, 1940–1970," *Journal of Interdisciplinary History* 34, 2 (2003): 297–8.

8 On Stopes see McLaren and McLaren, *The Bedroom and the State*, 24–8. On Sanger see Beth Light and Ruth Roach Pierson (eds.), *No Easy Road: Women in Canada, 1920s–1960s* (Toronto: New Hogtown Press, 1990), 122–4. For Sackville and Eaton's see Ellen Joyce Trott, "Attitudes towards Birth Control: Canada 1885–1935," MA thesis, Carleton University, 1984, 103–6,

109, 142, 147. Alfred Henry Tyrer, *Sex, Marriage and Birth Control* (Toronto: Marriage Welfare Bureau, 1936), 37.

9 *NHPW* 28, 5 (May 1922): 274.

10 Dodd, "The Canadian Birth Control Movement 1929–1939," 111, 138.

11 For example see Bailey, *For the Public Good*, 7.

12 For more information on the Palmer trial see McLaren and McLaren, *The Bedroom and the State*, 116–19.

13 *Saturday Night* 14 (1 March 1901): 4.

14 For opponents see *Woman's Century* (March 1920): 22; United Church Archives, Hugh Dobson Papers, B 10, file M1, Committee on the Integrity of the Family, "A Statement on Christian Marriage," c 1930; file Q, "Sterilization," United Church Commission on Sterilization and Birth Control. For Sackville see Ellen Joyce Trott, "Attitudes towards Birth Control: Canada, 1885–1935," 105–6. For class and ethnic involvement see *Vancouver Sun* (27 August 1932), 5.

15 For Quebec and methods used throughout Canada see Gérard Bouchard, "La sexualité comme pratique et rapport chez les couples paysans du Saguenay (1860–1930)," *Revue Histoire de l'Amérique française* 56, 2 (Automne 2000): 183–217; Gervais and Gauvreau, "Women, Priests and Physicians," 293–314. For the Alberta woman's story see Eliane Leslau Silverman, *The Last Best West – Women on the Alberta Frontier 1880–1939* (Montreal: Eden Press, 1984), 60, 65.

16 For breast feeding see Memorial University of Newfoundland, Folklore and Language Archive, Barbara Doran, collector, "There was no one but myself": The Life of a Midwife in Outport Newfoundland," 82-326, 3. For pessaries see Chapman, "Women, Sex and Marriage in Western Canada 1890–1920," 8. For other items found in the wild see Lewis, "Goose Grease and Turpentine," 79. For Eaton's see the Clio Collective, *Quebec Women: A History*, trans. Roger Gannon and Rosalind Gill (Toronto: The Women's Press, 1987), 138.

17 *CMR* 28, 11 (November 1900): 475; Charles A.L. Reed (ed.), *A Text-Book of Gynecology* (New York: D. Appleton and Company, 1901), 10; see also J. Bland-Sutton and Arthur E. Giles, *The Diseases of Women: A Handbook for Students and Practitioners* (London: Rebman, 1906), 114; *MMN* 21, 2 (February 1909): 72; Comyns Berkeley, "Diseases of the Vagina," in Thomas Watts Eden and Cuthbert Lockyer (eds.), *The New System of Gynaecology*, vol. 2 (Toronto: The Macmillan Company of Canada Ltd., 1917), 76–7.

18 Latex introduced in the early 1930s resulted in a decline in condom prices. Linda Gordon, *Woman's Body, Woman's Right: A Social History of Birth Control* (New York: Viking, 1976), 317. For other methods see Bouchard,

"La sexualité comme pratique et rapport chez les couples paysans du Saguenay," 208, 203, 211–12; *UTMJ* 14, 6 (April 1937): 239; Arthur Hale Curtis and John William Huffman, *A Textbook of Gynecology* (Philadelphia: W.B. Saunders, [1950] 1951), 98; interviews with Drs Mackay and Hespeler, 29 October 1993.

19 For Toronto clinic and others see Dodd, "The Canadian Birth Control Movement 1929–1939," 68, 128 and McLaren, *A History of Contraception from Antiquity to the Present Day*, 236. For sterilizations see Dodd, "The Canadian Birth Control Movement 1929–1939," 58; Mary Bishop, "A.R. Kaufman: Father of Birth Control in Canada," unpublished paper, n.d., 37. For Eaton's see Trott, "Attitudes towards Birth Control, 147, 142.

20 Bouchard, "La sexualité comme pratique et rapport chez les couples paysans du Saguenay," 208, 203. Dodd, "The Canadian Birth Control Movement 1929–1939," 127.

21 For listing of methods see Henry C. Chapman, *A Manual of Medical Jurisprudence and Toxicology* (Philadelphia: W.B. Saunders, 1896), 128; Andrée Lévesque, *La Norme et les déviantes: Des femmes au Québec pendant l'entre-deux-guerres* (Montréal: Les Éditions du remue-ménage, 1989), 102.

22 For exertion see Frederick C. Irving, *A Textbook of Obstetrics – for Students and Practitioners* (New York: The Macmillan Co., 1936), 208; McGill University Archives, Montreal General Hospital, RG 96, vol. 200, patient casebook 45-95, 1950, Mrs George Youthers, admitted 3 January 1950, discharged 17 January 1950. For emmenagogues see *CMAJ* 12, 3 (March 1922): 166 and J.S. Fairbairn, *Gynaecology with Obstetrics: A Text-Book for Students and Practitioners* (London: Humphrey Milford, Oxford University Press, 1924), 141–2.

23 *CMAJ* 22, 6 (June 1930): 794.

24 McGill University Archives, Royal Victoria Hospital, RG 95, medical casebooks, patient Mrs Ruggoso, admitted 6 November 1901, died 12 November 1901; Eleanor Whelan, admitted 16 April 1905, n.d. discharge; for more on pills see *CMAJ* 22, 6 (June 1930): 796; interview with Velma Messinger, 14 July 1993; Archibald Donald Campbell and Mabel A. Shannon, *Gynaecology for Nurses* (Philadelphia: F.A. Davis Co., 1946), 64–5.

25 For Metis women see Silverman, *The Last Best West*, 62. For Cree women see Joan Kerik, compiler, *Living with the Land: Use of Plants by the Native People of Alberta* (Edmonton: Alberta Culture, Youth and Recreation, Provincial Museum of Alberta, 1975), 17. For women at Cape Smythe see Vilhjalmus Stefansson, "The Stefansson-Anderson Arctic Expedition of the American Museum: Preliminary Ethnological Report," *Anthropological Papers of the American Museum of Natural History* XIV,

Part 1 (New York: AMS Press, 1914): 201. For Finnish women see Varpu
Lindstrom-Best, *Defiant Sisters: A Social History of Finnish Immigrant Women
in Canada* (Toronto: Multicultural History Society of Ontario, 1988), 82.

26 Mary-Ellen Kelm, *Colonizing Bodies: Aboriginal Health and Healing in British
Columbia, 1900–50* (Vancouver: UBC Press, 1998), 6; Kristin Burnett,
"The Healing Work of Aboriginal Women in Indigenous Newcomer
Communities," in Jayne Elliott, Meryn Stuart, and Cynthia Toman
(eds.), *Place and Practice in Canadian Nursing History* (Vancouver: UBC
Press, 2008), 40–52. On birth control and abortion in native life see also
Kim Anderson, *A Recognition of Being: Reconstructing Native Womanhood*
(Toronto: Second Story Press, 2000), 87–8.

27 For various methods see: E.C. Dudley, *The Principles and Practice of
Gynecology for Students and Practitioners* (Philadelphia: Lea & Febiger,
1908), 752; *CL* 49, 8 (April 1916): 338; Berkeley, "Diseases of the Vagina,"
in Eden and Lockyer (eds.), *The New System of Gynaecology* vol. 2, 77;
CMAJ 12, 3 (March 1922): 166; *CMAJ* 22, 6 (June 1930): 796; J. Munro
Kerr et al., *Combined Textbook of Obstetrics and Gynaecology for Students
and Medical Practitioners* (Edinburgh: E. & S. Livinstone, 1933), 229; J.M.
Munro Kerr with Donald McIntyre and D. Fyfe Anderson, *Operative
Obstetrics: A Guide to the Difficulties and Complications of Obstetric Practice*
(London: Bailliere, Tindall and Cox, 1937), 629; *NSMB* 16, 4 (April 1937):
208; *DMJ* 4, 1 (February 1939): 43; William A. Brend, *A Handbook of Medical
Jurisprudence and Toxicology* (London: Griffin, 1941), 119; Percy E. Ryberg,
Health, Sex and Birth Control (Toronto: The Anchor Press, 1942), 56–7; *CMAJ*
63, 5 (November 1950): 493. For the 1930 study see McLaren, "Illegal
Operations," 800–1.

28 For Dafoe see *CMAJ* 22, 6 (June 1930): 794.

29 McGill University Archives, Montreal General Hospital, RG 96, vol. 102,
patient casebook 3701-3750, 1935, patient Miss Cynthia Moore, admitted
6 August 1935, discharged 12 August 1935.

30 *CJMS* 18, 2 (August 1905): 115–117; *MMJ* 32, 12 (December 1903): 889.

31 *PHJ* 7, 3 (March 1916): 139; Wendy Mitchinson, *Giving Birth in Canada
1900–1950* (Toronto: University of Toronto Press, 2002), 160–5.

32 *CJMS* 22, 2 (August 1908): 79.

33 *NHPW* 28, 5 (May 1922): 274.

34 *NSMB* 10, 5 (May 1931): 328; *NSMB* 10 7 (July 1931): 403; for quote see
NSMB 10, 9 (September 1931): 662.

35 For Lacoste see Provincial Board of Health, Ontario 1925, Ontario *Sessional
Papers*, no. 20, 49; Angus McLaren, *Our Own Master Race: Eugenics in
Canada, 1885–1945* (Toronto: McClelland & Stewart, 1990), 82–3.

36 For Haitre see Gerald Stortz, "Of Tactics and Prophylactics," *Canadian Lawyer* (March 1982): 6; for Couture see Dodd, "The Canadian Birth Control Movement 1929–1939," 42.

37 Bailey, *For the Public Good*, 9.

38 For Wickett see Mariana Valverde, "'When the Mother of the Race Is Free': Race Reproduction and Sexuality in First-Wave Feminism," in Franca Iacovetta and Mariana Valverde (eds.), *Gender Conflicts: New Essays in Women's History* (Toronto: University of Toronto, 1992), 17. For blaming women see *MMJ* 32, 12 (December 1903): 889. For an overview of eugenics see McLaren, *Our Own Master Race*.

39 *CMAJ* 13, 9 (September 1923): 677–8.

40 For Chisholm see Dodd, "The Canadian Birth Control Movement 1929–1939," 49; on race suicide see also *CJMS* 54, 6 (December 1923): 182; Fairbairn, *Gynaecology with Obstetrics*, 739; *CMAJ* 22, 1 (January 1930): 91; and *CN* 27, 6 (June 1932): 354.

41 *The Hospital, Medical and Nursing World* 30, 3 (September 1926): 68.

42 Houston, *The Art of Treatment*, 479.

43 *CD* 6, 10 (October 1940): 18.

44 Ontario *Sessional Papers* no. 20, Provincial Board of Health, Ontario 1925, 49; *MMB* 99 (November 1929): 4.

45 For prevention see *NSMB* 11, 4 (April 1932): 462; *CPHJ* 23, 12 (December 1932): 562; *NSMB* 15, 7 (July 1936): 452. For its safety see Fairbairn, *Gynaecology with Obstetrics*, 741, 739, 740.

46 Dodd, "The Canadian Birth Control Movement 1929–1939," 43; Herbert A. Bruce, *Varied Operations* (Toronto: Longmans, Green and Company, 1958), 248, 247.

47 For advertisements see *ManMR* 23, 8 (August 1943) 198; *MMC* 1, 3 (December 1946): 75; interview with Dr Mackay, 29 October 1993; Ryberg, *Health, Sex and Birth Control*, 54, 146–8, 167.

48 For University of Toronto see Dodd, "The Canadian Birth Control Movement 1929–1939," 57; interview with Dr Richards, 9 August 1993.

49 William Albert Scott and H. Brookfield Van Wyck, *The Essentials of Obstetrics and Gynecology* (Philadelphia: Lea & Febiger, 1946), 353.

50 Frank Winthrop Draper, *A Text-book of Legal Medicine* (Philadelphia: W.B. Saunders and Co., 1905), 168; *CL* 53, 12 (August 1920): 560; Fred L. Adair (ed.), *Obstetrics and Gynecology*, vol. 1 (Philadelphia: Lea & Febiger, 1940), 673.

51 Reed (ed.), *A Text-Book of Gynecology*, 10. For an estimate of court cases see Tracy Penny, "'Getting Rid of My Trouble': A Social History of Abortion in Ontario, 1880–1929," MA thesis, Laurentian University, 1995.

52 *CMAJ* 12, 3 (March 1922): 163. For the Depression see S.A. Cudmore et al., *A Study in Maternal, Infant and Neo-Natal Mortality* (Ottawa: Dominion Bureau of Statistics, 1945), 45.

53 *CPHJ* 31, 7 (July 1940): 313; Ryberg, *Health, Sex and Birth Control*, 56.

54 Curtis and Huffman, *A Textbook of Gynecology*, 205.

55 D.W. Cathell, *The Physician Himself and Things That Concern His Reputation and Success* (Philadelphia: The F.A. Davis Co., 1898), 77; Joseph B. DeLee, *The Principles and Practice of Obstetrics* (Philadelphia: W.B. Saunders Co., 1913), 1017–18; *CL* 49, 8 (April 1916): 337.

56 *CL* 42, 9 (May 1909): 648–9; see also *CJMS* 27, 2 (February 1910): 81.

57 *CL* 49, 8 (April 1916) 337–8.[59] McGill University Archives, Faculty of Medicine, RG 38, c12, folder 310, Examinations, Toxicology, and Medical Jurisprudence, 1 December 1944.

58 *Saturday Night* 37 (3 December 1921): 1; interview with Verda McDonald, 14 July 1993.

59 *CPHJ* 25, 3 (March 1934): 116.

60 *Canadian Hospital* 11, 2 (February 1934): 7; *CMAJ* 34, 5 (May 1936): 520; *AMB* 3, 4 (October 1938): 16; *CPHJ* 31, 7 (July 1940): 315; *ManMR* 21, 11 (November 1941): 211; Ryberg, *Health, Sex and Birth Control*, 56.

61 Cathell, *The Physician Himself*, 79.

62 For single women of both groups see Cathell, *The Physician Himself*, 79; *CL* 42, 9 (May 1909): 648–9; *CJMS* 27, 2 (February 1910): 79; DeLee, *The Principles and Practice of Obstetrics*, 1017–18; *CL* 49, 8 (April 1916): 337.

63 See Victoria General Hospital, Halifax, Archives, Evelyn Royter, patient no. 1650, register 1527, surgical department, admitted 18 February 1931, discharged 2 March 1931; Martha McNamara, patient no. 1205, register no. 1087, surgical department, admitted 9 January 1931, discharged 20 January 1931.

64 See *Maclean's* 60 (1 April 1947): 61.

65 Victoria General Hospital, Halifax, Archives, patient no. 1205, register no. 1087, surgical department, Martha McNamara, admitted 9 January 1931, discharged 20 January 1931.

66 Cathell, *The Physician Himself*, 77. For aborting a legitimate child see McLaren, "Illegal Operations," 799.

67 Cathell, *The Physician Himself*, 77; *DMM* 23, 5 (November 1904): 321; DeLee, *The Principles and Practice of Obstetrics*, 1017–18; *CL* 49, 8 (April 1916): 337.

68 *CMAJ* 19, 6 (December 1933): 631; Letter from Dr Richards, August 1993; interviews with Geraldine Mitchell, 8 June 1993; Betsy Lawrence, 30 August 1993; Esther Thomas, 21 July 1993.

69 DeLee, *The Principles and Practice of Obstetrics*, 1017–18; *PHJ* 7, 3 (March 1916): 139; British Columbia Archives and Records Service, *British Columbia Royal Commission on State Health Insurance and Maternity* Benefits (Victoria: King's Printer, 1932), GR 707, box 4, file 4, "Digest of Evidence," 843; *CPHJ* 28, 12 (December 1937): 592–3; Adair (ed.), *Obstetrics and Gynecology*, vol. 1, 672.

70 *UTMJ* 25, 2 (November 1947): 54.

71 Victoria General Hospital, Halifax, Archives, patient number 1024, register no. 957, surgical department, Mrs Mavis Denton, admitted 30 December 1930, discharged 11 January 1931.

72 J. Clifton Edgar, *The Practice of Obstetrics ... for the Use of Students and Practitioners* (Philadelphia: P. Blakiston's Son & Co., 1907), 37–9; Henry H. Morton, *Genito-Urinary Diseases and Syphilis* (Philadelphia: F.A. Davis, 1906), 90.

73 For breast feeding see J. Clarence Webster, *A Textbook of Obstetrics* (Philadelphia: W.B. Saunders and Co., 1903), 615; W. Blair Bell, "Disorders of Function," in Eden and Lockyer (eds.), *The New System of Gynaecology*, vol. 1, 415.

74 Reed (ed.), *A Text-Book of Gynecology*, 10.

75 Barton Cooke Hirst, *A Text-Book of Obstetrics* (Philadelphia: W.B. Saunders Company, 1912), 89. For Murphy see *MMN* 21, 2 (February 1909): 72.

76 Fairbairn, *Gynaecology with Obstetrics*, 740–1. For cervical stems and intra-uterine rings see also *UTMJ* 14, 6 (April 1937): 239; Curtis and Huffman, *A Textbook of Gynecology*, 98.

77 Harry Sturgeon Crossen and Robert James Crossen, *Diseases of Women* (St. Louis: The C.V. Mosby Co., 1930), 880 (quote), 235. On coitus inter-ruptus see Sir James Purves-Stewart, *The Diagnosis of Nervous Diseases* (London: Edward Arnold and Company, 1937), 659; *UTMJ* 14, 6 (April 1937): 235–6.

78 For breast feeding see Ten Teachers, *Diseases of Women* (London: Edward Arnold & Co., 1935), 79.

79 Ryberg, *Health, Sex and Birth Control*, 149, 153, 157–8, 161–3. On condoms see also Emil Novak, *Textbook of Gynecology* (Baltimore: The Williams & Wilkins Company, 1943), 513–14; Scott and Van Wyck, *The Essentials of Obstetrics and Gynecology*, 354. Others, too, distrusted the stem pessaries because of their tendency to cause infection. See Campbell and Shannon, *Gynaecology for Nurses*, 59. For rejection of the safe period see *CMAJ* 59, 2 (August 1948): 172.

80 *CMAJ* 59, 2 (August 1948): 172.

81 For infections see Reed (ed.), *A Text-Book of Gynecology*, 10; *CL* 45, 6 (February 1912): 450; *PHJ* 7, 3 (March 1916): 139. For other results of instruments see Berkeley, "Diseases of the Vagina," in Eden and Lockyer (eds.), *The New System of Gynaecology*, vol. 2, 77.

82 Brend, *A Handbook of Medical Jurisprudence and Toxicology*, 119.

83 *CMAJ* 12, 3 (March 1922): 165; *CMAJ* 22, 6 (June 1930): 794; *CPHJ* 25, 12 (December 1934): 571; *AMB* 3, 4 (October 1938): 16; *ManMR* 21, 11 (November 1941): 211; *BAM* 20, 10 (July 1947): 210.

84 For douches see *CMAJ* 22, 6 (June 1930): 794. For various drugs see *CMAJ* 12, 3 (March 1922): 165; *NSMB* 11, 4 (April 1932): 462; Kerr with McIntyre and Anderson, *Operative Obstetrics*, 629; Curtis and Huffman, *A Textbook of Gynecology*, 562. For potassium permanganate see *CMAJ* 30, 6 (June 1934): 629.

85 David M. Eddy, "Variations in Physician Practice: The Role of Uncertainty," *Health Affairs* 3 (1984): 85.

86 Harry Oxorn, *Harold Benge Atlee M.D.: A Biography* (Hantsport, Nova Scotia: Lancelot Press, 1983), 123; see also letter from Dr Richards, 9 August 1993.

87 *CPMR* 27, 2 (February 1902): 92; for consultations see also Alfred Lewis Galabin and George Blacker, *The Practice of Midwifery* (London: J. & A. Churchill, 1910), 804; *CMAJ* 7, 5 (May 1917): 413.

88 *MMJ* 30, 5 (May 1901): 387; see also *CL* 34, 12 (August 1901): 663.

89 *CPMR* 34, 2 (February 1909): 71; *DMM* 34, 6 (June 1910): 223; *CMAJ* 7, 5 (May 1917): 413.

90 Lewis Galabin and Blacker, *The Practice of Midwifery*, 1077; *CL* 44, 10 (June 1911): 771; McGill University Archives, Royal Victoria Hospital Papers, RG 95, vol. 108, gynaecological case charts, 1914, patient Mrs Harriet Scott, admitted 18 June 1914, discharged n.d. For Stewart and Wright see *Annual Report of the Canadian Association for the Prevention of Tuberculosis 1917*, 49.

91 *CMAJ* 39, 4 (October 1938): 402.

92 See *CL* 53, 12 (August 1920): 557; *CJMS* 54, 4 (October 1923): 135; *CMAJ* 13, 4 (April 1923): 249; *CMAJ* 19, 5 (November 1928): 574; Thomas H. Cherry, *Surgical and Medical Gynecologic Technic* (Philadelphia: F.A. Davis Company, 1929), 344–5; *CLP* 80, 4 (April 1933): 116; *CMAJ* 24, 4 (April 1931): 618; *CN* 27, 6 (June 1932): 289; *CMAJ* 28, 1 (January 1933): 107; Ten Teachers, *Midwifery* (London: Edward Arnold & Co., 1935), 218; Irving, *A Textbook of Obstetrics*, 473; *NSMB* 16, 5 (May 1938): 374; Adair (ed.), *Obstetrics and Gynecology*, vol. 1, 189.

93 Interview with Gertrude Roswell, 16 August 1993.

94 For quote see *ManMR* 21, 3 (March 1941): 47; see also Ten Teachers, *Midwifery*, 695.

95 *CPHJ* 21, 5 (May 1930): 222.

96 For Henry see *ManMR* 18, 8 (August 1938): 148; letter from Dr Richards, 9 August 1993; Kitchener-Waterloo Hospital, patient no. 217, Mrs Wallace Williams, admitted 20 January 1945. The institutions examined were not Catholic ones so the situation was most likely quite different in those hospitals.

97 Interviews with Gertrude Roswell, 16 July 1993; Jane Rutherford 28 July 1993; Geraldine Mitchell, 8 June 1993; Betty Mackenzie, 19 August 1993; Dorothy Atkinson, 15 June 1993.

98 Adair (ed.), *Obstetrics and Gynecology*, vol. 1, 345; Novak, *Textbook of Gynecology*, 513; *MMC* 1, 3 (December 1946): 75; Curtis and Huffman, *A Textbook of Gynecology*, 98; *MMC* 1, 2 (November 1946): 88; interview with Betsy Lawrence, 30 August 1993.

Chapter 8

1 *CJMS* 11, 1 (January 1902): 3.

2 Charles A.L. Reed (ed.), *A Text-Book of Gynecology* (New York: D. Appleton and Company, 1901), 3.

3 For obstetrician/gynaecologist debate see Barton Cooke Hirst, *A Text-Book of Obstetrics* (Philadelphia and London: W.B. Saunders, 1912), 9; Joseph B. DeLee, *The Principles and Practice of Obstetrics* (Philadelphia and London: W.B. Saunders, 1913), xii; J.S. Fairbairn, *Gynaecology with Obstetrics: A Text-Book for Students and Practitioners* (London: Humphrey Milford, Oxford University Press, 1924), 22; *CMAJ* 20, 6 (June 1929): 646; J.M. Munro Kerr, J. Haig Ferguson, James Young, and James Hendry, *Combined Textbook of Obstetrics and Gynaecology for Students and Medical Practitioners* (Edinburgh: E.& S. Livinstone, 1933), 687.

4 *DMM* 15, 4 (October 1900): 178; G. Tod Gilliam, *A Text-book of Practical Gynecology* 2nd ed.(Philadelphia: F.A. Davis Co., 1907), 1. For histories of gynaecology see Ornella Moscucci, *The Science of Woman: Gynaecology and Gender in England* (Cambridge: University of Cambridge Press, 1990); Michael J. O'Dowd, *The History of Obstetrics and Gynaecology* (New York: Pantheon, 1994); Deborah Kuhn McGregor, *From Midwives to Medicine: The Birth of American Gynaecology* (New Brunswick, NJ: Rutgers University Press, 1998).

5 For Smith see *CMR* 28, 11 (November 1900): 474. For Gardner see *MMJ* 29, 9 (September 1900): 649.

6 Quote in *DMM* 35, 2 (August 1910): 55. On the surgical orientation see *CPMR* 30, 2 (February 1905): 92; *DMM* 35, 2 (August 1910): 42. On fees see Henry J. Garrigues, *Gynecology, Medical and Surgical: Outlines for Students and Practitioners* (Philadelphia: J.B. Lippincott, 1905): 51. On perception of women see *DMM* 23, 5 (November 1904): 321; ignoring the skills of others see *MMN* 16, 5 (May 1904): 182.

7 *CMAJ* 14, 9 (September 1924): 797; *CMAJ* 17, 3 (March 1927): 285; William R. Houston, *The Art of Treatment* (New York: Macmillan Co., 1936), 481; Harry Sturgeon Crossen and Robert James Crossen, *Diseases of Women* 7th ed. (St. Louis: The C.V. Mosby Co., 1930), 208; *CMAJ* 29, 6 (December 1933): 585; Emil Novak, *Textbook of Gynecology* 2nd ed. (Baltimore: The Williams & Wilkins Co., 1944), viii; Helen Flanders Dunbar, *Emotions and Bodily Changes* 3rd ed. (New York: Columbia University Press, 1947), 318.

8 For women's reproductive organs see *CJMS* 11, 1 (January 1902): 3. For ovaries see *CPMR* 31, 10 (October 1906): 557. W. Blair Bell, "Disorders of Function," in Thomas Watts Eden and Cuthbert Lockyer (eds.), *The New System of Gynaecology*, vol. 1, (Toronto: The Macmillan Co. of Canada, 1917), 415.

9 Gilliam, *A Text-book of Practical Gynecology*, 401.

10 American Authors, *The Practice of Obstetrics* 2nd ed. (New York and Philadelphia: Lea Brothers, 1901), 172. See also John Hoberman, "The Primitive Pelvis: The Role of Racial Folklore in Obstetrics and Gynecology during the Twentieth Century," in Christopher E. Forth and Ivan Crozier (eds.), *Body Parts: Critical Explorations in Corporeality* (Lanham, MD: Lexington Books, 2005): 85–104.

11 Nelly Oudshoorn, "The Decline of the One-Size-Fits-All Paradigm, or How Reproductive Scientists Try to Cope with Modernity," paper presented at the conference "Between Mothers, Goddesses, Monsters, and Cyborgs – Feminist Perspectives on Science, Technology and Health Care," Odense University, Denmark, November 1–5 1994, 4–5. On estrogen and discovery of its effects and chemical make-up see *CMAJ* 47, 5 (November 1942): 424; *UTMJ* 25, 3 (December 1947): 88–9. On the chemical makeup and complexity see *CMAJ* 34, 3 (March 1936): 294; *CMAJ* 47, 1 (July 1942): 12. On pelvic types see *NSMB* 19, 3 (March 1940): 25–6.

12 For Atlee see *NSMB* 19, 3 (March 1940): 25–6; *Saturday Night* 64 (1 February 1949): 16.

13 *Annual Report of the Vancouver General Hospital, 1912*, 49; *Annual Report of the Vancouver General Hospital, 1918*, 92–113; McGill University Archives, *Annual Report of the Royal Victoria Hospital, Montreal, Year Ending December*

*1925, 7*0, 110–11; Royal Victoria Hospital, RG 95, file 187, gynaecological reports, 1933, n.p.; *Annual Report of the Royal Victoria Hospital, Montreal Year Ending December 1940,* 102–4.

14 For an early example see *CMR* 30, 8 (August 1902): 340; Harry Oxorn, *Harold Benge Atlee M.D.: A Biography* (Hantsport, Nova Scotia: Lancelot Press, 1983), 128–9.

15 McGill University Archives, *Annual Report of the Montreal General Hospital, Year Ending 30 April 1901,* 112, 114.

16 Reed (ed.), *A Text-Book of Gynecology,* 5.

17 For Morton see *NSMB* 6, 2 (February 1927): 15. For Montreal General Hospital see McGill University Archives, *Annual Report of the Montreal General Hospital, 1928,* 89. For Alvarez see Queen's University Archives, Faculty of Medicine, Series VI, Notes and Lectures, box 5, Walter C. Alvarez, *The Book of the Post Graduate Course,* "Diagnostic Time Savers for Overworked Physicians," November 1945, 4.

18 Reed (ed.), *A Text-Book of Gynecology,* 728–9. See also E.C. Dudley, *The Principles and Practice of Gynecology for Students and Practitioners* 5th ed. (Philadelphia and New York: Lea & Febiger, 1908), 20.

19 Thomas Clifford Allbutt, W.S. Playfair, and Thomas Watts Eden (eds.), *A System of Gynaecology* (London: Macmillan, 1906), 738; J. Bland-Sutton and Arthur E. Giles, *The Diseases of Women: A Handbook for Students and Practitioners* (London and New York: Rebman, 1906), 410; Clifton Edgar, *The Practice of Obstetrics ... for the Use of Students and Practitioners* 3rd ed. (Philadelphia: P. Blakiston's Son & Co., 1907), 36.

20 For alcoholism see Kerr, Ferguson, Young, and Hendry, *Combined Textbook of Obstetrics and Gynaecology,* 360; for other issues see *UTMJ* 23, 3 (December 1945): 110. *CMAJ* 57, 5 (November 1947): 475; *CMAJ* 57, 5 (November 1947): 475; Dunbar, *Emotions and Bodily Changes,* 342.

21 For childbirth dangers see Charles Penrose, *A Text-Book of Diseases of Women* 5th ed. (Philadelphia: W.B. Saunders, 1904), 18; *CMAJ* 1, 2 (February 1911): 132; DeLee, *The Principles and Practice of Obstetrics,* xii; A.H.F. Barbour and B.P. Watson, *Gynecological Diagnosis and Pathology* (Edinburgh and London: William Green & Sons, 1913), 4.

22 David James Evans, *Obstetrics: A Manual for Students and Practitioners* (Philadelphia and New York: Lea Brothers, 1900), 119; Victoria General Hospital, Halifax, Archives, patient no. 650/05 Box 87, Mrs Terrance Moore, admitted July 21 1905; McGill University Archives, RG 95, vol. 25, gynaecology case charts, 1906, patient no. 2484, Mrs Joan Slater, admitted 30 April 1906.

23 *NSMB* 14, 3 (March 1935): 172. For criticism of obstetrics see also *CMAJ* 14, 9 (September 1924): 797; *UTMJ* 5, 5 (March 1928): 141; *CJMS* 75, 2 (February 1934): 40; Fred L. Adair (ed.), *Obstetrics and Gynecology*, vol. 2 (Philadelphia: Lea and Febiger, 1940), 358.

24 Quoted in R.W. Garrett, *Textbook of Medical and Surgical Gynaecology* (Kingston, 1897), 62. For dirty instruments see *MMJ* 29, 9 (September 1900): 649; *CL* 50, 6 (February 1917): 263. For dirty hands see *CPMR* 25, 3 (March 1900): 115; *CMR* 29, 6 (June 1901): 144. For sounds see *MMJ* 29, 9 (September 1900): 649; *CMAJ* 1, 12 (December 1911): 1128.

25 Reed (ed.), *A Text-Book of Gynecology*, 4.

26 *CMAJ* 34, 2 (February 1936): 223.

27 For earlier period see *CMR* 28, 2 (February 1900): 53. For concern about examining a virgin see *CL* 34, 9 (May 1901): 460; W. Blair Bell, *The Principles of Gynaecology* (London: Longmans, Green and Co., 1910), 95; H. Beckwith Whitehouse, "Methods of Examination," in Eden and Lockyer (eds.), *The New System of Gynaecology* vol. 1, 119. For a modern-day look see Joan Emerson, "Behavior in Private Places: Sustaining Definitions of Reality in Gynecological Examinations," in Hans Peter Freitzel (ed.), *Patterns of Communicative Behavior* (New York: Macmillan, 1970), 74–97.

28 For the rectal exam see *CL* 33, 9 (May 1900): 519; Garrigues, *Gynecology, Medical and Surgical*, 35. For using the mother see *CPMR* 26, 5 (May 1901): 248. For use of anaesthesia see Bland-Sutton and Giles, *The Diseases of Women*, 33; Bell, *The Principles of Gynaecology*, 95; Whitehouse, "Methods of Examination," in Eden and Lockyer (eds.), *The New System of Gynaecology*, vol. I, 126. For the perceived painfulness of and the moral objection to the examination see Garrigues, *Gynecology, Medical and Surgical*, 35.

29 Terms used in *CPMR* 25, 3 (March 1900): 115, and Garrigues, *Gynecology, Medical and Surgical*, 9.

30 *CPMR* 38, 6 (June 1903): 343; *DMM* 34, 2 (February 1910): 82; Whitehouse, "Methods of Examination," in Eden and Lockyer (eds.), *The New System of Gynaecology*, vol. 1, 119, 126.

31 For verbal examination see Garrigues, *Gynecology, Medical and Surgical*, 9. For Gardner see *MMJ* 29, 9 (September 1900): 648.

32 *CMAJ* 32, 5 (May 1935): 518–19.

33 Interview with Gertrude Roswell, 16 August 1993.

34 For Atlee see *CMAJ* 32, 5 (May 1935): 518. For Atlee's poem see Oxorn, *Harold Bengee Atlee M.D.*, 121–2; interview with Dr Hespeler, 19 October 1993.

35 Letter from Dr Richards to author, 9 August 1993; interview with Dorothy Atkinson, 15 June 1993.

36 *MMN* 16, 5 (May 1904): 183.

37 McGill University Archives, Royal Victoria Hospital, RG 95, vol. 104, gynaecological case charts, 1913, Mrs Leitia Danvers, patient no. 6429, admitted 24 November 1913. For noncompliance see also *MMN* 16, 5 (May 1904): 181.

38 Howard A. Kelly and Collaborators, *Gynecology* (New York and London: D. Appleton, 1928), 103. For patients disliked see Ten Teachers, *Diseases of Women* (London: Edward Arnold, 1935), 488.

39 *ManMR* 19, 11 (November 1939): 221; *CMAJ* 44, 2 (February 1941): 141. For VD see Victoria General Hospital, Halifax, Archives, register 1563, surgical department, patient no. 65, patient Karen Lang, admitted 12 September 1921, discharged 16 October 1921; register 1527, surgical department, patient no. 1650, patient Evelyn Royter, admitted 18 February 1931, discharged 2 March 1931.

40 Crossen and Crossen, *Diseases of Women*, 589.

41 Henry C. Chapman, *A Manual of Medical Jurisprudence and Toxicology* 2nd ed. (Philadelphia: W.B. Saunders, 1896), 104.

42 Bland-Sutton and Giles *The Diseases of Women*, 226, 372. See also Wendy Mitchinson, *Giving Birth in Canada, 1900–1950* (Toronto: University of Toronto Press, 2002), 121–3.

43 American Authors, *The Practice of Obstetrics* 2nd ed. (New York and Philadelphia: Lea Brothers, 1901), 172.

44 *CMR* 28, 9 (September 1900): 407; McGill University Archives, *Annual Report of the Montreal General Hospital for the Year Ending April 30 1901*, 115. The normal position is accepted as both anteflexed and antiverted.

45 Whitehouse, "Methods of Examination," in Eden and Lockyer (eds.), *The New System of Gynaecology*, vol. 1, 119.

46 See Mitchinson, *Giving Birth in Canada, 1900–1950*, 123–4.

47 *CMAJ* 42, 6 (June 1940): 567.

48 *CMAJ* 13, 11 (November 1923): 791; *CMAJ* 19, 2 (August 1928): 228; *CMAJ* 27, 5 (November 1932): 513; *CMAJ* 38, 6 (June 1938): 576; *CMAJ* 42, 2 (February 1940): 146; *CMAJ* 48, 6 (June 1943): 514. For questioning displacements see *DMM* 56, 6 (June 1921): 5; *CMAJ* 48, 6 (June 1943): 515–16.

49 Henricus J. Stander, *Williams Obstetrics: A Textbook for the Use of Students and Practitioners* 7th ed. (New York and London: D. Appleton-Century, 1936), 17; see also *UTMJ* 14, 3 (January 1937): 97; *NSMB* 19, 3 (March 1940): 25.

50 Garrigues, *Gynaecology, Medical and Surgical*, 9; Kelly and Collaborators, *Gynecology*, 392; Crossen and Crossen, *Diseases of Women*, 201.

51 *DMJ* 4, 2 (April 1939): 6; Novak, *Textbook of Gynecology*, 471.

52 Sarah Stage, *Female Complaints: Lydia Pinkham and the Business of Women's Medicine* (New York: W.W. Norton and Co., 1979), 173; *DMJ* 3, 3 (November 1938): 32.

53 For Gordon see *CL* 34, 9 (May 1901): 460. For douching see *CMAJ* 39, 4 (October 1938): 413. For sedatives see *MMN* 12, 5 (May 1900): n.p.

54 For sedatives see *DMM* 55, 1 (July 1920): 6, advertisement. For Morse see *NSMB* 15, 1 (January 1936): 32. For experience see Julie Vandervoort, *Tell the Driver: A Biography of Elinor F.E. Black, M.D.* (Winnipeg: University of Manitoba Press, 1992), 46–7.

55 Crossen and Crossen, *Diseases of Women*, 201.

56 For bloodletting see E.E. Montgomery, *Practical Gynecology* (Philadelphia: Blakiston, 1912), 106. For leeching see *CL* 36, 3 (November 1902): 185; Allbut, Playfair, and Eden (eds.), *A System of Gynaecology*, 750. For electricity see *CL* 34, 5 (January 1901): 258; Garrigues, *Gynaecology, Medical and Surgical*, 51. For pessaries see Bland-Sutton and Giles, *The Diseases of Women*, 114; *MMN* 21, 11 (November 1909): 412; *CMAJ* 1, 12 (December 1911): 1130; *CMAJ* 27, 5 (November 1932): 513; *CMAJ* 41, 2 (August 1939): 117; *NSMB* 28, 10 (October 1949): 237.

57 *CPMR* 37 10 (October 1912): 567; *CL* 46, 3 (November 1912): 197; *CL* 46, 3 (November 1912): 198.

58 *Canadian Practitioner* 47, 9 (September 1922): 397; *CN* 26, 5 (May 1930): 244; *CMAJ* 13, 11 (November 1932): 793; *CMAJ* 28, 2 (February 1933): 221; *Annual Report, Victoria General Hospital, Halifax, 1929–1930*, 18–19; see also Charles Hayter, "Seeds of Discord: the Politics of Radon Therapy in Canada in the 1930s," *Bulletin of the History of Medicine* 77, 1 (Spring 2003): 88.

59 *The Hospital, Medical and Nursing World* 28, 3 (September 1925): 86–7; *CMAJ* 25, 5 (November 1931): 584; *UWOMJ* 16 (March 1946): 80; *ManMR* 27, 3 (March 1947): 145.

60 *CL* 33, 12 (August 1900): 676–7; *CMAJ* 1, 6 (June 1911): 485–7; *CL* 46, 3 (November 1912): 215; *CMAJ* 5, 8 (August 1915): 668.

61 *NSMB* 10, 7 (July 1931): 437.

62 For bandwagon effect see Houston, *The Art of Treatment*, 480; for cancer see *CMAJ* 37, 3 (September 1937): 236.

63 *CMAJ* 51, 5 (November 1944): 444.

64 *CMAJ* 45, 3 (September 1941): 253.

65 *CMAJ* 44, 2 (February 1941): 136.

66 For Cockburn see *CPMR* 33, 12 (December 1908): 757. For conservative stance and too much surgery see *MMN* 16, 5 (May 1904): 182; *DMM* 34, 2 (February 1910): 81; *CL* 39, 1 (September 1905): 90; Allbutt, Playfair, and Eden (eds.), *A System of Gynaecology*, 2.

67 *CPMR* 30, 9 (September 1905): 477.

68 R.W. Garrett, *Textbook of Medical and Surgical Gynaecology* ([s.n.] Kingston, 1897), 176.

69 For Atlee see *CMAJ* 53, 2 (August 1945): 122; Oxorn, Harold Benge Atlee M.D., 136. For Best see *CMAJ* 57, 5 (November 1947): 474, 477. For too much surgery see also *CMAJ* 14, 9 (September 1924): 798; Crossen and Crossen, *Diseases of Women*, 208; *CMAJ* 35, 6 (December 1936): 625; *CMAJ* 48, 6 (June 1943): 519; *MMC* 4, 1 (January 1949): 44.

70 Public Archives of Nova Scotia, Victoria General Hospital papers, patient records, box 42, 869/00, patient Miss Bertha Crandell, admitted 17 September 1900. On maintaining an ovary and the ability to conceive see *CL* 34, 9 (May 1901): 460–1; *CPMR* 31, 10 (October 1906): 559; *DMM* 33, 3 (September 1909): 92; *CL* 44, 5 (January 1911): 378; Archibald Donald, "Ovariotomy," in Eden and Lockyer (eds.), *The New System of Gynaecology*, vol. 1, 431.

71 For Hay see *CL* 37, 6 (February 1904): 538–9. For aging and sense of self-worth see *CPMR* 31, 10 (October 1906): 557; *CPMR* 33, 12 (December 1908): 760; Winfield Scott Hall, *Sexual Knowledge* (Philadelphia: The International Bible House, 1913), 109. For sexuality see Reed (ed.), *A Text-Book of Gynecology*, 588; *CMR* 30, 8 (August 1902): 339; *CL* 37, 3 (November 1903): 247; Bland-Sutton and Giles, *The Diseases of Women*, 508.

72 *CL* 34, 1 (September 1900): 23. See also *CPMR* 30, 2 (February 1905): 92; *CPMR* 31, 10 (October 1906): 557–8; *CPMR* 36, 10 (October 1911): 610; *The Canadian Medical Quarterly* 4, 1 (April 1918): 26.

73 *CMAJ* 1, 6 (June 1911): 488.

74 For Smith see *CL* 37, 3 (November 1903): 247–8; *CMR* 30, 8 (August 1902): 340; *The Vermont Medical Monthly* 9 (September 1903): 217–18. For support of radicalism see *MMN* 16, 5 (May 1904): 182; *DMM* 35, 2 (August 1910): 44.

75 Kelly and Collaborators, *Gynecology*, 654; *Chatelaine* 21, 4 (April 1948): 75; *CN* 45, 7 (July 1949): 517.

76 For discussion on sex see Charles Herbert Best and Norman Burke Taylor, *The Physiological Basis of Medical Practice: A University of Toronto Text in Applied Physiology* (Baltimore: William Wood, 1937), 1166; Adair (ed.), *Obstetrics and Gynecology*, vol. 2, 854–5; Sir Comyns Berkeley and Victor

Bonney, *A Textbook of Gynaecological Surgery* 4th ed. (London, New York, Toronto, Melbourne: Cassell, 1942), 229.

77 *CMAJ* 58, 2 (February 1948): 152.

78 For Smith see *CPMR* 28, 10 (October 1903): 563; *CL* 37, 3 (November 1903): 245; *CJMS* 11, 4 (April 1902): 231; *CMR* 28, 5 (May 1900): 195; *MMN* 12, 5 (May 1900): 165–6.

79 *CMAJ* 32, 6 (June 1935): 667.

80 *UTMJ* 27, 6 (March 1950): 242, 244.

81 For Watts see *UTMJ* 16, 3 (January 1939): 196. For postmenopausal bleeding see *CMAJ* 60, 5 (May 1949): 452.

82 Reed (ed.), *A Text-Book of Gynecology*, 464.

83 Both cases are discussed in *MMJ* 34, 5 (May 1907): 317–19.

84 *CPMR* 36, 5 (May 1911): n.p.

85 *The University of Toronto Medical Bulletin* 1, 3 (April 1913): 59.

86 Kitchener-Waterloo Hospital Records, patient no. 3230, admitted 14 October 1943. On consent see Aleck William Bourne, *Synopsis of Midwifery and Gynaecology* (Toronto: The Macmillan Co., 1925), 229; D. Harcourt Kitchin, *Legal Problems in Medical Practice* (London: Edward Arnold & Co., 1936), 31, 29, 32; *ManMR* 16, 8 (August 1936): 162; Adair (ed.), *Obstetrics and Gynecology*, vol. 2, 736.

87 McGill University Archives, *Annual Report of the Royal Victoria Hospital, Montreal, 1930*, 107–9; for Burnside see *CMAJ* 44, 3 (March 1941): 283.

88 Ten Teachers, *Midwifery* (London: Edward Arnold, 1935), 671; J.M. Munro Kerr with Donald McIntyre and D. Fyfe Anderson, *Operative Obstetrics: A Guide to the Difficulties and Complications of Obstetric Practice* (London: Bailliere, Tindall and Cox, 1937), 532–3; Berkeley and Bonney, *A Textbook of Gynaecological Surgery*, 454.

89 Gérard Bouchard, "La sexualité comme pratique et rapport chez les couples paysans du Saguenay (1860–1930)," *Revue d'histoire de l'Amérique française* 56, 2 (2000): 203. Andrea Smith has discussed the use of hysterectomies as birth control without consent against native women. See *Conquest: Sexual Violence and American Indian Genocide* (Cambridge, MA: South End Press, 2005), Chapter 4.

90 McGill University Archives, Montreal General Hospital, RG 96, vol. 200, patient casebook 45-95,1950, Mrs Gaeton Laforce, patient no. 59, admitted 3 January 1950, discharged 19 January 1950.

91 Victoria General Hospital, Halifax, Archives, register no. 1303, Aurora Cameron, patient no. 1401, surgical department, admitted 3 July 1921, discharged 8 August 1921.

92 Berkeley and Bonney, *A Textbook of Gynaecological Surgery*, 76.

93 McGill University Archives, Montreal General Hospital, RG 96, vol. 163, patient casebook, gynaecology, 1902–4, Jane Granger, patient no. 2, admitted 6 January 1902, discharged 19 February 1902.

94 *Chatelaine* 22, 5 (May 1949): 34, 82, 84.

95 McGill University Archives, Royal Victoria Hospital, RG 95, vol. 5, gynaecology case charts, 1903, Mrs Perle George, patient no. 1459, admitted 9 June 1903; Kitchener-Waterloo Hospital Records, Mrs Annette Mobley, patient no. 138, admitted 13 January 1943. See Sally Wilde, "Truth, Trust and Confidence in Surgery, 1890–1919: Patient Autonomy, Communication, and Consent," *Bulletin of the History of Medicine* 83, 2 (Summer 2009): 302–330.

Chapter 9

1 Quotes from Thomas Wilson, "Cancer of the Uterus," in Thomas Watts Eden and Cuthbert Lockyer (eds.), *The New System of Gynaecology*, vol. 2 (Toronto: The Macmillan Co., 1917), 421, 491–2; *CPMR* 36, 10 (October 1911): 619; and *MMJ* 29, 11 (November 1900): 812; 817; for fear of it see *Chatelaine* 3, 11 (November 1930): 15; *Health* (September–October 1947): 15. For a discussion of images of cancer and people's reactions to them see Susan Sontag in her book *Illness as Metaphor* (New York: Farrar, Straus and Giroux, 1978).

2 For a more lengthy version of the discussion of breast cancer see Wendy Mitchinson, "Breast Cancer in Canada: Medical Response and Attitudes, 1900–1950," *Histoire Sociale* 76 (November 2005): 399–432.

3 Barbara Clow, *Negotiating Disease: Power and Cancer Care, 1900–1950* (Montreal and Kingston: McGill-Queen's University Press, 2001), ix, xi, 10, 40. For other work on the history of cancer see A.D. Kelly, *The Cancer Movement in Canada, 1930–1980* (Toronto: National Cancer Institute of Canada, n.d.); Robert Proctor, *The Cancers Wars: How Politics Shapes What We Know and What We Don't Know about Cancer* (New York: Basic Books, 1995); David E. Shepherd, "First in Fear and Dread: Cancer Control in Saskatchewan, The First Decade – 1929–1939," *Canadian Bulletin of the History of Medicine* 20, 2 (2003): 323–42; Ernesta A. McCullough, *The Ontario Cancer Institute: Successes and Reverses at Sherburne Street* (Montreal and Kingston: McGill-Queen's University Press, 2003); Patricia Jasen "Malignant Histories: Psychosomatic Medicine and the Female Cancer Patient in Postwar Era," *Canadian Bulletin of Medical History* 20, 2 (2003): 265–98.

4 *CL* 40, 5 (January 1907): 452; for class see *CPMR* 38, 1 (January 1913): 5; for race see John Davis Hartley, *A System of Gynaecology* (New York: J.B. Flint, 1899), 222 and also Keith Wailoo, *How Cancer Crossed the Color Line* (New York: Oxford University Press, 2001); for diet see E.E. Montgomery, *Practical Gynecology* (Philadelphia: Blakiston, 1912), 705; Wilson, "Cancer of the Uterus," 421.

5 For diet see E.E. Montgomery, *Practical Gynecology* (Philadelphia: Blakiston, 1912), 705; *CMAJ* 39 (August 1938): 175–6. For class see *CL* 40, 5 (January 1907): 452; *CPMR* 38, 1 (January 1913): 5. For heredity see *CMAJ* 19 (July 1928): 114–15. For race see John Davis Hartley, *A System of Gynaecology* (New York: J.B. Flint, 1899), 222. For civilization see *Saturday Night* 50 (1 June 1935): 3. For sex, gender, and age see Milton J. Rosenau, *Preventative Medicine and Hygiene* (New York: A. Appleton and Co., 1927), 424; *CPHJ* 24, 11 (November 1933): 539; *CJMS* 35, 4 (April 1914): 199.

6 Robert A. Macbeth, "The Origin of the Canadian Cancer Society," *Canadian Bulletin of Medical History* 22, 1 (2005): 158–9; H.E. MacDermot, *History of the Canadian Medical Association Volume 2* (Toronto: Murray Printing Co., 1958), 127; *NSMB* 11, 4 (April 1932): 209; Queen's University Archives, *Annual Report, Kingston General Hospital, Year Ending September 30, 1933*, 8; Provicial Board of Health, Ontario, 1937. Ontario *Sessional Papers*, no. 14, 165; B.C. Archives, Add Mss, 313, vol. 242; *Annual Report, Provincial Royal Jubilee Hospital, 1944*, 9.

7 For early treatments see *CPMR* 38, 1 (January 1913): 9. For alternative treatment see Clow, *Negotiating Disease*; for new treatment see *CMAJ* 30, 5 (May 1934): 573.

8 Sigismund Peller, *Cancer Research since 1900: An Evaluation* (New York: Philosophical Society, 1979), 224; Barron H. Lerner, "Inventing a Curable Disease: Historical Perspectives on Breast Cancer," in Anne S. Kasper and Sarah J. Ferguson (eds.), *Breast Cancer: Society Shapes an Epidemic* (New York: St. Martin's Press, 2000), 29; Daniel De Moulin, *A Short History of Breast Cancer* (The Hague: Martinus Nijhoff, 1983), 88. Barbara Clow in her book confirms that the local view dominated in Canada and elsewhere but that other theories such as contagion or systemic origin were also put forward. See Clow, *Negotiating Disease*, 43–5.

9 Ruth Brecher and Edward Brecher, *The Rays: A History of Radiology in the United States and Canada* (Baltimore: Williams and Wilkins, 1969), 271–2; Charles R.R. Hayter, "'To the relief of malignant diseases of the poor': The acquisition of radium for Halifax, 1916–1926," *Journal of the Royal Nova Scotia Historical Society* 1 (1998): 131; Kelly, *The Cancer Movement in Canada, 1930–1950*, 8–10, 17–19; Charles R.R. Hayter, Günes N. Ege, and Peter J.

Fitzpatrick, "Rays of Hope: The Establishment of Radiation Oncology in Canada, 1895–1976," in Jon E. Aldrich and Brian C. Lentle (eds.), *A New Kind of Ray: The Radiological Sciences in Canada 1895–1995* (Vancouver: Canadian Association of Radiologists, 1995), 50. For the most definitive history of the use of radiation for cancer see Charles Hayter, *An Element of Hope: Radium and the Response to Cancer in Canada, 1900–1940* (Montreal and Kingston: McGill-Queen's University Press, 2005). See also Edward Shorter, *A Century of Radiology in Toronto* (Toronto: Wall & Emerson, 1995).

10 Charles Hayter, "Seeds of Discord: the Politics of Radon Therapy in Canada in the 1930s," *Bulletin of Medical History* 77, 1 (Spring 2003): 97; Charles Hayter, "Tarnished Adornment: The Troubled History of Quebec's Institut du Radium," *Canadian Bulletin of Medical History* 20 (2003): 355, 357.

11 *CPMR* 47, 9 (September 1922): 387; *CMAJ* 43, 6 (December 1940): 580; *ManMR* 27, 1 (January 1947): 15; *AMB* 14, 4 (October 1949): 4; Shepherd, "First in Fear and Dread," 336.

12 *CL* 43, 4 (May 1909): 177; *PHJ* 6, 6 (June 1915): 290; *CMAJ* 32, 6 (June 1935): 647–8.

13 *CMR* 30, 6 (June 1902): 262–3.

14 *CMAJ* 55, 4 (September 1946): 237. For mortality see *UTMJ* 8, 4 (February 1931): 128–9.

15 Peller, *Cancer Research since 1900*, 155. See also Proctor, *Cancer Wars*, 3; *CN* 4, 6 (June 1908): 264; *DMM* 34, 2 (February 1910): 66; *CJMS* 35, 4 (April 1914): 199; *CMAJ* 10, 5 (May 1920): 425; *UTMJ* 8, 4 (February 1931): 128–9.

16 See J. Clifton Edgar, *The Practice of Obstetrics ... for the Use of Students and Practitioners* (Philadelphia: P. Blakiston's Son & Co., 1907), 465; David Tod Gilliam, *A Text-book of Practical Gynecology* (Philadelphia: F.A. Davis, 1907), 246.

17 For quotes see Thomas Clifford Allbutt, W.S. Playfair, and Thomas Watts Eden (eds.), *A System of Gynaecology* (London: Macmillan, 1906), 331. For being older and well nourished see Gilliam, *A Text-book of Practical Gynecology*, 247; Thomas Watts Eden, *A Manual of Gynaecology* (London: J. & A. Churchill, 1911), 287–8; A.H.F. Barbour and B.P. Watson, *Gynecological Diagnosis and Pathology* (Edinburgh: William Green & Sons, 1913), 73.

18 For trauma see *CMAJ* 20, 2 (February 1929): 181; *UTMJ* 12, 1 (November 1934): 22; *CMAJ* 33, 4 (October 1935): 374; *ManMR* 25, 4 (April 1945): 146. For infection see *UTMJ* 8, 4 (February 1931): 128–9. For reference to Jewish women see *CMAJ* 33, 4 (October 1935): 374 and Archibald Donald Campbell and Mabel A. Shannon, *Gynaecology for Nurses* (Philadelphia: F.A. Davis, 1946), 127. For endocervicitis see *CMAJ* 30, 5 (May 1934): 522. For heredity see *CMAJ* 40, 1 (January 1939): 44; *CMAJ* 32, 6 (June 1935):

648. For age see *CMAJ* 32, 5 (May 1935): 499; Campbell and Shannon, *Gynaecology for Nurses*, 33–4.

19 *CPMR* 36, 10 (October 1911): 619; *CL* 46, 3 (November 1912): 196; *CMAJ* 33, 4 (October 1935): 375; *NSMB* 18, 10 (October 1939): 587; *CMAJ* 44, 2 (February 1941): 133; *CMAJ* 59, 5 (November 1948): 458; *AMB* 15, 2 (April 1950): 32.

20 *CJMS* 8, 4 (October 1900): 243; *CMAJ* 32, 5 (May 1935): 499–500.

21 For how women saw bleeding see Wilson, "Cancer of the Uterus," in Eden and Lockyer (eds.), *The New System of Gynaecology*, vol. 2, 491–2; *CMAJ* 32, 6 (June 1935): 647–68; *ManMR* 27, 1 (January 1947): 15; *AMJ* 15, 2 (April 1950): 32. For lack of pain see *CMAJ* 33, 4 (October 1935): 375; Dalhousie University Archives, Oxorn Fonds MS-13-58, H.B. Atlee, *The Problem of Being a Woman*, 200. For pelvic exams see *CMAJ* 32, 6 (June 1935): 647–8. For Atlee see *NSMB* 13, 9 (September 1934): 449–50. For an article on the concern about early detection see Ilana Löwy, "'Because of Their Praiseworthy Modesty, They Consult Too Late': Regime of Hope and Cancer of the Womb, 1800–1910," *Bulletin of the History of Medicine* 85, 3 (Fall 2011): 356–83.

22 Kelly, *The Cancer Movement in Canada 1930–1950*, 8. For rarity in coming across cervical cancer in practice in Toronto see Edward Shorter, *Bad Manners: The Troubled History of Doctors and Patients* (New York: Simon and Schuster, 1985), 163–4.

23 William Blair Bell (ed.), *Some Aspects of the Cancer Problem* (New York: William Wood & Company, 1930), 216.

24 For regular examinations see Howard A. Kelly et al., *Gynecology* (New York: D. Appleton, 1928), 589–90. For precancerous conditions see Thomas H. Cherry, *Surgical and Medical Gynecologic Technic* (Philadelphia: F.A. Davis, 1929), 589; *UTMJ* 8, 4 (February 1931): 128–9; *UTMJ* 12, 1 (November 1934): 22; *CMAJ* 33, 4 (October 1935): 374; *CPHJ* 27, 3 (March 1936): 120; *ManMR* 25, 4 (April 1945): 146; *Health* 16 (September–October 1948): 13; Bell, *Some Aspects of the Cancer Problem*, 217.

25 Quoted in Clow, *Negotiating Disease*, 97.

26 Shepherd, "First in Fear and Dread," 335; W.G. Cosbie, *The Toronto General Hospital, 1819–1965: A Chronicle* (Toronto: Macmillan, 1975), 206–7.

27 *Health* 16 (September–October 1948): 13.

28 *AMB* 7, 2 (April 1942): 44. Biopsy is mentioned as early as 1906. *CJMS* 19, 5 (May 1906): 289. See also Vayena, "Cancer Detectors," 46.

29 Clow, *Negotiating Disease*, 98.

30 For information on the Pap smear see *CMAJ* 62, 2 (February 1950): 158; D. Erkshire Carmichael, *The Pap Smear: Life of George N. Papanicolaou*

(Springfield, IL: Charles C. Thomas, 1973), 60–1. For further information on the Pap smear see Eftychia Vaynena, "Cancer Detectors: An International History of the Pap Test and Cervical Cancer Screening, 1928–1970," PhD diss., University of Minnesota, 1999; Maria Papanicolaou-Kokkori, *George N. Papanicolaou: M.D., Ph.D.: Life and Career, The Way to the Pap Smear* (New York: Hellenic Medical Society of New York, 2008); Kirsten E. Gardner, "Controlling Cervical from Screening to Vaccination: An American Perspective," in Cheryl Krasnick Warsh (ed.), *Gender, Health, and Popular Culture: Historical Perspectives* (Waterloo: Wilfrid Laurier University Press, 2011), 109–26.

31 *CN* 41, 8 (August 1946): 650.

32 For screening in Canada see Vaynena, "Cancer Detectors," 11, 63–5, 90–1, 100, 164, 212; *CMAJ* 58, 5 (May 1948): 520; Dorothy Henderson, *For the Greater Glory: Biographical Sketches of Six Humanitarians Whose Lives Have Been for the Greater Glory* (Toronto: Ryerson, 1958), 40. For cost see *UTMJ* 27, 1 (October 1949): 20. See also Alexandra Howson, "Surveillance, Knowledge and Risk: The Embodied Experience of Cervical Screening," *Health* 2, 2 (1998): 195–215; Mandy Hadenko, "The Challenge of Developing and Publicizing Cervical Cancer Screening Programs," in Warsh (ed.), *Gender, Health, and Popular Culture*, 127–149. Hadenko argues that Canada was behind in the screening programs compared to the United States but she doesn't address the problem of them from the woman's perspective and the "problem" of that even today.

33 *AMB* 15, 2 (April 1950): 32.

34 For what to remove see *CMR* 30, 6 (June 1902): 265; J. Clarence Webster, *A Text-book of Diseases of Women* (Philadelphia: W.B. Saunders, 1907), 570; *CL* 43, 3 (May 1909): 182; *CPMR* 37, 10 (October 1912): 572–3; Wilson, "Cancer of the Uterus," in Eden and Lockyer (eds.), *The New System of Gynaecology*, vol. 2, 506. For a modern critique of treatment see Sandra Coney, *The Unfortunate Experiment* (Auckland, NZ: Penguin Books, 1988).

35 For mortality statistics see J. Bland-Sutton and Arthur E. Giles, *The Diseases of Women: A Handbook for Students and Practitioners* (London: Rebman, 1906), 245; for letting the disease run its course see *CJMS* 33, 3 (March 1913): 214. For palliative care see *CMR* 30, 6 (June 1906): 262–3; *CL* 43, 3 (May 1909): 182.

36 Wilson, "Cancer of the Uterus," in Eden and Lockyer (eds.), *The New System of Gynaecology*, vol. 2, 506.

37 *CPMR* 37, 10 (October 1912): 86; *CL* 46, 3 (November 1912): 196; *CL* 47 (June 1914): 747–8.

38 *Annual Report of the Royal Victoria Hospital, Montreal, Year Ending December 1929*, n.p.; for the Toronto General History see Cosbie, *The Toronto General Hospital, 1819–1965*, 189; Shorter, *A Century of Radiology*, 37, 40. For Manitoba see Hayter, "Seeds of Discord," 87, 89, 96.

39 For Kirkland see *CN* 26, 5 (May 1930): 246. For Cosbie see *UTMJ* 8, 4 (February 1931): 130.

40 For support of radium treatment see *CMAJ* 29, 3 (September 1933): 292; J.M. Munro Kerr et al., *Combined Textbook of Obstetrics and Gynaecology for Students and Medical Practitioners* (Edinburgh: E. & S. Livinstone, 1933), 874; *ManMR* 14, 8 (August 1934): 11–12; Emil Novak, *Textbook of Gynecology* (Baltimore: The Williams & Wilkins Company, 1944), 239; *ManMR* 25, 4 (April 1945): 146; William Albert Scott and H. Brookfield Van Wyck, *The Essentials of Obstetrics and Gynecology* (Philadelphia: Lea & Febigeer, 1946), 265; *CMAJ* 33, 4 (October 1935): 375; CMAJ 32, 6 (June 1935): 651.

41 For Richards see Hayter, Günes, Ege, and Fitzpatrick, "Rays of Hope," 49. For Bloodgood see *NSMB* 14, 5 (May 1935): 237. For exaggeration see *NSMB* 18, 10 (October 1939): 587, 602.

42 *McMJ* 17, 3 (October 1948): 329.

43 Geoffrey Chamerlain, *Victor Bonney, The Gynaecological Surgeon of the Twentieth Century* (New York: Pantheon, 2000), vii; Kerr et al., *Combined Textbook of Obstetrics and Gynaceology*, 874; *UTMJ* 12, 1 (November 1934): 27–8.

44 For Meigs see *MMC* 3, 8 (August 1948): 23. For Lederman see *McMJ* 17, 3 (October 1948): 331.

45 Harry Sturgeon Crossen and Robert James Crossen, *Diseases of Women* (St. Louis: The C.V. Mosby Co., 1930), 623. For impact on marital relations see Sir Comyns Berkeley and Victor Bonney, *A Textbook of Gynaecological Surgery* (London: Cassell, 1942), 891.

46 *ManMR* 14, 8 (August 1934): 12; see also *NSMB* 15, 6 (June 1936): 331; *ManMR* 25, 4 (April 1945): 146.

47 Clow, *Negotiating Disease*, 98.

48 *CMAJ* 46, 4 (April 1942): 394–5.

49 *CMAJ* 30, 1 (January 1934): 24, 28.

50 For commonness of breast cancer see Hartley, *A System of Gynaecology*, 221; *Annual Report of the Victoria General Hospital, Halifax, 1948/49*, 20–1. For mortality see *PHJ* 16 (June 1925): 259; *PHJ* 16, 2 (August 1925): 353, 359; *Surgery, Gynecology and Obstetrics* 96, 5 (May 1953): 509. For Richards see *British Journal of Radiology* NS 21 (March 1948): 109. Richards, hired at the Toronto General Hospital in 1917, was Canada's leading radiologist. See Shorter, *A Century of Radiology in Toronto*, 10, 18; Manitoba Cancer Relief

and Research Institute quoted in Kelly, *The Cancer Movement in Canada, 1930–1980*, 8.

51 Patricia Jasen, "Breast Cancer and the Language of Risk, 1750–1950," *Social History of Medicine* 15, 1 (2002): 17–43. For trauma see Clow, *Negotiating Disease*, 58; *CL* 40, 5 (January 1907): 452.

52 *CJMS* 35, 4 (April 1914): 198–9; *UTMJ* 5, 7 (May 1928): 203.

53 *NSMB* 13, 9 (September 1934): 505.

54 *CMAJ* 40, 5 (May 1939): 476–8.

55 For estrogen link see *CMAJ* 17 (August 1937): 112–17; Charles Herbert Best and Norman Burke Taylor, *The Physiological Basis of Medical Practice: A University of Toronto Text in Applied Physiology* (Baltimore: William Wood, 1937), 1175; *CMAJ* 37, 3 (September 1937): 236; *UWOQ* 8, 4 (1938): 169; *CMAJ* 44, 1 (January 1941): 1; *UWOQ* 10, 2 (January 1940): 77–9. For CMA see Clow, *Negotiating Disease*, 47. For warnings see *McMJ* 15, 3 (October 1946): 247–8.

56 *CN* 44, 4 (April 1948): 262. Such removal had a long history. See *CPR* 39, 10 (October 1914): 619; Moulin, *A Short History of Breast Cancer*, 102–3; James S. Olson, *Bathsheba's Breast: Women, Cancer and History* (Baltimore and London: Johns Hopkins University Press, 2002), 80–1.

57 Barbara Clow found a similar dynamic in her general study of cancer in Ontario. See Clow, *Negotiating Disease*, 59.

58 *CMAJ* 31, 1 (July 1934): 9.

59 *CMAJ* 32 (April 1935): 384; *UWOQ* 18, 1 (January 1948): 33.

60 For age see *ManMR* 24, 6 (June 1944): 165; *NSMB* 7 (1928): 247; and *NSMB* 13 9 (September 1934): 505.

61 For biopsy see *UWOMJ* 18, 1 (January 1948): 33 and *CMAJ* 32 (April 1935): 387. Clow in *Negotiating Disease* does not distinguish between the two types of biopsy (see 52).

62 *NSMB* 13 (October 1934): 513–14.

63 For Primrose see *UTMJ* 1, 5 (April 1924): 9–10; for Bloodgood see *NSMB* 14, 6 (June 1935): 309.

64 For McKinnon see *CJPH* 40, 6 (June 1949): 262. Clow has cited Canadian pathologist William Deadman as acknowledging that 10 percent of tissue samples (in general) that underwent analysis posed significant diagnosis problems for the best pathologist. Clow, *Negotiating Disease*, 27.

65 For Primrose see *UTMJ* 1, 5 (April 1924): 9–10. For MacDougall see *CMAJ* 40, 6 (June 1939): 569.

66 Iris Marion Young, *Throwing Like a Girl and Other Essays in Feminist Philosophy and Social Theory* (Bloomington, IN: Indiana University Press, 1990), 203–4. See also Sue Wilkinson and Celia Kitzinger, "Whose Breast

Is It Anyway?: A Feminist Consideration of Advice and 'Treatment' for Breast Cancer," in *Women's Studies International Forum* 16, 3 (May 1993): 229–38; Linda Sue Heuser, "A Content Analysis of Emotion Words Used in Mass Media Periodicals and Professional Journals to Describe Women's Emotional Reactions to Breast Cancer," PhD diss., University of Oregon, 1989, 15, 13; Fiona Giles, "The Tears of Lacteros: Integrating the Meanings of the Human Breast," in Christopher E. Forth and Ivan Crozier (eds.), *Body Parts: Critical Explorations in Corporeality* (Lanham, MD: Lexington Books, 2005), 123–41.

67 Clow, *Negotiating Disease*, 97.

68 *CMAJ* 31, 1 (July 1934): 10.

69 For examples of delay see Mary Rubio and Elizabeth Waterson (eds.), *The Selected Journals of L.M. Montgomery, Volume 2: 1910–1921* (Toronto: Oxford University Press, 1987), 240–1; Victoria General Hospital, Halifax, Archives, surgical department, patient no. 290, register no. 207, Mrs Rachel Fitzroy, admitted 11 November 1920, discharged 6 December 1920; patient no. 670, register no. 607, Angie Carrothers, admitted 21 November 1930, discharged 27 November 1930; patient no. 1574, register no. 1655, Mrs Amy Sullivan, admitted 1 April 1937, discharged 20 April 1937; *CMAJ* 31, 1 (July 1934): 9; *NSMB* 14, 6 (June 1935): 309; *CMAJ* 40, 3 (March 1939): 232.

70 *MMJ* 29, 11 (November 1900): 814; *CL* 43, 4 (May 1909): 177; *PHJ* 6, 6 (June 1915): 290; *CMAJ* 37, 6 (December 1937): 557.

71 See Sharon Batt, *Patient No More: The Politics of Breast Cancer* (Charlottetown: Gynergy Books, 1994); Rose Kushner, *Why Me?* (Cambridge, MA: The Kensington Press, 1982) and her updated version, *Alternatives* (Cambridge MA: The Kensington Press, 1984); Anne S. Kasper and Sarah J. Ferguson (eds.), *Breast Cancer: Society Shapes an Epidemic* (New York: St. Martin's Press, 2000); Ellen Leopold, *A Darker Ribbon: Breast Cancer, Women, and Their Doctors in the Twentieth Century* (Boston: Beacon Press, 1999); Patricia A. Kaufert, "Women, Resistance, and the Breast Cancer Movement," in Margaret Lock and Patricia A. Kaufert (eds.), *Pragmatic Women and Body Politics* (Cambridge: Cambridge University Press, 1998), 287–309; Pamela Sanders-Goebel, "Crisis and Controversy: Historical Patterns in Breast Cancer Surgery," *Canadian Bulletin of Medical History* 8, 1 (1991): 85–6; Moulin, *A Short History of Breast Cancer;* Chapter 7, "The Medical Breast: Life-Giver and Life-Destroyer," in MarilynYalom, *A History of the Breast* (New York: Ballantine, 1997), 205–240; Joan Austoker, "The 'Treatment of Choice': Breast Cancer Surgery 1860–1985," *The Bulletin for the Society of the Social History of Medicine* 37 (December 1985): 100–7; Olson, *Bathsheba's Breast;* Robert A. Aronowitz,

Unnatural History: Breast Cancer and American Society (Cambridge: Cambridge University Press, 2007); Jasen, " Breast Cancer and the Language of Risk, 1750–1950," 17–43.

72 Olson, *Bathsheba's Breast*, 185; Hayter, "Seeds of Discord," 76; Leopold, *A Darker Ribbon*, 84, 177; Barron Lerner, *The Breast Cancer Wars: Hope, Fear, and the Pursuit of a Cure in Twentieth-Century America* (Oxford and New York: Oxford University Press, 2001), 4; Robert Aronowitz, "Do Not Delay: Breast Cancer and Time, 1900–1970," *Milbank Quarterly* 79, 3 (2001): 376–8.

73 For descriptions of Halsted and his surgery see Sanders-Goebel, "Crisis and Controversy," 77, 82–3; Sherwin Nuland, "A Very Wide and Deep Dissection," review of Lerner, *The Breast Cancer Wars*, in *New York Review of Books* 20 September 2001, 14, 51; Leopold, *A Darker Ribbon*, 51, 53. For Kirkland see *CN* 26, 5 (May 1930): 245.

74 *MMJ* 29, 11 (November 1900): 815.

75 Batt, *Patient No More*, 58. The side effects emerged in the general literature comparing surgery and radiation therapy. My thanks to an anonymous reader for pointing this out.

76 McGill University Archives, *Annual Report of the Royal Victoria Hospital, Montreal, Year Ending December 1901*, 61–2; for depressed nipples see RG 95, vol. 88, obstetric casebook, Mrs I., patient no. 352, admitted 9 April 1902, discharged 12 May 1902.

77 *MMJ* 29, 11 (November 1900): 812–17.

78 For side effects see Victoria General Hospital, Halifax, Archives, patient no. 290, register no. 207, Mrs Rachel Fitzroy, admitted 11 November 1920, discharged 6 December 1920; Victoria General Hospital, Halifax, Archives, register 1619, surgical department, Mrs Martha MacDonald, patient no. 258, admitted 24 September 1921, discharged 1 December 1921. For need for surgery see *CMAJ* 14, 10 (October 1924): 917–18; *NSMB* 7 (1928): 149; *CMAJ* 30, 1 (January 1934): 24, 28; *UWOMJ* 8, 4 (1938): 167; *CMAJ* 52, 1 (January 1945): 18.

79 Harold Burrows, *Mistakes and Accidents of Surgery* (Toronto: McClelland and Stewart, 1923), 76; for Ontario woman see Clow, *Negotiating Disease*, 28.

80 Sanders-Goebel," Crisis and Controversy," 83–4; Clow, *Negotiating Disease*, xvii; *CMAJ* 30, 1 (January 1934): 24.

81 For early years see Hayter, Günes, Ege, Fitzpatrick, "Rays of Hope," 46; statistics based on *Annual Reports of the Superintendent* for the respective years. For Toronto General Hospital see Cosbie, *The Toronto General Hospital, 1819–1965*, 189; Shorter, *A Century of Radiology in Toronto*, 42–4.

82 For Peters see *CMAJ* 51, 4 (October 1944): 338–9. Quoted in Clow, *Negotiating Disease*, 91.
83 Shorter, *A Century of Radiology in Toronto*, 37, 40.
84 *NSMB* 13, 9 (September 1934): 510. For other discussions of preoperative and postoperative radiation see *NSMB* 14, 3 (March 1935): 127; *UWOMJ* 8, 4 (1938): 169; *CMAJ* 51, 1 (January 1945): 18; *MMC* 3, 1 (January 1948): 23; *AMB* 14, 4 (October 1949): 4.
85 *CMAJ* 40, 6 (June 1939): 569.
86 *CMAJ* 30, 1 (January 1934): 24, 28; see also Keynes in *Acto Radiologica* 10, 2 (1929): 393, 397; *Annals of Surgery* 106 (October 1937): 619, 623, 625–7. For other support see Olson, *Bathsheba's Breast*, 90–2.
87 *ManMR (MMR)* 14, 9 (September 1934): 4.
88 *CMAJ* 51 (October 1944): 335–6, 339, 343; M. Vera Peters, "Cutting the 'Gordian Knot' in Early Breast Cancer," *Annals of the Royal College of Physicians and Surgeons of Canada* 8 (1975): 192. For more on Peters see Batt, *Patient No More*, 60. In the 1960s, when Peters presented her findings in the United States, they were rejected – she was a "foreigner," a radiologist, and a woman. Lerner, *The Breast Cancer Wars*, 7, 132–3.
89 *CMAJ* 31 (July 1934): 9; *ManMR* 24, 6 (June 1944): 116. Lerner, "Inventing a Curable Disease," 25–50.

Chapter 10

1 Harry Oxorn, *Harold Bengee Atlee M.D.: A Biography* (Hantsport, Nova Scotia: Lancelot Press, 1983), 142.
2 Edward Shorter, *From Paralysis to Fatigue: A History of Psychomatic Illness in the Modern Era* (New York: The Free Press, 1992), 201. For reflex theory see Daniel Clark, *Mental Disease. A Synopsis of Twelve Lectures Delivered at the Hospital for the Insane, Toronto, to the Graduating Medical Classes* (Toronto: William Briggs, n.d.), 38.
3 *Saturday Night* 17 (16 January 1904): 9; *Canadian Magazine* 26, 1 (November 1905): 78; *CN* 25, 6 (October 1905): 578; *CL* 39, 11 (July 1906): 1051; *Chatelaine* 1, 2 (April 1928): 42; *Saturday Night* 60 (16 June 1945): 39.
4 *CL* 34, 5 (January 1901): 256; *CL* 43, 12 (August 1910): 912; *CPMR* 34, 12 (December 1909), 755–6; see also Cheryl Krasnick Warsh, *Moments of Unreason: The Practice of Canadian Psychiatry and the Homewood Retreat, 1883–1923* (Montreal and Kingston: McGill-Queen's University Press, 1989); David G. Schuster, "Personalizing Illness and Modernity: S. Weir

Mitchell, Literary Women, and Neurasthenia 1870–1914," *Bulletin of Medical History* 79, 4 (Winter 2005): 695–722; Shorter, *From Paralysis to Fatigue*; Megan Barke, Rebecca Fribush, and Peter Stearns, "Nervous Breakdown in 20th-Century American Culture," *Journal of Social History* 33, 3 (Spring 2000): 565–84.

5 Victoria General Hospital, Halifax, Archives, Medical Department, no. 188, register no. 150, Barbara Grosvenor, admitted 1 February 1921, discharged 9 May 1921; no. 365, register 362, Moira Webster, admitted 22 July 1921, discharged 28 July 1921; no. 635, register no. 413, Mrs Eleanor Ritchie, admitted 16 March 1931, discharged 10 June 1931.

6 For differences of opinion see Charles A.L. Reed (ed.), *A Text-Book of Gynecology* (New York: D. Appleton and Co., 1901), 856; Judson S. Bury, *Diseases of the Nervous System* (Manchester: The University Press, 1912), 704; Frank A. Craig (ed.), *Diseases of Middle Life: The Prevention, Recognition and Treatment of the Morbid Processes of Special Significance in This Critical Period*, vol. 2 (Philadelphia: F.A. Davis, 1924), 455; *UTMJ* 10, 1 (November 1932): 46. For MacIntosh see *DMJ* 4, 2 (April 1939): 39–41.

7 On hysteria see McGill University Archives, *Annual Report of the Montreal General Hospital, Year Ending April 1901*, 87; *Annual Report, Royal Victoria Hospital 1911*, 51; George Alexander Gibson (ed.), *Practice of Medicine, vol. 2* (Philadelphia: J.B. Lippincott, 1901), 846; *BOHI* 5, 3 (April 1912): 27. On hysteria in men see *CL* 39, 9 (May 1906): 807; Woods Hutchinson, *Common Diseases* (Toronto: McClelland and Goodchild, 1913), 401; Tom Brown, "Shell-Shock in the Canadian Expeditionary Force, 1914–1918: Canadian Psychiatry in the Great War," in Charles G. Roland (ed.), *Health, Disease and Medicine: Essays in Canadian History* (Toronto: Clarke Irwin for the Hannah Institute for the History of Medicine, 1984), 308–23.

8 Gibson (ed.), *Practice of Medicine, vol. 2*, 846.

9 *OJNP* 1, 1 (1921): 65; McGill University Archives, *Annual Report of the Royal Victoria Hospital, Montreal 1925*, 47; William Osler, *The Principles and Practice of Medicine* 10th ed. (New York and London: D. Appleton and Co., 1926), 1121. For women dominating see Sir James Purves-Stewart, *The Diagnosis of Nervous Diseases* 8th ed. (London: Edward Arnold and Co., 1937), 145; Edward Billings, *A Handbook of Elementary Psychobiology and Psychiatry* (New York: The Macmillan Co., 1939), 113.

10 See Victoria General Hospital, Halifax, Archives, surgical department, no. 3558, register no. 3399, Mrs Ellice Erickson, admitted 7 August 1931, discharged 20 August 1931; Kitchener-Waterloo Hospital Records, Mrs Oswald Fuger, admitted 20 March 1943.

11 Clark, *Mental Diseases*, 64; W.H.B. Stoddart, *Mind and Its Disorders; A Textbook for Students and Practitioners of Medicine* 3rd ed. (Philadelphia: P. Blakiston's Son & Co., 1919), 172, 278.
12 *CMAJ* 25, 2 (August 1931): 140–1.
13 For modern period see Diane Saibil, "Widespread Use of SSRI Antidepressants Drives Soaring Health Care Costs in Canada," *Canadian Women's Health Network* 8 3/4 (Spring 2006): 507; Canadian Population Health Initiative, *Women's Health Surveillance Report: A Multi-dimensional Look at the Health of Canadian Women* (Ottawa: Canadian Institute for Health Information, 2003), iv. For menopause and depression see W. Blair Bell, "Disorders of Function," in Thomas Watts Eden and Cuthbert Lockyer (eds.), *The New System of Gynaecology*, vol. 1 (Toronto: The Macmillan Co. of Canada Ltd., 1917), 385; *CPHJ* 23, 3 (March 1932): 123; *CPHJ* 23, 10 (October 1932): 479. Margaret Lock, *Encounters with Aging: Mythologies of Menopause in Japan and America* (Berkeley: University of California Press, 1992), 333; Ellen M. Gee and Meredith M. Kimball, *Women and Aging* (Toronto and Vancouver: Butterworths, 1987), 42; Laura D. Hirshbein, "Gender, Age, and Diagnosis: The Rise and Fall of Involutional Melancholia in American Psychiatry, 1900–1980," *Bulletin of Medical History* 83, 4 (Winter 2009): 710–45.
14 Clark, *Mental Disease*, 42; for Hattie see *MMN* 14, 10 (October 1902): 362.
15 *CMAJ* 28, 6 (June 1933): 626. For mental illness and retardation see *Vancouver Sun* (3 September 1932): 3; *Vancouver Sun* (10 September 1932), 4; *CMAJ* 29, 3 (September 1933): 260.
16 Quoted in *Chatelaine* 21, 4 (April 1948): 74.
17 Bury, *Diseases of the Nervous System*, 716.
18 *CMAJ* 32, 5 (May 1935): 509.
19 *CL* 40, 11 (July 1907): 974; *Report of the Royal Commission on a Dispute Respecting Hours of Employment between the Bell Telephone Company of Canada Ltd. and Operators at Toronto, Ont.* (Ottawa: Government Printing Bureau, 1907), 74.
20 *CL* 37, 4 (December 1903): 309; *CPMR* 31, 6 (June 1906): 317; *CL* 44, 10 (June 1911): 748.
21 *Vancouver Sun* 3 September 1932, 3; *American Journal of Psychiatry* 91, 5 (January 1935): 900–1.
22 *CMAJ* 29, 4 (October 1933): 443–4.
23 *MMN* 14, 12 (December 1902): 437–440. See also J. Clarence Webster, *A Text-Book of Diseases of Women* (Philadelphia and London: W.B. Saunders Co., 1907), 144; *BOHI* 5, 3 (April 1912): 27; Bell, "Disorders of Function," in Eden and Lockyer (eds.), *The New System of Gynaecology*, vol. 1, 301.

24 J.S. Fairbairn, *Gynaecology with Obstetrics: A Text-Book for Students and Practitioners* (London: Humphrey Milford, Oxford University Press, 1924), 679; Osler, *The Principles and Practice of Medicine*, 1123.

25 H. MacNaughton-Jones, *Practical Points in Gynaecology* (London: Bailliere Tindall and Cox, 1901), 88–9; for link between menstruation and mental illness see also *CL* 33, 9 (May 1900): 518; *CPMR* 30, 5 (May 1905): 291, 294; W. Blair Bell, *The Principles of Gynaecology* (London: Longmans, Green and Co., 1910), 197; Maurice Craig, *Psychological Medicine: A Manual on Mental Diseases for Practitioners and Students* 3rd ed. (London: J. & A. Churchill, 1917), 34–5, 87.

26 Mary-Ellen Kelm, '"The only place likely to do her any good': The Admission of Women to British Columbia's Provincial Hospital for the Insane," *BC Studies* 96 (Winter 1992–93): 83.

27 *CPMR* 26, 3 (March 1901): 123.

28 For link see Fairbairn, *Gynaecology with Obstetrics*, 671; William P. Graves, *Gynecology* (Philadelphia and London: W.B. Saunders, 1929), 148; *CMAJ* 58, 2 (February 1948): 188. For lack of connection see Ten Teachers, *Diseases of Women* 5th ed. (London: Edward Arnold & Co., 1935): 82.

29 MacNaughton-Jones, *Practical Points in Gynaecology*, 84; Webster, *A Text-Book of Diseases of Women*, 144; Alfred Lewis Galabin and George Baker, *The Practice of Midwifery* (London: J. & A. Churchill, 1910), 1077; *BOHI* 4, 4 (July 1911): 37; David Berry Hart, *Guide to Midwifery* (London: Rebman 1912), 574; Clark, *Mental Diseases*, 910–2.

30 *CL* 34, 12 (August 1901): 657; *BOHI* 4, 4 (July 1911): 37.

31 Fairbairn, *Gynaecology with Obstetrics*, 671; Ten Teachers, *Midwifery* 5th ed. (London: Edward Arnold & Co., 1935), 215; *CMAJ* 43, 6 (December 1940): 571. For "toxic exhaustion" see *OJNP* 2, 2 (March 1933): 72.

32 *UWOMJ* 2, 3 (1931): 82; Ten Teachers, *Midwifery*, 215; *CMAJ* 43, 6 (December 1940): 571.

33 Clark, *Mental Diseases*, 88; *CL* 34, 12 (August 1901): 658–9; Webster, *A Text-Book of Diseases of Women*, 144; Ten Teachers, *Diseases of Women*, 490; William A. Brend, *A Handbook of Medical Jurisprudence and Toxicology* (London: Griffin, 1941), 150.

34 Clark, *Mental Diseases*, 88; *CL* 34, 12 (August 1901): 658–9; *CL* 37, 4 (December 1903): 306; Hart, *Guide to Midwifery*, 574; Craig, *Psychological Medicine*, 34–5; Fairbairn, *Gynaecology with Obstetrics*, 671; Ten Teachers, *Diseases of Women*, 490; Brend, *A Handbook of Medical Jurisprudence and Toxicology*, 150.

35 Clark, *Mental Diseases*, 87. For Hattie see *MMN* 14, 10 (October 1902): 362.

36 For MacKenzie see *CL* 36, 7 (March 1903): 471. For sepsis see *CMR* 28, 2 (March 1900): 119; *CL* 37, 4 (December 1903): 306; *BOHI* 5, 1 (October 1911), 29; Thomas Watts Eden, *A Manual of Midwifery* (Toronto: The Macmillan Co. of Canada, 1915), 612; Sir James Purves-Stewart, "Nervous Diseases Associated with Morbid Conditions of the Pelvic Organs in Women," in Eden and Lockyer (eds.), *The New System of of Gynaecology*, vol. 1, 742. For social and physical factors see American Authors, *The Practice of Obstetrics* 2nd ed. (New York and Philadelphia: Lea Brothers & Co., 1901), 576–7; *MMN* 21, 12 (December 1909): 425–6; Barton Cooke Hirst in *A Text-Book of Obstetrics* (Philadelphia and London: W.B. Saunders, 1912), 421.

37 Fairbairn, *Gynaecology with Obstetrics*, 679; see also Aleck William Bourne, *Synopsis of Midwifery and Gynaecology* 3rd ed. (Toronto: The Macmillan Co. of Canada, 1925), 190; *UWOMJ* 2, 3 (1931): 82; Ten Teachers, *Midwifery*, 215; *CMAJ* 43, 6 (December 1940): 571.

38 *CMAJ* 19, 3 (September 1928): 294–5; *CN* 41, 5 (May 1945): 354.

39 *CMAJ* 43, 6 (December 1940): 571; see also Brend, *A Handbook of Medical Jurisprudence and Toxicology*, 150; *CN* 41, 5 (May 1945): 354.

40 Fairbairn, *Gynaecology with Obstetrics*, 679: Ten Teachers, *Diseases of Women*, 490; Ten Teachers, *Midwifery*, 695.

41 Kelm, "The only place likely to do her any good," 82–3.

42 *DMM* 14, 3 (March 1900): 127. See also *CPMR* 26, 3 (March 1901): 123; "Annual Report of the Superintendent, The Provincial Hospital, St. John, N.B, 1910," in *Journals of the House of Assembly of N.B., 1911*, 43; Craig, *Psychological Medicine*, 34–5.

43 For Smith see *CL* 34, 12 (August 1901): 658–9. For Craig see his *Psychological Medicine*, 181–2.

44 *CMAJ* 26, 1 (January 1932): 59; Carl Henry Davis (ed.), *Gynecology and Obstetrics*, vol. 3 (Hagerstown, MD: W.F. Prior Co., 1935), Chapter 11, 8; Purves-Stewart, *The Diagnosis of Nervous Diseases*, 659; *CMAJ* 43, 6 (December 1940): 57; *CMAJ* 58, 2 (February 1948): 188.

45 *American Journal of Psychiatry* 10 (May 1931): 1032; *Canadian Home Journal* 40 (August 1943): 10–11, 50.

46 *Chatelaine* 21, 4 (April 1948): 30.

47 For patient reaction see *CMAJ* 26, 1 (January 1932): 61; *CMAJ* 43, 5 (November 1940): 459.

48 For drink being gendered male see *CL* 36, 11 (July 1903): 845; Craig, *Psychological Medicine*, 254–5; *HW* 22, 5 (November 1922): 180.

49 *CL* 37, 4 (December 1903): 306. See also Daniel B. Brower and Henry M. Bannister, *A Practical Manual of Insanity for Medical Student and General*

Practitioner (Philadelphia and London: W.B. Saunders & Co., 1902), 235; Craig, *Psychological Medicine*, 254–5.

50 Victoria General Hospital, Halifax, Archives, surgical department, no. 496, register no. 423, Gail Pritchard, admitted 5 November 1930, discharged 9 November 1930; see also medical department, no. 605, register 598, Mrs Mavis Saunders.

51 Victoria General Hospital, Halifax, Archives, surgical department, no. 496, register no. 423, Gail Pritchard, admitted 5 November 1930, discharged 9 November 1930.

52 *CMAJ* 28, 6 (June 1933): 625; *CMAJ* 36, 2 (February 1937): 155; *UTMJ* 21, 1 (October 1943): 24; Edwin H. Hirsch, *Sex Power in Marriage with Case Histories: A Realistic Analysis Concerning the Sexual and Emotional Problems of Marriage* (Toronto: McClelland and Stewart, 1948), 71.

53 For Hanna see *QMQ* 5, 4 (July 1908): 158–161; Bell, *The Principles of Gynaecology*, 396–7.

54 *PHJ* 15, 7 (July 1924): 307.

55 Quoted in Oxorn, *Harold Bengee Atlee M.D.*, 142; for Atlee see also *NSMB* 12, 4 (April 1933): 243; *Chatelaine* 10, 1 (January 1937): 13. For stress on women see also Fairbairn, *Gynaecology with Obstetrics*, 671; *CMAJ* 34, 4 (April 1936): 424.

56 For nerves see *Canadian Magazine* 26, 1 (November 1905): 78; *Saint John Globe* (4 April 1914): 5.

57 For electrostatic treatment see *CL* 34, 5 (January 1901): 258 and McGill University Archives, *Annual Report of the Royal Victoria Hospital, Montreal, Year Ending December 1905*, 81. For X-rays see McGill University Archives, *Annual Report of the Royal Victoria Hospital, Montreal Year Ending December 1905*, 82.

58 For rest cure see Henry T. Byford, *Manual of Gynecology* (Philadelphia: P. Blakiston's Son & Co., 1895), 144; *CL* 33, 9 (May 1900): 505; *CL* 39, 1 (September 1905): 95; Bell, *The Principles of Gynaecology*, 396. For criticism see *CL* 38, 11 (July 1905): 995.

59 J. Bland-Sutton and Arthur E. Giles, *The Diseases of Women: A Handbook for Students and Practitioners* (London and New York: Rebman, 1906) 410; see also *Report of the Royal Commission on a Dispute Respecting Hours of Employment between the Bell Telephone Company of Canada, Ltd. and Operators at Toronto, Ont.*, 73; *CPMR* 35, 5 (May 1910): 299.

60 Ludwig Hirt, *The Diseases of the Nervous System* (New York: D. Appleton and Co., 1893), 527.

61 McGill University Archives, *Annual Report of the Royal Victoria Hospital Year Ending December 1905*, 81–2; Bury, *Diseases of the Nervous System*, 734.
62 Kitchener-Waterloo Hospital Records, Mrs Frances Fitzgerald, patient no. 51, admitted 5 January 1943.
63 For Dr Mile's Nervine see *Chatelaine* 5, 3 (March 1932): 61. For Eskaphen B Elixir see *MMC* 5, 6 (June 1950): 66.
64 Victoria General Hospital, Halifax, Archives, medical department, no. 75, register no. 58, Mrs Deborah Feist, admitted 23 November 1920, discharged 9 December 1920; see also surgical department, Mrs Abigal Lowry, no. 2983, register no. 2809, admitted 17 June 1931, discharged 1 July 1931.
65 Harry Sturgeon Crossen and Robert James Crossen, *Diseases of Women* 7th ed. (St. Louis: The C.V. Mosby Co., 1930), 946.
66 *CMAJ* 80, 6 (December 1936): 169.
67 For patent medicine see R.V. Pierce, *Dr. Pierce's Neighbourhood Gossip Dream Book*, (Bridgeburg, ON: Dr. Pierce Laboratory, 1930), 31. For exerting will see Crossen and Crossen *Diseases of Women*, 210, 946. For counseling see *CJMS* 80, 6 (December 1936): 169.
68 McGill University Archives, Montreal General Hospital papers, RG 96, vol. 182, patient casebook 3701-3750, 1935, patient no. 3722, Miss Mary Johnston, admitted 7 August 1935, discharged 24 August 1935; Kitchener-Waterloo Hospital, patient records, no. 3837, Miss Verity Momaner, admitted 14 December 1941, discharged n.d.
69 McGill University Archives, Montreal General Hospital papers, RG 96, vol. 100, patient casebook 45-95, 1950, patient no. 61, Mrs Gorman, admitted 3 January 1950, discharged 17 January 1950.
70 For hormone therapy see *OJNP* 2, 2 (March 1933): 62. For shock treatment see *CMAJ* 47, 4 (October 1942): 311–12. For statistics on shock treatment see L.S. Penrose, "Results of Special Therapies in the Ontario Hospitals ... up to November 1944" (Ontario: Department of Health, 1944).
71 Edward Shorter, *Bad Manners: The Troubled History of Doctors and Patients* (New York: Simon and Schuster, 1985), 152.
72 Clark, *Mental Diseases*, 88. For Smith see *CL* 34, 12 (August 1901): 660.
73 Bourne, *Synopsis of Midwifery and Gynaecology*, 192; see also *CLP* 80, 4 (April 1932): 116 *CMAJ* 42, 6 (June 1940): 559.
74 *CN* 41, 5 (May 1945): 354.
75 MacNaughton-Jones, *Practical Points in Gynaecology*, 88; *CL* 46, 2 (October 1912): 128–9.
76 For his reluctance to remove both ovaries see Bell, *The Principles of Gynaecology*, 192; Bell, "Disorders of Function," in Eden and Lockyer (eds.), *The New System of Gynaecology*, vol. 1, 300.

77 *Proceedings of the American Medico-Psychological Association* 11 (1900): 99–101.

78 Quoted in *CL* 34, 4 (December 1900): 169. See also *CL* 34, 3 (November 1900): 122.

79 *MS* (December 1900), n.p. For more on Hall see *CPMR* 33, 3 (March 1908): 150; *CL* 37, 4 (December 1903): 307–8.

80 Quoted in *CL* 37, 4 (December 1903): 311; *CL* 44, 10 (June 1911): 745–52; see also *DMM* 22, 2 (February 1904): 72; *CPMR* 31, 6 (June 1906): 312–319; *MS* (December 1900), n.p.; *CL* 39, 7 (March 1906): 603; *UWOMJ* 1, 4 (April 1907): 145.

81 Quoted in *CMR* 28, 11 (November 1900): 477. For Smith see also *CL* 34, 12 (August 1901): 662.

82 McGill University Archives, Royal Victoria Hospital, RG 95, vol. 45, gynaecological case charts, 1908, patient no. 3480, Mrs Ruth Graftberg, admitted 27 August 1908.

83 Clark, *Mental Diseases*, 177. For Stand see *BOHI* 6, 3 (April 1913): 133–5.

84 *OJNP* 1, 1 (1921): 65.

85 *OJNP* 2, 2 (March 1933): 64, 72. For such surgery continuing see Fred L. Adair (ed.), *Obstetrics and Gynecology* vol. 2 (Philadelphia: Lea and Febiger, 1940), 569.

86 William R. Houston, *The Art of Treatment* (New York: Macmillan, 1936), 507. See also Graves, *Gynecology*, 155; Crossen and Crossen, *Diseases of Women*, 210; Ten Teachers, *Diseases of Women*, 488; Sir Comyns Berkeley and Victor Bonney, *A Textbook of Gynaeoclogical Surgery* 4th ed. (London, New York, Toronto, Melbourne: Cassell, 1942), 863.

87 Harvey Simmons, "Psychosurgery and the Abuse of Psychiatric Authority in Ontario," *Health Politics and Law* 12, 3 (1987): 540. For the United States see Dorothy Nelkin, *Selling Science: How the Press Covers Science and Technology* (New York: W.H. Freeman and Co., 1987), 48; Jeffrey Masson, *A Dark Science: Women, Sexuality and Psychiatry in the Nineteenth Century* (New York: Farrar, Straus and Giroux, 1986), 19; Elliot Valenstein, *Great and Desperate Cures: The Rise and Decline of Psychosurgery and Other Radical Treatments for Mental Illness* (New York: Basic Books, 1986).

88 *CJP* 4 (1950): 125.

Chapter 11

1 Alice Stockham, *Tokology: A Book for Every Woman* (Toronto: McClelland, Goodchild, and Stewart, 1916), 280.

2 For literature on menopause see Patricia A. Kaufert and Penny Gilbert, "Women, Menopause, and Medicalization," in *Culture, Medicine, and Psychiatry* 10, 1 (March 1980): 7–21; Kathleen I. MacPherson, "Menopause as Disease: The Social Construction of a Metaphor," *ANS, Advances in Nursing Science* 3 (1981): 95–113; Susan E. Bell, "Changing Ideas: The Medicalization of Menopause," *Social Science and Medicine* 24, 6 (1987): 535–42; Joy Webster Barbre, "From 'Goodwives' to Menoboomers: Reinventing Menopause in American History," PhD diss., University of Minnesota, 1991; Renate Klein and Lynette J. Dumble, "Disempowering Midlife Women: The Science and Politics of Hormone Replacement Therapy (HRT)," *Women's Studies International Forum* 17 (1994): 327–43; Margaret Morganroth Gullette, "Menopause as a Magic Marker: Discursive Consolidation in the United States, and Strategies for Cultural Combat," in Paul A. Komesaroff, Philipa Rothfield, and Jeanne Daly (eds.), *Reinterpreting Menopause: Cultural and Philosophical Issues* (New York: Routledge, 1997), 176–199; Judith A. Houck, "Common Experiences and Changing Meanings: Women, Medicine, and Menopause in the United States, 1897–1980," PhD diss., University of Wisconsin, 1998. See also her published version, *Hot and Bothered: Women, Medicine, and Menopause in Modern America* (Cambridge: Harvard University Press, 2006); Elizabeth Siegel Watkins, *The Estrogen Elixir: A History of Hormone Replacement Therapy in America* (Baltimore: The Johns Hopkins University Press, 2007); Cheryl Krasnick Warsh, *Prescribed Norms: Women and Health in Canada and the United States since 1800* (Toronto: University of Toronto Press, 2010), Chapter 2, 47–75.
3 For culturally determined understandings of menopause see Margaret Lock, *Encounters with Aging: Mythologies of Menopause in Japan and America* (Berkeley: University of California Press, 1992) and Yewoubdar Beyene, *From Menarche to Menopause: Reproductive Lives of Peasant Women in Two Cultures* (Albany: State University of New York Press, 1989.
4 See especially Lock, *Encounters with Aging*, xxxvi.
5 Robert A. Wilson, *Feminine Forever* (New York: M. Evans, 1966).
6 Watkins, *The Estrogen Elixir*, 2007.
7 Patricia Kaufert, "Menopause as Process or Event: The Creation of Definitions in Biomedicine," in Margaret Lock and Deborah Gordon, (eds.), *Biomedicine Examined* (Dordrecht, Boston, London: Kluwer Academic Publishers, 1988), 333: Susan E. Bell, "Gendered Medical Science: Producing a Drug for Women," *Feminist Studies* 21 (1995): 493.
8 Henry T. Byford et al., *An American Text-book of Gynaecology, Medical and Surgical, for Practitioners and Students* (Philadelphia: W.G. Saunders Co.,

1896), 84. For lack of emphasis on menstruation see *CL* 43, 9 (May 1910): 682; Winfield Scott Hall, *Sexual Knowledge* (Philadelphia: The International Bible House, 1913), 204–5; Arthur E. Giles, "Hysterectomy," in Thomas Watts Eden and Cuthbert Lockyer (eds.), *The New System of Gynaecology*, vol. 1 (Toronto: Macmillan Co., 1917), 511. For emphasis on menstruation see Charles A.L. Reed (ed.), *A Text-Book of Gynecology* (New York: D. Appleton and Company, 1901), 738; J. Clarence Webster, *A Text-Book of Diseases of Women* (Philadelphia and London: W.B. Saunders Co., 1907), 115; *CL* 48, 2 (October 1914): 79.

9 For "critical period" see J. Bland-Sutton and Arthur E. Giles, *The Diseases of Women: A Handbook for Students and Practitioners*, 5th ed. (London and New York: Rebman, 1906), 22; E.C. Dudley, *The Principles and Practice of Gynecology for Students and Practitioners* 5th ed. (Philadelphia and New York: Lea & Febiger, 1908), 29; *PHJ* 4, 12 (December, 1913): 649. For use of the word "climacteric" see Daniel R. Brower and Henry M. Bannister, *A Practical Manual of Insanity for Medical Student and General Practitioner* (Philadelphia and London: W.B. Saunders & Co., 1902), 290; Thomas Clifford Allbutt, W.S. Playfair, and Thomas Watts Eden (eds.), *A System of Gynaecology* 2nd ed. (London: Macmillan and Co., 1906), 893; Thomas Watts Eden, *A Manual of Gynaecology* (London: J. & A. Churchill, 1911), 79. For use of the phrase "change of life" see Brower and Bannister, *A Practical Manual of Insanity for Medical Student and General Practitioner*, 290; Henry J. Garrigues, *Gynecology, Medical and Surgical: Outlines for Students and Practitioners* (Philadelphia: J.B. Lippincott Co., 1905), 2; *CL* 45, 3 (November 1911): 213–14; W. Blair Bell, "Disorders of Function," in Thomas Watts Eden and Cuthbert Lockyer (eds.), *The New System of Gynaecology*, vol. 1 (Toronto: Macmillan Co., 1917), 381.

10 Houck, "Common Experiences and Changing Meanings," 20.

11 Byford et al., *An American Text-book of Gynaecology, Medical and Surgical*, 85.

12 Frank A. Craig (ed.), *Diseases of Middle Life: The Prevention, Recognition and Treatment of the Morbid Processes of Special Significance in This Critical Life Period*, vol. 2 (Philadelphia: F.A. Davis Co., 1924), 363. For examples of menopause used in the broader context see *OJNP* 1, 2 (July 1922): 23; Harry Sturgeon Crossen and Robert James Crossen, *Diseases of Women* 7th ed. (St. Louis: The C.V. Mosby Co., 1930), 831; Ten Teachers, *Diseases of Women* 5th ed. (London: Edward Arnold, 1935), 59. For Tew see *CMAJ* 34, 4 (April 1936): 405. For use of "critical" see *CPHJ* 23, 3 (March, 1932): 118; *CMAJ* 37, 4 (October 1937): 350. For use of the word "dangerous" see *CJMS* 61, 2 (February 1927): 39; *CMAJ* 37, 4 (October 1937): 350. For use of the word "climacteric" see *CMAJ* 10, 5 (May 1920): 425; P. Brooke

Bland, *Practical Obstetrics for Students and Practitioners* (Philadelphia: F.A. Saunders, 1932), 39; Charles Herbert Best and Norman Burke Taylor, *The Physiological Basis of Medical Practice: A University of Toronto Text in Applied Physiology* 2nd ed. (William Wood & Co., 1937), 1195.

13 Percy E. Ryberg, *Health, Sex and Birth Control* (Toronto: The Anchor Press, 1942), 182; *McMJ* 15, 3 (October 1946): 240; *CN* 46, 11 (November 1950): 879.

14 For the former connection see Byford et al., *An American Text-book of Gynaecology, Medical and Surgical*, 86 and Hall, *Sexual Knowledge*, 204. For the latter connection see Webster, *A Text-Book of Diseases of Women*, 115; J. Clifton Edgar, *The Practice of Obstetrics ... for the Use of Students and Practitioners* 3rd ed. (Philadelphia: P. Blakiston's Son & Co., 1907), 25; and *SMJ* 2, 4 (April 1910): 99.

15 *CJMS* 61, 2 (February 1927): 41.

16 For an early puberty leading to an early menopause see Luigi Luciani, *Human Physiology, vol. 5* (London: Macmillan and Co., 1921), 292; Carl Henry Davis (ed.), *Gynecology and Obstetrics*, vol. 1 (Hagerstown, MD: W.F. Prior Co., 1935), Chapter 2, 16. For an early puberty leading to a late menopause see J.M. Munro Kerr, J. Haig Ferguson, James Young, and James Hendry, *Combined Textbook of Obstetrics and Gynaecology for Students and Medical Practitioners* 2nd ed. (Edinburgh: E. & S. Livinstone, 1933), 52; *CMAJ* 37, 4 (October 1937): 350–1; Fred L. Adair (ed.), *Obstetrics and Gynecology*, vol. 1 (Philadelphia: Lea & Febiger, 1940), 531; Emil Novak, *Textbook of Gynecology* 2nd ed. (Baltimore: The Williams & Wilkins Co., 1944), 114; Alfred C. Beck, *Obstetrical Practice*, 4th ed. (Baltimore: The Williams & Wilkins Co., 1947), 18.

17 Ten Teachers, *Diseases of Women*, 80; for Gibson see *CN* 46, 11 (November 1950): 880. For age of menopause and number of children see *UTMJ* 24, 3 (December 1946): 71; William Scott and H. Brookfield Van Wyck, *The Essentials of Obstetrics and Gynecology* (Philadelphia: Lea & Febiger, 1946), 32; Arthur Hale Curtis and John William Huffman, *A Textbook of Gynecology* (Philadelphia: W.B. Saunders Co., 1951), 102.

18 For climate see Byford et al., *An American Text-book of Gynaecology, Medical and Surgical*, 84; Webster, *A Text-Book of Diseases of Women*, 115; Dudley, *The Principles and Practice of Gynecology*, 29. For race see Webster, *A Text-Book of Diseases of Women*, 115. For heredity see Byford et al., *An American Text-book of Gynaecology, Medical and Surgical*, 86.

19 *CN* 46 (November 1950): 880.

20 For social factors see Webster, *A Text-Book of Diseases of Women*, 115; *CL* 43, 9 (May 1910): 682. For marital relations and childbearing, etc., see *CL* 43, 9

(May 1910): 682; Willaim Blair Bell, *The Principles of Gynaecology: A Manual for Students and Practitioners* (London: Longmans, Green & Co., 1910), 87.

21 For positive influences see Luciani, *Human Physiology, vol. 5*, 292; William P. Graves, Gynecology 4th ed. (Philadelphia and London: W.B. Saunders, 1929), 37; Davis (ed.), *Gynecology and Obstetrics*, vol. 1, Chapter 2, 16; *CMAJ* 37, 4 (October 1937): 350–1. For negative influences see Luciani, *Human Physiology, vol. 5*, 292; Aleck William Bourne, *Synopsis of Midwifery and Gynaecology* 3rd ed. (Toronto: Macmillan, 1925), 272; Davis (ed.), *Gynecology and Obstetrics*, vol. 1, Chapter 2, 16.

22 For delay see Craig (ed.), *Diseases of Middle Life*, 363–4; Bourne, *Synopsis of Midwifery and Gynaecology*, 272; Graves, *Gynecology*, 37. Some believed the reverse, that reproductive disease resulted in early menopause. See *McMJ* 15, 3 (October 1946): 242; *CN* 46 (November 1950): 880.

23 Graves, *Gynecology*, 37; Ryberg, *Health, Sex and Birth Control*, 184. For others see Robert William Johnstone, *A Text-Book of Midwifery for Students and Practitioners* (A. & C. Black, 1934), 37; Davis (ed.), *Gynecology and Obstetrics*, vol. 1, Chapter 2, 16; Frederick Carpenter Irving, *A Textbook of Obstetrics for Students and Practitioners* (New York: Macmillan, 1936), 28; Novak, *Textbook of Gynecology*, 114.

24 Bell in "Changing Ideas," 536, 538.

25 Davis (ed.), *Gynecology and Obstetrics*, vol. 1, Chapter 2, 16. For Shute see *CMAJ* 37, 4 (October 1937): 352; for blaming women see also *UTMJ* 24, 3 (December 1946): 71; Archibald Donald Campbell and Mabel A. Shannon, *Gynaecology for Nurses* (Philadelphia: F.A. Davis Co., 1946), 45–6; *UTMJ* 27, 2 (November 1949): 45. For an even more recent "blaming of women" see Joel Wilbush, "Climacteric Disorders – Historical Perspectives," in John W.W. Studd and Malcolm I. Whitehead (eds.), *The Menopause* (Oxford: Blackwell Scientific Publications, 1988), 7.

26 Emily Martin, *The Woman in the Body: A Cultural Analysis of Reproduction* (Boston: Beacon Press, 1989), 45; see also her "Is There a Woman in the Text?," *John Hopkins Magazine* (October 1987): 35; and "The Woman in the Menopausal Body," in Komesaroff, Rothfield, and Daly (eds.), *Reinterpreting Menopause*, 239–54.

27 Margaret Blackman, *During My Time: Florence Edenshaw Davidson, A Haida Woman* (Vancouver and Toronto: Douglas and McIntyre, 1982), 32; Edward A. Strecker, *Fundamentals of Psychiatry* 5th ed. (Philadelphia and Montreal: J.B. Lippincott, 1952), 131; Kim Anderson, *Life Stages and Native Women: Memory, Teaching, and Story Medicine* (Winnipeg: University of Manitoba Press, 2011), 129–30.

28 Brower and Bannister, *A Practical Manual of Insanity for Medical Student and General Practitioner*, 290; see also *CL* 43, 9 (May 1910): 682.
29 Webster, *A Text-Book of Diseases of Women*, 117.
30 *CL* 48, 2 (October 1914): 79.
31 Public Archives of Nova Scotia, Victoria General Hospital, Halifax, RG 25, Series B, III.141, Clinical Records, patient Joan Roberts, admitted 5 October 1911.
32 *CMAJ* 25, 3 (September 1931): 361; *CPHJ* 23, 3 (March 1932): 124.
33 Campbell and Shannon, *Gynaecology for Nurses*, 44; Poovey, quoted in Gullette, "Menopause as a Magic Marker," 180.
34 For Cleghorn and Stern see Beth Light and Ruth Roach Pierson (eds.), *No Easy Road: Women in Canada 1920s to 1960s* (Toronto: New Hogtown Press, 1990), 328.
35 *PHJ* 10, 11 (November 1919): 491. See also *CMAJ* 26, 1 (January 1932): 59; *CPHJ* 23, 10 (October 1932): 479. J.C. Connell, *The Book of Life: From Generation to Generation* (Toronto: Ryerson Press, 1935), 135.
36 Byford et al., *An American Text-book of Gynaecology, Medical and Surgical*, 86; Hall, *Sexual Knowledge*, 206.
37 Public Archives of Nova Scotia, Oxorn Fonds MS-13-58, H.B. Atlee, "Medical Lecture Notes – Gynaecology," 10; Bourne, *Synopsis of Midwifery and Gynaecology*, 239; Bland, *Practical Obstetrics*, 39; Crossen and Crossen, *Diseases of Women*, 830; Johnstone, *A Text-Book of Midwifery*, 37; Best and Taylor, *The Physiological Basis of Medical Practice*, 1195; *McMJ* 15, 3 (October 1946): 240; Scott and Van Wyck, *The Essentials of Obstetrics and Gynecology*, 33; *AMB* 13, 1 (January 1948): 64.
38 *McMJ* 15, 3 (October 1946): 240. Not as positive but recognizing that the rate of atrophy varied was J.C. Goodwin, *UTMJ* 24, 3 (December 1946): 71.
39 Edgar, *The Practice of Obstetrics*, 26.
40 For breasts see David Tod Gilliam, *A Text-book of Practical Gynecology* (Philadelphia: F.A. Davis Co., 1907), 66; Dudley, *The Principles and Practice of Gynecology*, 29. For skin see Byford et al., *An American Text-book of Gynaecology, Medical and Surgical*, 84. For weight gain see *CL* 33, 12 (August 1900): 676–7; Garrigues, *Gynecology, Medical and Surgical*, 3; Bell, *The Principles of Gynaecology*, 89; Bland-Sutton and Giles, *The Diseases of Women*, 22; Hall, *Sexual Knowledge*, 206.
41 Craig (ed.), *Diseases of Middle Life*, 365. For weight gain see *CMAJ* 19, 6 (December 1928): 680; *CMAJ* 29, 6 (December 1933): 588; *CMAJ* 34, 4 (April 1936): 406.

42 Ryberg, *Health, Sex and Birth Control*, 185–6; for Cleghorn see *Chatelaine* 21, 4 (April 1948): 30; see also *Saturday Night* (16 May 1950): 30.

43 *AMB* 15, 1 (January 1950): 13.

44 Houck, "Common Experiences and Changing Meanings," 101, 103.

45 Ryberg, *Health, Sex and Birth Control*, 77.

46 Gilliam, *A Text-book of Practical Gynecology*, 65; see also Garrigues, *Gynecology, Medical and Surgical*, 3; Eden, *A Manual of Gynaecology*, 79; R.H. Cole, *Mental Diseases: A Textbook of Pyschiatry for Medical Students and Practitioners* (London: University of London Press, 1913), 207; *CMAJ* 5, 5 (May 1915): 397; Eden and Lockyer (eds.), *The New System of Gynaecology*, vol. 3, 511.

47 Oxorn Fonds MS-13-58, H.B. Atlee, "Medical Lecture Notes – Gynaecology," 9, 11; *AMB* 13, 1 (January 1948): 64.

48 See Lock, *Encounters with Aging*, and Beyene, *From Menarche to Menopause*, 128, for the Mayans.

49 Warsh, *Prescribed Norms*, 49.

50 For different views see Garrigues, *Gynecology, Medical and Surgical*, 3; Gilliam, *A Text-book of Practical Gynecology*, 65; Bell, *The Principles of Gynaecology*, 91; Charles C. Norris, *Gonorrhea in Women* (Philadelphia: W.B. Saunders, 1913), 388; Maurice Craig, *Psychological Medicine: A Manual on Mental Diseases for Practitioners and Students* (London: Churchill, 1917), 181.

51 See *UTMJ* 24, 3 (December 1946): 71; *CMAJ* 58, 3 (March 1948): 253; *AMB* 15, 1 (January 1950): 13.

52 For increase in sex drive see *CJMS* 61, 2 (February 1927): 39; Davis (ed.), *Gynecology and Obstetrics*, vol. 3 (Hagerstown, MD: W.F. Prior, 1935), Chapter 8, 11; Adair (ed.), *Obstetrics and Gynecology*, vol. 2, 541; *McMJ* 15, 3 (October 1946): 240.

53 *Chatelaine* 21, 4 (April 1948): 31.

54 For various problems see Bland-Sutton and Giles, *The Diseases of Women*, 22; Gilliam, *A Text-book of Practical Gynecology*, 65; Garrigues, *Gynecology, Medical and Surgical*, 3; Craig, *Psychological Medicine*, 182; Cole, *Mental Diseases*, 207; Bell, *The Principles of Gynaecology*, 89; *CMAJ* 5, 5 (May 1915): 397; Hall, *Sexual Knowledge*, 204–5.

55 Byford et al., *An American Text-book of Gynaecology, Medical and Surgical*, 84; *MMJ* 29, 9 (September 1900): 655; Garrigues, *Gynecology, Medical and Surgical*, 3; Victoria General Hospital, Halifax, Archives, patient records, box 89, 346/05, patient Majorie Pritchard.

56 For various symptoms see *OJNP* 1, 2 (July 1922): 23; *CJMS* 61, 2 (February 1927), 41; *CMAJ* 29, 6 (December 1933): 588; *CMAJ* 37, 3 (September 1937):

225; *Chatelaine* 13, 10 (October 1940): 34; *ManMR* 24, 4 (April 1944): 104; *AMB* 15, 1 (January 1950): 13–14.

57　For "malady" see *McMJ* 15, 3 (October 1946): 239; for "ovarian amenorrhoea" see *UTMJ* 27, 2 (November 1949): 43.

58　Barbre, in "From 'Goodwives' to Menoboomers," 18.

59　Lock argues that physicians saw it as a disease in the interwar years. See her *Encounters with Aging*, 342–3.

60　McGill University Archives, Montreal General Hospital, RG 96, vol. 190, patient casebook 4725-4769, Mrs Anna Stevens, admitted 17 July 1945, discharged 2 August 1945.

61　For Oborne see *AMB* 15, 1 (January 1950): 14. For cancer see *CMAJ* 10, 5 (May 1920): 425; *CN* 39, 5 (May 1943): 337; *AMB* 15, 1 (January 1950): 14. For Mitchell see *CMAJ* 17, 1 (July 1932): 100; Patricia Jasen, "Menopause and Historical Construction of Cancer Risk," *Canadian Bulletin of Medical History* 28, 1 (2011): 43–70.

62　Fiona Mackie, "The Left Hand of the Goddess: The Silencing of Menopause as a Bodily Experience of Transition," in Komesaroff, Rothfield, and Daly (eds.), *Reinterpreting Menopause*, 17; see also Philipa Rothfield, "Menopausal Embodiment," 32–53, in the same collection.

63　*CPMR* 26, 3 (March 1901), 123.

64　Craig, *Psychological Medicine*, 182; Bell, "Disorders of Function," in Eden and Lockyer (eds.), *The New System of Gynaecology*, vol. 1, 385; Bland-Sutton and Giles, *The Diseases of Women*, 509.

65　Jessie L. Beattie, *A Walk Through Yesterday: The Memoirs of Jessie L. Beattie* (Toronto: McClelland and Stewart, 1976), 29; Reed (ed.), *A Text-Book of Gynecology*, 741; Stockham, *Tokology*, 276; Hall, *Sexual Knowledge*, 205.

66　See *CJMS* 61, 2 (February 1927); 41; *CPHJ* 23, 10 (October 1932): 483–4; *CMAJ* 34, 5 (May 1936): 597; *CMAJ* 40, 1 (January 1939): 40; *CN* 39, 5 (May 1943): 337; *ManMR* 24, 4 (April 1944): 104; *CMAJ* 56, 4 (April 1947): 402; *AMB* 15, 1 (January 1950): 13.

67　For Baragar see *CPHJ* 23, 10 (October 1932): 479; for McGeachy see *ManMR* 30, 5 (May 1950): 291. For mention of depression see also *CJMS* 61, 2 (February 1927); 41; *CN* 26, 5 (May 1930): 247; *CMAJ* 34, 4 (April 1936): 406; *CN* 39, 5 (May 1943): 337; *AMB* 15, 1 (January 1950): 13.

68　Scholars seem not to realize that some physicians in a much earlier period were willing to refute the link. See Ellen M. Gee and Meredith M. Kimball, *Women and Aging* (Toronto and Vancouver: Butterworths, 1987), 42; Lock, *Encounters with Aging*, 333. Cheryl Krasnick Warsh in *Prescribed Norms* tends to emphasize "menopause as Madness," a concept that some physicians were trying to overcome.

69 Warsh refers to it as a craze by 1947. See *Prescribed Norms*, 67.

70 Byford et al., *An American Text-book of Gynaecology, Medical and Surgical*, 89.

71 For various nostrums see *MMN* 13, 10 (October 1901): 351; for dangers of alcohol and sedatives see Eden, *A Manual of Gynaecology*, 82. For ergot see *CMAJ* 5, 5 (May 1915): 397.

72 For Smith see *MMN* 13, 10 (October 1901): 351. See also *CL* 33, 12 (August 1900): 676–7; *CMAJ* 5, 8 (August 1915): 669; Bell, "Disorders of Function," in Eden and Lockyer (eds.), *The New System of Gynaecology*, vol. 1, 385.

73 Interview with Drs Mackay and Hespler, 29 October 1993, Halifax.

74 Craig (ed.), *Diseases of Middle Life*, 366.

75 Novak, *Textbook of Gynecology*, 538.

76 *Chatelaine* 7, 10 (October 1938): 50. For a fascinating description of the fortunes of the Pinkham company in the United States with respect to advertising its effectiveness with menopausal symptoms see Sarah Stage, *Female Complaints: Lydia Pinkham and the Business of Women's Medicine* (New York: W.W. Norton and Co., 1979), 196, 198, 242.

77 For Whitehouse see *CMAJ* 29, 6 (December 1933): 590; for Shute see *CMAJ* 37, 4 (October 1937): 354.

78 Lock, *Encounters with Aging*, 329.

79 *CJMS* 61, 2 (February 1927): 42. For a discussion of this kind of tension see Alexandria Dundas Todd, *Intimate Adversaries: Cultural Conflict between Doctors and Their Women Patients* (Philadelphia: University of Pennsylvania Press, 1989), 118.

80 For Atlee see Public Archives of Nova Scotia, Medical Archives Collection, "Medical Society of Nova Scotia," Executive Meeting, 1936, 23-4. For development of DES see Bell, "Gendered Medical Science," 474; Roberta J. Apfel and Susan M. Fisher, *To Do No Harm: DES and the Dilemmas of Modern Medicine* (New Haven: Yale University Press, 1984), 14; Barbara Brookes, "'The Glands of Destiny': Hygiene, Hormones and English Women Doctors in the First Half of the Twentieth Century," *Canadian Bulletin of Medical History* 23, 1 (2006): 49–68.

81 For references to Emmenin see *OJNP* 2, 2 (March 1933): 62; *CMAJ* 34, 5 (May 1936): 597; *CMAJ* 42, 6 (June 1940): 585; *CMAJ* 49, 2 (August 1943): 151. For history of Premarin, an estrogen product, see Alison Li, "Marketing Menopause: Science and the Public Reclations of Premarin," in Georgina Feldberg et al., *Women, Health, and Nation* (Montreal and Kingston: McGill-Queen's University Press, 2003), 101–120.

82 For Goodwin see *UTMJ* 24, 3 (December 1946): 72; for Atlee see Dalhousie University Archives, Oxorn Fonds MS-13-58, H.B. Atlee, "Medical Lecture Notes – Gynaecology," 11; for Hilliard see *CMAJ* 37, 3 (September 1937): 225; for Sangster see *Chatelaine* 22, 5 (May 1949): 84.

83 For Whitehouse see *CMAJ* 29, 6 (December 1933): 590; William R. Houston, *The Art of Treatment* (New York: Macmillan, 1936), 480; For Shute see *CMAJ* 40, 1 (January 1939): 40; for Black see Julie Vandervoort, *Tell the Driver: A Biography of Elinor F.E. Black* (Winnipeg: University of Manitoba Press, 1992), 156–7.

84 *NSMB* 24, 5 (May 1945): 224; *CMAJ* 53, 1 (July 1945): 33.

85 For Darragh see *McMJ* 15, 3 (October 1946): 247–8. For Harris see *CMAJ* 58, 3 (March 1948): 253. See also France B. McCrea and Gerald E. Markle, "The Estrogen Replacement Controversy in the USA and UK: Different Answers to the Same Question," *Social Studies of Science* 14 (1984): 3.

86 Reed (ed.), *A Text-Book of Gynecology*, 738, 741; Cole, *Mental Diseases*, 207. See also Elizabeth Siegel Watkins, "The Medicalization of Male Menopause in America," *Social History of Medicine* 20, 2 (2007): 369–88.

87 Stall, quoted in Mike Featherstone and Mike Hepworth, "The History of the Male Menopause, 1848–1936," *Maturitas* 7 (1985): 253. On decline of virility see Henry H. Morton, *Genito-Urinary Diseases and Syphilis* (Philadelphia: F.A. Davis Company, 1906), 477. See also Cole, *Mental Diseases*, 207.

88 Nelly Oudshoorn, "United We Stand: The Pharmaceutical Industry, Laboratory, and Clinic in the Development of Sex Hormones into Scientific Drugs, 1920–1940," *Science, Technology, & Human Values* 18, 1 (Winter 1993): 19. On male menopause duration and age see *OJNP* 1, 2 (July 1922): 23. See also Luciani, *Human Physiology, vol. 5*, 292.

89 For Baragar see *CPHJ* 23, 10 (October 1932): 483–4. For psychological and mental problems see *OJNP* 1, 2 (July 1922): 23; *CMAJ* 26, 1 (January 1932): 59; Ryberg, *Health, Sex and Birth Control*, 183.

90 For Cumberland see *OJNP* 1, 2 (July 1922): 23; Ryberg, *Health, Sex and Birth Control*, 187–9.

91 For Stern see *Chatelaine* 21, 4 (April 1948): 75; Edwin H. Hirsch, *Sex Power in Marriage with Case Histories – A Realistic Analysis Concerning the Sexual and Emotional Problems of Marriage* (Toronto: McClelland and Stewart, 1948), 136.

92 Quote comes from *Maclean's* 62 (15 October 1949): 15. For various symptoms see *CMAJ* 55, 5 (November 1946): 441–2; *Health* 16

(May–June 1948): 8; *CN* 46 (November 1950): 901. For virility see *Health* 16 (December 1948): 20; *Chatelaine* 22, 6 (June 1949): 27; *Maclean's* 62 (15 October 1949): 36; *CN* 46 (November 1950): 901.

93 Julia Rechter, "The Glands of Destiny: A History of Popular Medical and Scientific Views of the Sex Hormones in the 1920s," PhD diss., University of California, Berkeley, 1997, 176.

94 For connection with hormones see *Health* 16 (December 1948): 20; Hirsch, *Sex Power in Marriage with Case Histories*, 136; *Chatelaine* 22, 6 (June 1949): 27. For Katz see *Maclean's* 62 (15 October 1949): 36. For Cleghorn see *MMC* 4, 6 (June 1949): 27.

95 Mary Rubio and Elizabeth Waterson (eds.), *The Selected Journals of Lucy Maud Montgomery Volume 3: 1921–29* (Toronto: Oxford University Press, 1992), 172.

Conclusion

1 Gerald Grob, "Presidential Address: Psychiatry Holy Grail: The Search for the Mechanisms of Mental Illness," *Bulletin of the History of Medicine* 72, 2 (Summer 1998): 189.

2 E. Melanie Dupuis, *Nature's Perfect Food: How Milk Became America's Drink* (New York: New York University Press, 2002), 161–2.

3 On measurements see Ian Hacking, quoted in Margaret Lock and Gilles Bibeau, "Healthy Disputes: Some Reflections on the Practice of Medical Anthropology in Canada," *Health and Canadian Society* 1, 1 (1993): 151.

4 Nelly Oudshoorn, *Beyond the Natural Body: An Archaeology of Sex Hormones* (Routledge: London and New York, 1994), 3.

5 Janice G. Raymond, "Medicine as Patriarchal Religion," *Journal of Medicine and Philosophy* 7, 2 (1982): 197–216.

6 David M. Eddy, "Variations in Physician Practice: The Role of Uncertainty," *Health Affairs* 3 (1984): 75.

7 Dr Helen Singer Kaplan, quoted in Janice M. Irvine, *Disorders of Desire: Sex and Gender in Modern American Sexology* (Philadelphia: Temple University Press, 1990), 229.

8 Susan Bordo, *Unbearable Weight: Feminism, Western Culture, and the Body* (Berkeley: University of California Press, 1993), 73.

9 Hazel Miriam Ross, "Women and Wellness: Defining, Attaining, and Maintaining Health in Eastern Canada," Ph.D. diss., University of Washington, 1982.

10 Alexandria Dundas Todd, *Intimate Adversaries: Cultural Conflict between Doctors and Their Women Patients* (Philadelphia: University of Pennsylvania Press, 1989), 103.
11 Leonore Tiefer, *Sex Is Not a Natural Act and Other Essays* (Boulder, CO: Westview Press, 1995), 32–3.
12 O'Brien, quoted in "Introduction," Dawn H. Currie and Valerie Raoul (eds.), *The Anatomy of Gender: Women's Struggle for the Body* (Ottawa: Carleton University Press, 1991), 12; Leonore Tiefer, *Sex Is Not a Natural Act and Other Essays*, 32.

Notes on Sources and Methodology

1 Mark T. Gilderhus, *History and Historians: A Historiographical Introduction* 5th ed. (Upper Saddle River, NJ: Prentice Hall, 2003), 137.
2 See Charles G. Roland and Paul Potter, *An Annotated Bibliography of Canadian Medical Periodicals 1926–1975* (Toronto: The Hannah Institute for the History of Medicine, 1979).
3 Dianna Scully and Pauline Bart, "A Funny Thing Happened on the Way to the Orifice: Women in Gynecology Textbooks," *American Journal of Sociology* 78, 4 (1972–3): 1945.
4 Cynthia Abeele, "'Nations Are Built of Babies': Maternal and Child Welfare in Ontario, 1914–1940," PhD diss., University of Guelph, 1987, Chapter 1, app. 1.1.
5 Nancy Cott, *Bonds of Womanhood* (New Haven: Yale University Press, 1977), 2.
6 The list of records used were: Faculty of Medicine, Queen's University, case histories 1913–14, 1916, 1920; Kingston General Hospital, death records, 1903–1919; Kingston General Hospital, operating room records, 1911–1919; Kingston General Hospital, register 1917–18; Kitchener-Waterloo Hospital, patient records, 1940s (mostly obstetrical); Montreal General Hospital, patient casebooks, medical and surgical, 1900–1946; Montreal General Hospital, gynaecological patient records, 1902–3; Owen Sound Hospital, 1895–41 statistical runs by David Gagan given to me from his research on his history of the hospital; Royal Jubilee Hospital, Vancouver (discharge books) 1891–1919, as well as the discharge books for 1925, 1935, and 1945; McGill University Archives, Royal Victoria Hospital, Montreal, gynaecological cases, 1903–21; Toronto Home for Incurables, register, 1900–1919; Victoria General Hospital, Halifax, Archives, operating ledger, 1920–22; Victoria General Hospital, Halifax, patient records, 1890–1920; Victoria

General Hospital, Halifax, patient records, medical and surgical 1905, 1910, 1920–1930; Women's College Hospital, register, 1917–1920.

7 David Flaherty, "Privacy and Confidentiality: The Responsibilities of Historians," *Reviews in American History* 8, 3 (September 1980): 419–29.

8 I looked at the following reports: Coburg Asylum, 1902–1948; General Hospital, St John, NB, 1901–1915; Halifax Visiting Dispensary, 1900–1950; Kingston General Hospital, 1906, 1912, 1917, 1927, 1928–47; Montreal General Hospital, 1900–1950; Montreal Maternity Hospital, 1900–49; Royal Victoria Hospital, Montreal, 1900–1950 (every fifth year); Royal Jubilee Hospital, Victoria, 1900–1917, 1920–1949; Vancouver General Hospital, 1905–1918; Victoria General Hospital, Halifax, 1900–1950.

9 See Jane Appleton, "Ethical Issues in Narrative Research in Palliative Care," in Peter L. Twohig and Vera Kalitzkus (eds.), *Making Sense of Health, Illness and Disease* (Amsterdam, New York: Rodopi, 2004), 259–76; Jonathan Gillis, "The History of the Patient History since 1850," Bulletin of the History of Medicine 80, 3 (Fall 2006): 490–512; Irving Zola, "Pathways to the Doctor: From Person to Patient," *Social Science and Medicine* 7, 9 (1973): 677–89; Richard Ivan Jobs and Patrick McDevitt, "Introduction: Where the Hell Are the People?" *Journal of Social History* 39, 2 (Winter 2005): 310. For an analysis of case files, including patient records, see Franca Iacovetta and Wendy Mitchinson (eds.), "Introduction: Social History and Case Files Research," in *On the Case: Explorations in Social History* (Toronto: University of Toronto Press, 1999), 3–21.

10 Unfortunately, there are few historical studies of marginalized women and medical treatment.

11 For an excellent description of the development of hospital record keeping see Barbara Craig, "Hospital Records and Record Keeping, c. 1850-c. 1950 Part I: The Development of Records in Hospitals," *Archivaria* 29 (Winter 1989–90): 57–87 and Part II *Archivaria* 30 (Summer 1990): 21–38. See also Guenter B. Risse and John Harley Warner, "Reconstructing Clinical Activities: Patient Records in Medical History," *Social History of Medicine* 5, 2 (August 1992): 183–206. Case histories as a form of medical discourse goes back to the period of Hippocrates. The form the case history takes, however, changes with the particular concerns and medical doctrines of the period. See Harriet Nowell-Smith, "Nineteenth-Century Narrative Case Histories: An Inquiry into Stylistics and History," *Canadian Bulletin of Medical History* 12, 1 (1995): 47–67.

12 On oral history and memory see Robert Perks and Alistair Thomson, *The Oral History Reader* 2nd ed. (New York: Routledge, 2004); on memory see

Patrizia Gentile, "Excavating Queer 'Stories': Archiving, Oral History, and Memory Studies," unpublished paper sent to the author; Pierre Nora, "Between Memory and History: Les Lieux de Memoire," *Representations* 26 (Spring 1989): 7–24; Kerwin Lee Klein, "On the Emergence of Memory in Historical Discourse," *Representations* 69 (Winter 2000): 127–150; Natalie Zemon Davis and Randolph Starn, "Introduction," *Representations* 26 (Spring 1989): 1–6; Chris Healy and Maria Tumarkin, "Social Memory and Historical Justice," *Journal of Social History* 44, 4 (Summer 2011): 1007–1018; Joy Parr, "'Don't Speak for Me': Practicing Oral History Amidst the Legacies of Conflict," *Journal of the Canadian Historical Association* N.S. 21, 1 (Montreal, 2010): 1–12.

13 For a discussion of the debate over experience as a way of understanding the past see Joan Sangster, "Invoking Experience as Evidence," *Canadian Historical Review* 92, 1 (March 2011): 135–62.

Index